Breastfeeding, Social Justice, and Equity

Praeclarus Press, LLC
2504 Sweetgum Lane
Amarillo, Texas 79124 USA
806-367-9950
www.PraeclarusPress.com

DISCLAIMER

The information contained in this publication is advisory only and is not intended to replace sound clinical judgment or individualized patient care. The author disclaims all warranties, whether expressed or implied, including any warranty as the quality, accuracy, safety, or suitability of this information for any particular purpose.

ISBN: 978-1-939807-76-2

Cover Design: Ken Tackett
Developmental Editing: Kathleen Kendall-Tackett
Copyediting: Chris Tackett
Layout & Design: Nelly Murariu

Breastfeeding, Social Justice, and Equity

Papers from the 10ᵗʰ Breastfeeding and Feminism International Conference

March 19 - March 20, 2015

Sheraton Chapel Hill, Chapel Hill, NC

EDITORS

Paige Hall Smith, MSPH, PhD Director Center for Women's Health and Wellness; Associate Professor, Department of Public Health Education, School of Health and Human Sciences, University of North Carolina at Greensboro

Miriam Labbok, MD, MMS, MPH, IBCLC, FACPM, FABM, FILCA Carolina Global Breastfeeding Institute Founding Professor and

Director; Department of Maternal and Child Health, Gillings School of Global Public Health, University of North Carolina at Chapel Hill

Brittany D. Chambers, MPH, CHES; Doctoral Student; Department of Public Health Education, School of Health and Human Sciences, University of North Carolina at Greensboro

Praeclarus Press, LLC

www.PraeclarusPress.com

Acknowledgements

With thanks to Melanie Pringle, 2015 Graduate Research Assistant, Center for Women's Health and Wellness, School of Health and Human Sciences, University of North Carolina at Greensboro to the Carolina Global Breastfeeding Institute Endowment for the contributions of Thea Calhoun-Smith, Business Services Coordinator, Carolina Global Breastfeeding Institute, Department of Maternal and Child Health, Global School of Public Health, University of North Carolina at Chapel Hill. We also thank the many participants and exhibitors who were the heart of the 2015 Breastfeeding and Feminism International Conference, and all those who contributed chapters to this book.

Remembering Miriam

Miriam first spoke at the Breastfeeding and Feminism International Conference in 2005, just before she took her position as Director of the Carolina Global Breastfeeding Institute at UNC Chapel Hill. The next year she joined me as our conference co-director and she remained in that position through the 2016 conference. Over that decade we became friends as well as colleagues and hers is a relationship I shall always hold dear. I have many fond memories of meeting Miriam at our Chapel Hill café "hangout" hashing out conference themes, guest speakers, calls for abstracts, galley proofs, and money. When I go there now I can still see her sauntering in, usually rushing from somewhere else, dragging her laptop roller bag behind her. I will miss both arguing with her and laughing together—probably in equal measure! She brought to our conference decades of experience, relationships with friends and colleagues around the world, and a fierce concern for the lives and wellbeing of women and children. The Breastfeeding and Feminism International Conference is not her only legacy but it is one of which she was proud—the four books we published together, three with Praeclarus Press, attest to the value we both placed on providing a space for people from different backgrounds, professions, life experiences, and viewpoints to come together with the shared goal of creating a world where breastfeeding was accepted as an essential aspect of health, nutrition, and human rights. I know I'm not alone when I say "I miss you Miriam." Hugs.

Table of Contents

Part 3
Advancing Strategies Across the Social Ecology

This section examines women's experiences with and prevention strategies to address challenges with breastfeeding across the social ecology.

Foreword

Since its inception in 2005, the voices at the annual Breastfeeding and Feminism International Conference have addressed the many injustices and inequities that prevent all women from being able to mother as they want, feed their babies the way they want, and live the life that supports them economically and nourishes their soul. We have discussed and described a wide variety of social, economic, legal, political, and medical inequities, as well as persistent injustices by race, class, education, gender, and sexuality that make breastfeeding inaccessible to so many women. We have also considered solutions that recognize the value of women's whole lives and the importance of the mother-child relationship. The 2015 conference was a special event, as it marked our 10th anniversary and provided the opportunity for us to reflect on where we have been and where we want to go.

Our conference themes over the decade have:

- highlighted the need for solutions that value and support employed mothers;
- recognized breastfeeding as a reproductive right;
- considered the importance of the "birthplace" and maternity-care practice
- highlighted the importance of having feminist and social justice thinking inform public health approaches;
- considered "frames" for breastfeeding that do not recreate moral morasses;
- recognized the need to "consider women" as we move forward with the *Surgeon General's Call to Action;*

- considered the role of the greater "village" in inspiring and engaging women to breastfeed;
- and promoted the forging of partnerships for a better tomorrow.

The theme for 2015, "Social Justice and Equity," pulled all of these previous ideas together to help us all with "Reflect, Reclaim, and Re-Vision" the next decade. At this time in U.S. history, as well as in many other places around the world, individual privilege and status, achieved by personal income, education, partnership, dominant sexuality, and/or race is nearly a prerequisite to having the agency and ability to navigate the cultural, social, and health care contradictions around breastfeeding. In some countries around the world, the opposite is occurring: as women gain status, they stop breastfeeding because it is a maternal behavior that is incompatible with emerging employment and living patterns. This means that millions of women are making infant feeding choices based on social or health care inequities, not personal preferences.

During the conference, our 70 presenters – in panels, discussion groups and posters – addressed this theme, as well as the broad context within which women made infant feeding decisions. In this volume, we are pleased to share with you 48 papers from this conference, organized into three broad sections. Our opening two chapters, from the conference organizers, address different aspects of changes over the past decade. Smith's words focus on the BFIC itself, while Labbok revisits changes in U.S. and global policy over the past decade. Part 2 focuses on a topic central to BFIC over the past decade, the importance of centering women's experiences in conversations about infant feeding; in this volume, we specifically highlight the ways women's experiences are shaped by race. Part 3 offers solutions and strategies across the social ecology.

We are pleased that this volume, as a reflection of the BFIC generally, presents papers from a wide diversity of disciplines and perspectives, from researchers, practitioners, and activists from established, as well as emerging professionals and scholars, and from voices around the globe. We want to thank all of the authors for their dedication to this effort to disseminate these ideas to a broad audience.

This volume of papers from the 2015 BFIC is the third book we have published with Praeclarus Press, LLC. Earlier volumes covered papers from the 2013 and 2014 conferences (Labbok & Smith, 2016; Smith & Labbok, 2015). This is the last of the series, at least for the present! We would like to extend an enthusiastic "thank you" to Kathleen Kendall-Tackett, Owner and Editor-in-Chief; Scott Sherwood, former Director of Operations, and their team for their support and hard work to make this series a reality.

We would also like to thank members of our planning and social media committees who helped review abstracts, plan the program, and have our voice present on social media: Jodine Chase; Ellen Chetwynd; Virginia Guidry; Eric Hodges; Jeanette McCullough; Aunchalee Palmquist; Rebecca Ruhlen; Jennifer Yourkavitch; Kristin Tully; and Abigail Smetana. Our hard-working staff also deserves our thanks and a hug for making this conference a reality: Melanie Pringle, Graduate Research Assistant, Center for Women's Health and Wellness, School of Health and Human Sciences, University of North Carolina at Greensboro; and Thea Calhoun-Smith, Business Services Coordinator, Carolina Global Breastfeeding Institute, Department of Maternal and Child Health, Gillings School of Global Public Health, University of North Carolina at Chapel Hill. Lastly, we welcome our new editor, Brittany Chambers, and want to acknowledge the significant contributions she made to organizing this volume and getting it to the press on time.

For more information to engage with others, visit our website (www.breastfeedingandfeminsm.org), and our Facebook page (Breastfeeding and Feminism).

We hope you enjoy this volume.
PAIGE HALL SMITH, MIRIAM H. LABBOK,
and BRITTANY D. CHAMBERS

References

Labbok, M.L., & Smith, P.H. (2016). *Advancing breastfeeding: Forging partnerships for a better tomorrow.* Amarillo, TX: Praeclarus Press.

Smith, P.H., & Labbok. M.L. (2015). *It takes village: The role of the greater community in inspiring and empowering women to breastfeed.* Amarillo, TX: Praeclarus Press.

Part 1
Reframing, Reclaiming, and Revisiting

This volume opens with a reflection on progress made in creating breastfeeding rates globally. The first chapter focuses on the critical scholarly contributions discussed over the past 10 years at the Breastfeeding and Feminism International Conference. The last chapter discusses changes in breastfeeding rates and international supports for breastfeeding.

CHAPTER 1

Revisiting, Reframing, and Re-visioning

Paige Hall Smith

Two little words can make a big difference—specifically, the two words "and Feminism," as in "Breastfeeding *and Feminism*." These two words mark the Breastfeeding and Feminism International Conference as a being quite different from other breastfeeding conferences. From its inception in 2005, the Breastfeeding and Feminism Symposium, renamed in 2013 as the Breastfeeding and Feminism International Conference (BFIC), was designed to bring feminist theory and feminist research on breastfeeding, together with research and practice illuminating women's experiences with breastfeeding in novel and exciting ways in order to stimulate a new feminist-voice informing, in supportive ways, breastfeeding research, practice, promotion, and support. To achieve this goal, BFIC brings together researchers, students, health care practitioners, policy makers, and those providing mother-to-mother support in order to share scholarship and experiences that investigate, identify, and improve the sociocultural, economic, political, and gendered context within which women make infant feeding decisions.

The feminist scholarship and voices at this conference are, although necessarily, and at times critical of current breastfeeding protection, promotion, and support practices, are hoping to contribute to an improved climate for breastfeeding mothers, and lower the costs to women of breastfeeding by reducing the constraints on breastfeeding (Smith, Labbok, & Hausman, 2012; Smith & Labbok, 2015). This is an emerging feminist perspective as the dominant feminist voice has, for the most part, been either neutral toward the infant feeding choices, or has framed breastfeeding itself as a "constraint" to women's advancement (Wolf, 2006).

Where We Have Been

At this conference, we have had presentations over the years that describe and illuminate the gendered context within which women make their decisions about how to feed their babies. This gendered context provides more resources, authority, and power to some ways of living, working, reproducing, and caring for young than it does to others. This imbalance often reduces the social and economic value of caregiving, and makes it challenging for women to choose or sustain breastfeeding and makes caregiving an impediment to women's full equality.

Over the years, presenters have described how this context plays out in important ways. We have discussed:

- How women's status, shaped by income, education, and race influences women's infant feeding experiences in ways that mean that. At this time in the U.S. and many other countries, women who are more marginalized find it more difficult to breastfeed;

- That, although, societies need for women to work and mother, they maintain policies and practices that make it difficult for them to do both; thus, women are forced to make choices that undermine both breastfeeding and women's economic progress;

- How society approves of images in public spaces that sexualize women's bodies and breasts, but find breastfeeding so sexual that women are denied this opportunity, or opt out for fear of being uncomfortable;

- How health care providers and institutions continue to medicalize and commercialize pregnancy and artificial milk, as well as human milk and breastfeeding, which too often undermine women's bodies and authority;

- How different forms of violence against women influences infant feeding choices;

- How various solutions to advance breastfeeding can recreate gender inequities and moral conundrums;

- How lactation's biological necessities give shape to some breastfeeding promotion strategies that re-create problems for breastfeeding women;

- The importance of building on women's experiences;

- How media distorts and misrepresents breastfeeding and breastfeeding mothers;

- The challenges women experience breastfeeding, pumping, and milk-sharing, and the impact that pumping and milk sharing has on women's experiences with breastfeeding;

We've also had presentations on a wide variety of interventions that span the social ecology, including strategies for improving women's knowledge and self-efficacy, advancing clinical interactions and support, helping women integrate mothering with employment, and building community, city, and country-wide responses, both in the U.S., and beyond our borders.

Where We Are Now

Over the decades governmental, health care, workplace, and social support for breastfeeding have risen substantially, and these supports make it easier for more women to actualize their own breastfeeding goals, thus breastfeeding longer. But one thing stands out: we continue to have a "breastfeeding problem" that emerges from the difficulty many women have reconciling the biological imperative of lactation, with the realities of their lives as they as productive members of the labor force and society. We have moved from being a society where women do not breastfeed because they do not want to, to being a society where most want to breastfeed, but find feeding at the breast to be so challenging so that they pump instead. Indeed, pumping is the normative practice (Labiner-Wolfe et al., 2008), and we often find that women use the word "breastfeeding" interchangeably with the word "pumping."

In 2010, British scholar Sally Johnson, presenting at this conference, reported results from her research suggesting that women pump because it helps them navigate the dilemmas that come from the varying cultural pressures and contradictions they experience when trying to be good breastfeeding mothers, good workers, good partners, and have good lives (Johnson, 2012). For most women, the dilemmas, pressures, and contradictions that come from trying to integrate breastfeeding and mothering with paid employment and breastfeeding in public, while maintaining status and quality of life, have been resistant to change. We have, however, implemented solutions that make it easier for some women to pump at work.

This trend toward pumping, as a solution to the "breastfeeding problem," highlights one of the fundamental issues we face in the breastfeeding world—one articulated by Penny Van Estrik (1989) in her classic book, *Beyond the Breast-Bottle Controversy:* do we focus our lens on breastfeeding as (1) a *product*—the product being human milk, or (2) as a *process*—that is, as a behavior that engages women in an interdependent relationship with their children? These two perspectives lead to different foci, solutions, and controversies.

The product-focused perspective has driven discourse on the value of human milk for health, and on how *not* breastfeeding is risky for women and infants. It leads to research on the content and benefits of human milk, and to practice and policy solutions that seek to increase access to human milk, such as advancing donor milk and milk sharing, and promoting workplace lactation rooms and polices. The product-focused perspective drives the counter feminist arguments that the science is faulty, and public health arguments are insufficient to warrant public intrusion into women's lives (see discussion in Hausman, Smith, & Labbok, 2012).

The process-focused perspective has driven research highlighting women's experiences, the value of skin to skin, the benefits of breastfeeding for women, and the social value of the maternal-child relationship and caregiving. The process-focused perspective seeks solutions that keep mothers and babies together in the hospital and beyond, such as co-located childcare, maternity leave, and those that make it easier for women to breastfeed in public. This perspective also fuels the counter-feminist arguments that breastfeeding is risky, as it demands too much from women, constrains gender equity, and boxes them into a "good mother" frame.

Where Do We Need to Go

As we go forward together over the next decade, we need to reflect on, reclaim, and re-vision two important, yet contradictory realities:

1. For breastfeeding to be successful, mothers and babies must be together.
2. Being with babies reinforces gender inequities in ways that undermine women's economic, political, and social development.

The tension between these two realities is one reason why breastfeeding is a contentious, emotion-filled issue. The biological necessity that mothers and babies be together is one that is difficult for most, and impossible for many, given the structures and policies affecting how we work, caregive, and live today. As the challenges are more difficult for women and families with fewer economic resources, these tensions play out in ways that recreate uncomfortable and unacceptable disparities in breastfeeding by race, class, culture, sexuality, and health status.

Over the next 10 years, these two realities much be reconciled in ways that do not undermine women's lives, are inclusive of different populations, and ensure good quality of life for breastfeeding mothers and healthy babies. This is a difficult challenge. This will require will a focus on both product and process—food and relationship—but it will also require us to ensure that our frame includes two other "Ps": breastfeeding as a gendered caregiving *practice*, and the impact of breastfeeding on *people*. It is critical that we build women's experiences, concerns, and hopes for their lives into our strategies that span the social ecology; we also have much to learn about breastfeeding and people by ensuring that our research and clinical practice encompasses the experiences of people of a wide ranges of gender identities, sexualities, ethnicities, and cultures. We need social agreement that breastfeeding is a socially valued activity, and is seen as a "worthy choice" (see Mann in this volume). We need to advance culturally embedded strategies that provide respect, status, and resources to caregiving and caregivers. The niggling thing is that in order to reduce the social, economic, legal, political, and medical obstacles to this worthy choice, we will need significant changes in the ways our societies organize gender, power, and labor.

References

Labiner-Wolfe, J., Fein, S., Shealy, K.R., & Wang, C. (2008). Prevalence of breastmilk expression and associated factors. *Pediatrics. 122* (suppl 2), S63-S68.

Hausman, B., Smith, P.H., & Labbok, M. (2012). Introduction: Breastfeeding constraints and realities. In Smith, P.H., Hausman, B.L., & Labbok, M. (Eds.) (2012). *Beyond health, beyond choice: Breastfeeding constraints and realities.* New Brunswick, NJ: Rutgers University Press.

Johnson, S., Lemming, D., Steven L., & Williamson, I. (2012). In Smith, P.H., Hausman, B.L., & Labbok, M. (Eds.) (2012). *Beyond health, beyond choice: Breastfeeding constraints and realities.* New Brunswick, NJ: Rutgers University Press.

Mann, H.S. (2017) Breastfeeding as embodied care: On its goodness, awfulness, and irreducible pleasure. In M. Labbok & P.H. Smith (Eds.), *Advancing breastfeeding: Forging partnerships for a better tomorrow.* Amarillo, TX: Praeclarus Press.

Smith, P.H., Hausman, B.L., & Labbok, M. (Eds.) (2012). *Beyond health, beyond choice: Breastfeeding constraints and realities.* New Brunswick, NJ: Rutgers University Press.

Smith, P.H., & Labbok, M. (Eds.). *It takes a village: The role of the greater community in inspiring and empowering women to breastfeed.* Amarillo, TX: Praeclarus Press.

Van Estrik, P. (1989). *Beyond the breast-bottle controversy.* New Brunswick, NJ: Rutgers University Press.

Wolf, J.H. (2006). What feminists can do for breastfeeding and what breastfeeding can do for feminism. *Signs: Journal of Women in Culture and Society, 36*(2), 397-424.

CHAPTER 2

Global and U.S. Policy and Programs: Reflecting, Reclaiming, Re-Visioning

Miriam H. Labbok

It is rare that one has the opportunity to freely expound on the past, present, and offer conjectures for the future of a trend in human behavior. Breastfeeding behaviors have changed rapidly in the last century, having been reasonably stable for millennia. Might it be possible to travel through the last 25 years, and project a possible trajectory into the future? Let's take this trip, with a guarded optimistic tour guide, and see where it might take us.

Twenty-five years ago, this year, I was privileged to serve as the Technical Secretariat for the preparatory work and for the program for an international meeting held in Florence, Italy at the UNICEF Innocenti Centre, the outcome of which was meeting proceedings (Labbok et al., 1988; 1990), a book (Saadeh, Labbok, Cooney, & Koniz-Booher, 1993), and a declaration (UNICEF, 2006). This declaration became known as the *1990 Innocenti Declaration*. This meeting emerged due to a confluence of occurrences: a growing attention to Women's and Children's (Human) Rights, an increased recognition of the importance and recent declines in breastfeeding, and interest on the part of UNICEF in more actively supporting the "B" in UNICEF's GOBI (Growth charting, Oral rehydration therapy, Breastfeeding, and Immunization) construct for child survival.

The Innocenti Declaration, signed by more than 30 countries, including the USA, included agreement that by 1995, every country would:

1. Establish a **National Oversight Authority** for breastfeeding
2. Fully implement the Ten Steps to Successful Breastfeeding
3. Legislate the **International Code of Marketing of Breastmilk Substitutes** and subsequent related resolutions
4. Establish universal **Guaranteed Paid Maternity Leave and Breastfeeding Breaks.**

Today, in 2015, we know that these promised changes have not been realized. However, there is some good news in that, by 2005, there had been the development and dissemination of the *WHO/UNICEF Global Strategy on Infant and Young Child Feeding*, and EU and U.S. (and NC) *Blueprints for Action to Support Breastfeeding*, as well as the *2005 Innocenti+15* meeting and outcomes (UNICEF, 2006). All of these documents reconfirmed all of the basic tenets of the Innocenti Declaration (exception: the U.S. did not support the Code), and added additional operational targets, including increased attention to issues such as emergencies, HIV, and infant feeding, and the necessity of community support, as well as demand creation to achieve breastfeeding goals.

This period of years also saw the end of the USSR, and as these nations emerged as individual, there was renewed support for implementation of the Ten Steps and the Code of Marketing, in part due to the work of Kramer and colleagues in Belarus on the Ten Steps, and in part due UNICEF support in response to the need to support breastfeeding while protecting against the rapid increase in commercial infant formula marketing. As a result of these efforts, BFHI advanced, breastfeeding became increasing acceptable in industrialized countries, and exclusive breastfeeding was increased in developing countries (see Table 1).

In the last decade, there also have been significant increases in the number of publications addressing breastfeeding issues, increases in the number of countries that have introduced legislation in support of the International Code of Marketing, growing U.S .Federal activity in support of breastfeeding, and, of course, we have had 10 Breastfeeding and Feminism International Conferences. There is also reason for optimism as we become more attuned to the environment as research into the "carbon footprint" of infant formula production and use continues (Tingling, et. al., 2011).

Table 1

Global and U.S. Policy: Reflecting, Reclaiming, Re-Visioning

[Note: 2015 and onwards are projections, based on previous progress. However, there is an assumption that global rate of increase stalled in from 2005-2015 due to reduction of organized global support.]

Year	Global	% BF<6 mo.	US	% initiation
1990	Innocenti Declaration	34	Surgeon General's Report	50
2005	Global Strategy for Infant and Young Child Feeding: Centralized funding diminished	39	U.S. Blueprint for Action Data collection	72
2015	WHO/UNICEF renewing activity	39	2011 Surgeon General's Call to Action being implemented	81
2025	Significantly renewed support for programs of protection, promotion and SUPPORT, and associated policy	42	Paid maternity leave, Increased pre-service clinician training, breastfeeding supported Beyond Health, Beyond Choice	87
2040	Accepted as essential aspect of Health and Nutrition and Human's Rights	47	Equity achieved and optimal breastfeeding is the normative behavior	92

Note:

UNICEF. 1990 – 2005 Celebrating the Innocenti Declaration on the Protection, Promotion and Support of Breastfeeding: Past Achievements, Present Challenges and the Way Forward for Infant and Young Child Feeding, UNICEF Innocenti Research Centre, Florence, Italy, 2006.

CDC Division of Nutrition, Physical Activity, and Obesity, accessed 2014, http://www.cdc.gov/breastfeeding/data/nis_data/index.htm

Labbok, M., Wardlaw, T., Blanc, A., Clark, D., & Terreri, N. (2006). Trends in exclusive breastfeeding: Findings. *Journal of Human Lactation, 22*(3), 272-276.

Not everything was positive for breastfeeding over these years. Misunderstandings concerning HIV and breastfeeding led to programs and families alike introducing barriers to breastfeeding. As a result, several countries, including the U.S., recommended not breastfeeding for women who might be HIV+ until they were tested. This message was inappropriate in most developing country settings, where formula use is unsafe, and women did not have easy access to testing. Today, testing is more readily available, and the infants of exclusively breastfeeding women, and women on HAART in developing countries settings, actually have better outcomes than the non-breastfed, or the mixed-fed infant (World Health Organization [WHO], 2006). Finally, the U.S. still lags far behind on the four Innocenti operational targets, along with many other countries. If we discussed the good and bad, perhaps we should also mention the "ugly." Funding by both UNICEF and WHO was substantially reduced starting early in the new millennium.

Today, we are reclaiming this issue across the globe. There has now been recognition that breastfeeding was major contributor to progress on the Millennium Development Goals related to maternal and child health and survival. This is reflected in UNICEFs *Promise Renewed* publication and the new global Breastfeeding Advocacy Initiative. More recently, the Gates Foundation funded a new post at WHO to support the Code and related issues. In the U.S., we are benefitting from the WK Kellogg Foundation First Food Builders initiative, funding many organizations interested in supporting breastfeeding with attention to equity. Also in the U.S., we are now working on the actions recommended by the *U.S. Surgeon General Call to Action* (2011). This is the first U.S. agenda reflecting international targets, and has catalyzed notable surges in U.S. federal support for improvements in the workplace, and for Baby-Friendly Hospital Initiative (BFHI).

These programs, policy, and trends lend optimism for the decade and for the 25 years ahead. This is a good time to re-vision what must be done to achieve a breastfeeding norm, both in the U.S., and across the globe. We will need several paradigm shifts in our perceptions, programs, and support for breastfeeding. We will need to move from seeing breastfeeding as sexual to seeing it as sensible; from classifying breastfeeding as a medical issue to recognizing it as a sociocultural issue; from in-service training to pre-service training; from considering BFHI a radical change to accepting its tenets as quality of care; from being defensive to being defended; from a being considered a new activity to being accepted as a normal activity; and, from "taboo" to "a fine tradition renewed."

It is essential that we create the environment for these changes. Table 1 illustrates where we might be if we succeed in creating the environment in which these changes are enabled. This table uses previous rates of change to project possible future rates of breastfeeding. In it, we also consider how programs have changed to date, and what we might hope to achieve in the future if we succeed in re-visioning breastfeeding with these paradigm shifts. We have the potential to see a breastfeeding norm in our lifetimes. But how will we achieve these paradigm shifts? Much will depend on the reality that we are progressing from the mothers of the 1990s, to the mothers of today, and on to the mothers of tomorrow, and those that have and will support them. It will be up to each of us to consider what we have done, what we are doing today, and what we must do in the future, so that a new vision will be achieved.

References

Centers for Disease Control and Prevention, [CDC]. (2014). *Breastfeeding data.* Division of Nutrition, Physical Activity, and Obesity, accessed 2014, http://www.cdc.gov/breastfeeding/data/nis_data/index.htm

Department of Health and Human Services. (2011). *The Surgeon General's Call to Action to Support Breastfeeding.* Washington, DC: Author.

Labbok, M.H., & McDonald, M. (1990). Proceedings of the Interagency workshop on health care practices related to breastfeeding. *International Journal of Gynecology & Obstetrics*, 31(Supplement 1), 1-191.

Labbok, M. H., Wardlaw, T., Blanc, A., Clark, D., & Terreri, N. (2006). Trends in exclusive breastfeeding: findings from the 1990s. *Journal of Human Lactation, 22*(3), 272-276.

Saadeh, R. J., Labbok, M. H., Cooney, K. A., & Koniz-Booher, P. (Eds.) (1993). *Breast-feeding: The technical basis and recommendations for action.* Geneva: The World Health Organization; 1993.

Tinling, M., Labbok, M.H., & West, J. (2011). *Greenhouse gas emissions of infant formula production: A lifecycle approach.* Presentation at One Asia Breastfeeding Partners Forum-89. Ulaanbaatar, Mongoial Setp. (pp. 14-16).

UNICEF. (1990 – 2005). *Celebrating the Innocenti Declaration on the Protection, Promotion and Support of Breastfeeding: Past achievements, present challenges and the way forward for infant and young child feeding.* UNICEF Innocenti Research Centre, Florence, Italy, 2006.

WHO. (2007). *HIV transmission through breastfeeding: A review of the evidence.* Retrieved from http://whqlibdoc.who.int/ publications/2008/9789241596596_eng.pdf.

Part 2

Centering Women's Experiences with Race, Gender, and Life

Consistent with research discussing disparities in breastfeeding, these chapters explore the unique nuances of gender, race, and social context as women navigate breastfeeding.

Section 1

Improving the Gendered Context

CHAPTER 3

Breastfeeding as Embodied Care: On Its Goodness, Awfulness, and Irreducible Pleasure

Hollie Sue Mann

Philosophers and political theorists have thought about care in a number of ways—as a moral attitude, a disposition, an orientation to the world, a kind of work, and a source of oppression. The ethics-of-care literature has largely been shaped by the work of feminists, and so it is not surprising that it has tended to focus attention on gender and care-work. This analysis is incomplete. It fails to get at other characteristics that contribute to care's undervalued status in society, characteristics that are certainly related to gender, but stand somewhat conceptually apart from it. Specifically, I am interested in the fact that the work of care so often is bodily intensive work, and perhaps nothing illustrates this more than breastfeeding.

A definition in two parts: embodied care is an *ethic* that understands individual and social morality as deeply bound up with the caring relationships and communities in which human beings are embedded. Care is also a set of practices where individuals take up the work of caring for the bodies of others predominantly with and through their own bodies, but in a deeply mindful way.[1] Finally, care, it seems to me, is a virtue that is choice-worthy because it is a context within which we become most fully human. Therefore, it should be chosen for its own sake.

Breastfeeding as an End in Itself, Like Friendship

What does it mean to say that breastfeeding is a kind of intrinsic good? Ancient Greek political philosopher Aristotle argued that our *telos*, the fullest expression of our being, is realized when we undertake right action, in the right way, and for the right reasons. And for him, there are certain activities and practices that are desirable for the way in which they help constitute the fullest expression of our humanity. Take friendships, for example. Friendships are sometimes a kind of external good for Aristotle, like money or power, but they are also the "form virtuous activity takes when it is especially fine and praiseworthy" (Sherman, 1989). Friendships are important for virtue precisely because they provide us with the opportunity for excellent action and desirable sentiments that would otherwise be unavailable to us (*NE* 1171b33-35; Sherman, 1989). Deeply embodied relationships of care, like breastfeeding, do very much the same thing. Friendships provide us with the necessary context to *learn* how to do well by others (*NE* 1155a8-10). Caregiving relationships, in particular those that arise within the contexts of childrearing and maternity, are most valuable because they form an important structure in which we learn

---

1   I do understand care to be one type of bodywork. Judith Twigg, "Carework as a Form of Bodywork," *Ageing and Society* 20 (2000). However, I view care as unique and distinct from other forms of bodywork, such as massage, beauty practices, physical therapy, and so on, because it is in and through relationships of care that we come to better understand, and to enact the widest range of our uniquely human capacities as moral agents. Indeed, it may be that other virtues or activities, like the practice of educating others, or of acting courageously in war, are equally fundamental to flourishing, but that would need to be textually demonstrated and/or philosophically argued, which is beyond the scope of this paper.

other-regarding thought and action, and they also become the enabling conditions for our own acting and doing well in life (*NE* 1169b9-16).

Breastfeeding as a Critical Practice, No Nature Worship

Exactly what sort of excellence is breastfeeding? Aristotle is helpful here, too. He suggests that those activities that constitute what he calls "the excellences": the things that contribute to our flourishing, do not emerge naturally, if what we mean by natural is an activity without habituation, practice, and judgment. Rather, we must be taught how to act courageously, be generous, live in friendship with others, and, of course, take care. This is particularly relevant for nursing mothers and those whose job it is, informally or formally, to assist and support them in the practice. Too often discourse around breastfeeding naturalizes and romanticizes it; "It's the most natural thing in the world!" "You'll know exactly what to do, and so will your baby!" "Just relax!" This way of glossing over nursing is dangerous—it sets women up to fail in all manner of ways, but it also completely gets wrong the sort of activity that breastfeeding is, which is one that demands a goodly bit of attention, effort, skill, fine discernment, receptivity, thoughtfulness, patience, judgment, self-care, and, when it's hard, a long view of why the work is worth it at all. This requires a tremendous amount of educative work on the part of political communities. If we simply conceive of breastfeeding as "the most natural thing in the world," then we miss its richness and value as a form of human excellence, as a form of *reflective* embodied care, with cognitive content, that goes a long way to shaping our ethical and political life.

Fashioning Nursing Bodies

Through cultivating a practice, we come to better grasp relevant particulars, and are able to exercise our capacities for finely tuned discernment and judgment based on what we have learned through the practice. What we want, then, when going about living a "good life," is to engage in a range of activities that reveal to us the unique kinds of creatures we are, possessing a plurality of possibilities and limitations. (To be clear, then, I am certainly not claiming that caregiving is the only activity we need engage in, or even that it is necessarily the one to which we should attach the most value.) This will also help us immensely in determining what sorts of things we need our political institutions to aim at accomplishing.

Breastfeeding very often forces us to confront and negotiate the radically vulnerable and contingent aspect of our lives. When we bring a baby to our breast, our animality is immediately present to us. Bodies in their most unsettling state—weak, leaky, violable, radically dependent—confront us.

Embodied care prompts us to identify certain desirable ends given our fragile and often tenuous state, and then to begin the difficult work of formulating political and ethical responses to facts of dependency and need. Even more concretely than a new awareness around human interdependence and finitude, nursing is incredibly fruitful for helping us to acquire the precise techniques and habits of caregiving more generally. We cannot develop the proper affective, physical, and cognitive skills appropriate to giving care if we are not first habituated to that activity. Mastering knowledge of the right tones of voice, forms of touch, methods and techniques for bathing, feeding, changing bedpans, cleaning and dressing wounds, and simply comforting the sick, requires participation in caring action. These are skills that must not only be developed and sharpened through habituation; they must be preserved in and through ongoing practice. I am not suggesting that women breastfeed for an eternity, but rather that while it is available to us, it is a deeply powerful resource for habituating us to other forms of care.

Breastfeeding also rather obviously offers us an opportunity to participate in recovering and affirming bodies that, by their very nature, violate "normal personhood." Breastfeeding moms use their senses to do their work, and they frequently interact with bodily fluids, waste, and material that many typically recoil from. Ongoing encounters with little bodies that may appear frightening or even contaminating to us can actually go a long way towards recalibrating our responses to those bodies and to our own when we find they fail us. Cultivating a critical practice of breastfeeding has the potential to alter reactions of disgust and fear of bodies in need of care. Another way of saying this is that nursing can function as an antidote to anti-democratic forms of normalization.

A concept of embodied care that acknowledges the power of norms to shape self-understandings points to the possibility of transforming those social imaginaries and "problematic" modes of inhabiting bodies. Bodily habits and corporeal styles are deeply connected to the socio-political realm we construct for ourselves. Taking this seriously would mean urging democratic transformations that work to relationships and modalities that reflect rather than contradict democratic values.

Two major criticisms are likely to be lurking out there at this point. First, isn't there a danger in presenting breastfeeding as the "right" choice for all women? My short answer to that question is this: of course. But I do hope to avoid running too far afoul of that sort of thing. I am by no means arguing that breastfeeding is THE only way to provide nourishment for a baby, or enjoy an enriching experience of motherhood. Such a claim would be ridiculous. Rather, I am claiming that embodied care is fundamental to a fully flourishing life, that it has certain necessary components (like the use of one's body to care for the body of another, reasoned judgment, interdependence, receptivity, technique, skill, etc.), and that breastfeeding is one very powerful practice of embodied care which many women are uniquely situated to take up. And so, they should, whenever possible. The idea that formula and donor milk are defensible and good decisions for some women should be obvious enough.

A second criticism I anticipate goes something like this: "Breast-feeding is miserable, time-consuming, boring, and a source of inequity in my household. I do it because it's good for the baby, but I don't see how it's good for me!" Here, I want to distinguish Aristotle's conception of doing well (*eudaimonia*) from a psychological state of happiness or a physical state of feeling good. Doing well, or flourishing, holds in view the entire of arc of a life, a life that, when all is said done, we could say was truly good. Such a life would have contained a range of experiences that gave it a sense of wholeness and authenticity, which will necessarily include many unpleasant or difficult things.

Breastfeeding as a Form of Shared Pleasure

Although it is true that breastfeeding is not physically enjoyable for all women, I want to conclude by turning to the fact that it is deeply pleasurable for some; pleasurable in ways we often don't like to talk about because of taboos regarding the asexuality and selfless service of motherhood, as well as physical intimacy between mother and child. But as Iris Marion Young (2005) has argued, when we are honest with ourselves and others about the sensual and pleasurable aspects of breastfeeding, we can see that it has the power to shatter the border between motherhood and sexuality. Perhaps then, women will have gone some way to reclaiming their own sexuality, as well as reimagining maternity. Conceiving of and talking about breastfeeding, then, as drudgery or merely "hard work" is troubling both because the "hard work" of care is not sufficient justification for the failure to perform it ourselves AND because this closes off the possibility of women claiming a right to breastfeed on the grounds that it is a deeply desired pleasure. It isn't simply that it is good for us, but it is also the case that, once we get the hang of it, it feels quite nice. As Young writes, "As feminists, we should affirm the value of nurturing; an ethic of caring does indeed hold promise for a more human justice, and political values guided by such an ethic would change the character of the public for the better. But we must also insist that nurturers need, that love is partly selfish, and that a woman deserves her own irreducible pleasures" (Young, 2005, p. 90).

References

Aristotle. (1999) *Nicomachean ethics.* (Terrance Irwin, Trans.) Cambridge: Hackett Publishing Company.

Sherman, N. (1989) *The fabric of character: Aristotle's theory of virtue.* Oxford, UK: Oxford University Press.

Twigg, J. (2000). Carework as a form of bodywork. *Ageing and Society,* 20(04), 389-411.

Young, I.M. (2005) Breasted experience: The look and the feeling. In *On female body experience.* Oxford: Oxford University Press.

CHAPTER 4

When Everyday Violence is a Barrier to Breastfeeding

Aunchalee E.L. Palmquist

Hawai'i is consistently ranked as the "healthiest" and "happiest" state in the nation. Indeed, for most population health indicators, Hawai'i comes out ahead of other states.

However, this picture of health looks quite different when population data are broken down by socioeconomic indicators, like race, ethnicity, household income, education, gender, and age are considered. Hawai'i may be the "healthiest" and "happiest" state, but for a privileged majority.

Native Hawaiian and other Pacific Islander (NHPI) groups experience significantly higher burdens of many diseases. For example, infant mortality, obesity, Type 2 diabetes, and infant mortality rates are higher among NHPI groups as compared with other racial and ethnic groups in Hawai'i (Centers for Disease Control and Prevention, 2012; Hawaii State Department of Health 2010a, 2010b, 2014). While breastfeeding initiation rates across race/ethnic categories are higher in Hawai'i than the national average, rates of recommended breastfeeding exclusivity and duration are significantly lower among NHPI groups. Likewise, perinatal mood disorders intimate partner violence, and illicit substance use are highest among NHPI. NHPI also comprise a segment of the State's population that experiences the highest rates of poverty and homelessness (Hawaii State Department of Health 2010b; Hayes et al. 2010; Schempf, Hayes, & Fuddy, 2010; U.S. Department of Health and Human Services, 2015).

Breastfeeding is integral to maternal-child health and well-being, and high rates of early breastfeeding cessation are undoubtedly related to NHPI health disparities. There is a substantial public Health and Human Services literature on the importance of cultural competency for promoting recommended Infant and Young Child Feeding (IYCF) practices within NHPI groups. But far less attention has been placed on gaining insight into how NHPI families who face chronic poverty and food insecurity navigate IYCF decisions. The purpose of this study was to explore the ways in which structural violence (Farmer et al., 2006) was tied to IFYCF strategies among homeless NHPI families through ethnographic inquiry and parent/caregiver narratives.

Method

After receiving ethics approval from the Elon University Institutional Review Board and collaborating agencies in Hawai'i, I traveled to Hawai'i, June-August 2012 to explore how social inequalities translated into everyday IYCF practices. I spent time in Honolulu and Hilo conducting participation observation with families who were either living part-time in an emergency shelter, or full-time in transitional housing. I focused my efforts on gathering exploratory data on the challenges these parents/caregivers face in nurturing their children through food. Field notes based on my participant observation were recorded daily (Bernard, 2011; Le Compte & Schensul, 2010). I also interviewed 41 participants, most of them parents/caregivers who were currently homeless, and with at least one child 0-5 years old in their care. Interviews were semi-structured, and prompts were designed specifically to elicit narratives of IYCF in the context of homelessness, food insecurity, and poverty.

Interviews were recorded and transcribed verbatim and checked for accuracy. Transcripts were imported into Dedoose for coding. A qualitative approach to data analyses was used consistent with ethnographic research in which narratives from within the interviews were identified, emergent themes were coded, and field notes from participant observation were used to further facilitate interpretation of these themes and to contextualize the narrative data (Bernard, 2011; Le Compte & Schensul, 2010; Riessman, 2007).

Key Themes

Common Breastfeeding Challenges: "I tried to, but ..."

Mothers who had initiated breastfeeding, but began supplementing with formula and/or ended breastfeeding before 6 months, cited issues commonly associated with disrupted breastfeeding: perceived insufficient milk, usually marked by an infant's fussiness following a feed; breast refusal; fussiness at the breast; sleeplessness; a baby's failure to thrive. Other reasons were that the baby "didn't like the breast." Hospital practices, like separating the mother and baby, prematurity, and early supplementation with formula, were also named as reasons why breastfeeding became difficult. Feeding a baby with a bottle of formula was sometimes described as the only way to satisfy a baby's hunger. Some parents talked about their baby's appetite as being insatiable, and the baby was only considered to be "full" or "happy" when they were quiet and fell asleep. Breastfeeding was described by at least one mother as a task that simply required "too much patience" and "too hard" for her to want to continue. Early supplementation was common, starting anywhere between 3 weeks and 6 months. Common weaning foods named included, *poi*, rice, fish, cereal, mashed fruits, and processed commercial baby foods.

A small number of mothers reported breastfeeding their infants exclusively for at least 6 months, and continuing into late infancy (2 to

3 years of age). These mothers were notably recent arrivals to Hawai'i from Micronesia (usually Marshall Islands or Chuuk), or who had come from families in which breastfeeding was valued, and where they were otherwise supported in their decision to continue breast-feeding. For these mothers, introducing complementary foods that they believed were healthy and appropriate for their child was the major challenge, and directly related to poverty, poor access to healthy foods, lack of transportation, and lack of strong systems of social support.

Violence, Trauma, and Infant and Young Child Feeding

Participants' narratives reveal that the circumstances in which they have enacted IYCF practices reflect historical trauma, social suffering, and structural violence. Intergenerational physical, sexual, and emotional abuse was a common theme throughout the narratives, along with stories that included mention of mental illness, alcoholism, addiction to illegal substances, intimate partner violence, child abandonment, and other forms of separation of parents and children, criminal activity and imprisonment, and teen pregnancy. In this way, these narratives are consistent with public health reports of neonatal maternal-child health disparities experienced by NHPI women.

Gaps in IYCF Support for Homeless Families

There was an absence of IYCF education and support in the overall configuration of social services provided to families within the two emergency and transitional housing settings. While pre-mixed infant formula was available, free of charge on site, breastfeeding support was not. Parents mentioned that the Women, Infant, and Children's (WIC) program offered breastfeeding peer counseling, but that these services were extremely difficult to access. The complementary foods that were available to parents to give older infants and young children were of poor nutritional quality, which was a major concern for parents. Parents also expressed anxiety and worry about being on the streets with their infants and young children, without access to safe shelter, food, or water during the hours in which the doors to the emergency housing shelter were closed, especially during inclement weather conditions.

Discussion

In order to get a handle on breastfeeding disparities in Hawai'i, one needs to examine the social context of everyday violence that leads to maternal and infant morbidity and mortality. Breastfeeding is not simply a behavior to support, but an integral component to improving maternal-child health outcomes. However, it is somewhat unrealistic to think that breastfeeding rates will be improved as long as high rates of perinatal intimate partner violence, substance abuse and addiction, child sexual abuse, and mental illness persist. There are many reasons why these mothers have decided to stop breastfeeding, including when it is medically contraindicated, or they believe that breastfeeding would put their child at risk of harm by violence, for example.

Physical healing will not be sustainable as long as the cycle of historical trauma remains unbroken. Eliminating health disparities requires addressing the causes of inequality and social suffering (Duran et al., 1998; Kleinman et al., 1997; Trask, 2004). This is no small task. Doing so requires structural interventions, not simply health interventions. It requires caring for physical health as well as well-being. It means that the balance of power needs to shift in such a way that health and healing begins within the community at the hands of those within the community to meet the goals and aspirations set by the community. It also needs to happen within a society that believes access to health services a basic human right, not a socioeconomic privilege.

Following recommendations for optimal IYCF requires recognizing the integral role of breastfeeding within the context of other health and social inequalities. Improving breastfeeding rates within low-income, food insecure NHPI communities must begin with preventative care. Preventing childhood trauma, neglect, childhood and adolescent overweight, substance use, preconception obesity and metabolic disorders, depression today might give the breastfeeding dyads of tomorrow the best chances of improved health.

When breastfeeding is not working out or is not possible, there must be universal access to safe donor human milk. There are currently no Human Milk Banking Association of North America (HMBANA) affiliated milk banks operating Hawai'i, and this is a travesty. Overall, breastfeeding rates are stellar in Hawai'i, and there is a great potential for donor human milk to positively impact NHPI neonatal morbidity and mortality.

Concluding Thoughts

The impact of historical trauma, structural violence, and poverty on the health trajectory of NHPI infants and young children must not be underestimated. Findings of this exploration raises important questions for community health in Hawai'i: What if it was possible to transform health disparities through effective family-centered breastfeeding promotion and universal access to donor human milk? What if community healing led to greater breastfeeding and better long-term health outcomes? What would public health interventions look like for homeless NHPI if services were more carefully coordinated to support families with infants and young children?

References

Bernard, H. R. (2011). *Research methods in anthropology: Qualitative and quantitative approaches*, Fifth Edition. Lanham, MD: Alta Mira Press.

Centers for Disease Control and Prevention. (2012). *Summary Health Statistics for U.S. Adults: 2011. Table 31.* Retrieved from http://www.cdc.gov/nchs/data/series/sr_10/srl0_256.pdf

Duran, E., Duran, B., Brave Heart, M. Y. H., & Yellow Horse-Davis, S. (1998). Healing the American Indian soul wound. In D. Yael (Ed.), *International handbook of multigenerational legacies of trauma* (pp. 341-354). New York: Plenum Press

Farmer, P.E., Nizeye, B., & Stulac, S. (2006). Structural violence and clinical medicine. *PLoS Medicine, 3*(10), e449.

Hawaii State Department of Health. (2010a). *Hawaii Health Data Warehouse, Behavior Risk Factor Surveillance System, Honolulu, HI.* Retrieved from http://health.hawaii.gov/brfss/files/2014/01/HBRFSS_2010results_12.pdf.

Hawaii State Department of Health. (2010b). *Hawaii PRAMS Trend Report 2004-2008, Hawaii State Department of Health, Honolulu, HI.* Retrieved from http://health.hawaii.gov/mchb/files/2013/05/pramstrendreport2010.pdf.

Hawaii State Department of Health. (2014). *Office of Health Status Monitoring (OHSM); Report Date: 04/01/2014.* Retrieved from http://www.hhdw.org/cms/uploads/Data%20Source_%20Vitals/Vitals_Infant%20Deaths_3AGG.pdf.

Hayes D., Donohoe-Mather, C,. Pager, S., & Fuddy, L. (2010). *Breastfeeding Fact Sheet.* Hawai'i Department of Health, Family Health Services Division, Honolulu, HI. Retrieved from www.health.hawaii.gov/mchb/files/2013/05/breastfeeding2010.pdf.

Kleinman, A., Das, V., & Lock, M. (Eds.) (1997) *Social suffering.* Berkeley, CA: UC Press.

Le Compte, M.D., & Schensul, J.J. (2010). *Designing and conducting ethnographic research,* Second Ed. Lanham, MD: Alta Mira Press.

Riessman, C.K. (2007). *Narrative methods for the human sciences.* Thousand Oaks, CA: Sage Publications.

Schempf, A., Hayes, D., & Fuddy, L. (2010). *Perinatal substance use fact sheet.* Hawai'i Department of Health, Family Health Services Division, Honolulu, HI. Retrieved from http://health.hawaii.gov/mchb/files/2013/05/perinatal2010.pdf.

Trask, H. K. (2004). The color of violence. *Social Justice, 31*(4), 8-16.

U.S. Department of Health and Human Services. (2015). *Profile: Native Hawaiian and Pacific Islanders, Office of Minority Health.* Retrieved from http://minorityhealth.hhs.gov/omh/browse.aspx?lvl=3&lvlID=65

CHAPTER 5

Emotional and Physical Trauma, and Its Impact on Breastfeeding Mothers

Dianne Cassidy

B reastfeeding has been the most common method of feeding babies since time began. In the 20th century, breastfeeding become something of a lost art, and increased acceptance of human milk substitutes quickly stepped in and claimed its place in the world of infant feeding. Medical professionals have recognized and identified breastfeeding as being the optimal choice for mothers and babies; nonetheless increasing breastfeeding initiation and duration rates has been a constant struggle.

When identifying reasons why women abandon breastfeeding, or refuse to initiate breastfeeding altogether, it is important to consider the role that emotional and physical trauma might play in women's decisions about infant feeding. Emotional and physical trauma suffered by women at a young age, during pregnancy, during labor and delivery, or in the immediate postpartum period can negatively impact a new mother's ability or desire to breastfeed her baby. Even when a woman agrees that breastfeeding is the best choice for her, past abuse, physical trauma or psychological impairment may impede her ability to initiate or continue with breastfeeding.

Although trauma can be a difficult subject to address, health care workers, support persons and family can be helpful to a new mother who is struggling with breastfeeding. By recognizing when trauma may be at the source of the issue, those working closely with the mother/baby dyad can assist in reinforcing the importance of breastfeeding, while being sensitive to a new mother's concerns.

Definition of Trauma

Pathologically, trauma is defined as a body wound or shock produced by sudden physical injury, as from violence or accident (dictionary. com). Psychologically, trauma is defined as an emotional wound or shock that creates substantial lasting damage to one's psychological development, often leading to neurosis (dictionary.com). A limited body of research has explored the relationships between intimate partner violence, sexual abuse in childhood and adulthood, and breastfeeding initiation and duration.

Child Sexual Abuse (CSA)

Child sexual abuse can be defined as sexual contact with a child by force, without consent, usually by someone who is in a position of authority or a caregiver. Sexual trauma is relatively common, affecting approximately 20% to 25% of women (Kendall-Tackett, 2005). International studies indicate that CSA can vary from 6% to 62% depending on the definition of abuse and methods used (Coles, 2009).

Childhood sexual abuse has many short and long term mental health consequences (English et al., 2005); the consequences vary, depending on the type of abuse, severity, age at onset, frequency, and duration of the abuse (English et al., 2005). Finklelhor and Browne (1986) hypothesize that the consequences of CSA begin with disempowerment, with sexual predators disempowering their victims by disregarding their needs and invading their body space (Browne & Finkelhor, 1986). Vulnerability, fear, loss of control intertwined with the intimacy of childbirth can resurface memories of past abuse.

Dissociation is a common reaction for women suffering from childhood sexual abuse (English et al., 2005). This coping strategy enables victims to mentally escape from the trauma that they are experiencing (English et al., 2005). In the context of motherhood, dissociation may lead some mothers to emotionally detach from their children (Silberg et al., 2003) and may interfere with the mother-child relationship (Bowman, Ryberg, & Becker, 2008). As Karl (2004) explained, "successful breastfeeding requires an intimate interactive connectedness between a mother and her infant for the mother to interpret infant cues and respond appropriately." These characteristics can conflict with mothers that are survivors of CSA (see Table 1).

Table 1
Factors that May Lead to Reduced Breastfeeding by Survivors of CSA

● Public exposure of the body
● Strong sensations as the baby feeds
● Uterine cramping, nipple pain
● Unwelcomed physical contact: (i.e., RN/LC touching breast)
● Increase in breast size that occurs with lactation
● Night time feedings

Adolescent Mothers

Adolescent motherhood has a strong link to childhood sexual abuse. The prevalence of childhood sexual abuse among adolescent mothers is close to 50% (Bowman, 2007). If adolescent mothers with histories of abuse are able to initiate breastfeeding, these babies are more likely to wean at an earlier age than babies of adolescent mothers who have not been abused (Bowman, 2007). There are several possibilities as to why adolescent mothers who are survivors of sexual abuse may decide not to breastfeed. Breastfeeding requires a close, intimate connection between mother and baby, which may be difficult for a survivor of sexual abuse. For these mothers, breastfeeding may feel intrusive and become a source of anxiety, disconnection, and trauma secondary to the abuse (Bowman, 2007).

Intimate Partner Violence

The term "intimate partner violence" describes physical, sexual, or psychological harm by a current or former partner or spouse (Centers for Disease Control and Prevention [CDC], 2014). IPV includes physical harm from a partner, emotional mistreatment that may be in the form of yelling, disrespect, and threats, sexual abuse including sabotaging the use of birth control, and economic abuse in the form of controlling money and property (see Table 2). Intimate partner violence (IPV) is a serious, preventable public health problem that affects millions of Americans; more than 20% of women experience IPV during their lifetime (Cerulli, Chin, Talbot, & Chaudron, 2010).

Although, we might expect that pregnancy would shield a woman from her partner's abusive behavior, in reality, it may have the opposite effect. There have been conflicting studies about how or whether IPV affects women's breastfeeding practices. However, amid mothers who choose not to initiate or sustain breastfeeding, victims of IPV are statistically overrepresented (Cerulli et al., 2010). There are a variety of reasons why women who experience violence might be less likely to initiate breastfeeding or have shorter duration (see Table 2).

Table 2

Factors that May Lead to Reduced Breastfeeding by Women Experiencing IPV

● Lack of support
● Power and support
● Lack of information
● Jealousy/sex
● Stress/disempowerment

Breastfeeding and trauma is a subject that does not discriminate. Health care providers, lactation consultants, and breastfeeding supporters can help support survivors by becoming familiar with dynamics of intimate partner violence and child sexual abuse, and strategies for working compassionately and supportively with abused women (Table 3). There are several important volumes that can help providers and researchers provide support and care for new mothers who may also have been abused (Chamberlain & Levenson 2013; Ellesburg & Heise, 2005; Stevens, 2001).

Table 3

Communicating with Survivors

● Responsibilities of providers
● Build a trusting relationship
● Non-judgmental attitude
● Address concerns
● Ethical responsibilities

References

Bowman, K.G., Ryberg, J.W., & Becker, H. (2009). Examining the relationship between a childhood history of sexual abuse and later dissociation, breast-feeding practices and parenting anxiety. *Journal of Interpersonal Violence, 24*(8), 1304-1317.

Browne, A., & Finkelhor, D. (1986). Impact of child sexual abuse: A review of the research. *Psychological Bulletin, 99*(1), 66-77.

Bureau of Justice Statistics. (2014). *National crime victimization survey.* Retrieved from http://www.data.gov/raw/1526/.

Cerulli, C., Chin, N., Talbot, N., & Chaudron, L. (2010). Exploring the impact of intimate partner violence on breastfeeding initiation: Does it matter? *Journal of Breastfeeding Medicine, 5*(5), 225.

Chamberlain, L., & Levenson, R. (2013, 3rd Edition). *Addressing Intimate Partner Violence, Reproductive and Sexual Coercion: A Guide for Obstetric, Gynecologic, Reproductive Health Care Settings.* Futures Without Violence.

Coles, J. (2009). Qualitative study of breastfeeding after childhood sexual assault. *Journal of Human Lactation, 25*(3), 317-324.

CDC. (2014). *Intimate partner violence.* Retrieved from www.cdc.gov/ViolencePrevention/intimatepartnerviolence/index.html.

Dictionary.com. (2014). *Trauma.* Retrieved from http://dictionary.reference.com/browse/trauma?s=t.

DiLillo, D. (2001). Interpersonal functioning among women reporting a history of childhood sexual abuse: Empirical findings and methodological issues. *Clinical Psychology Review, 21*(4), 553-576.

Ellsberg M., & Heise L. (2005). *Researching violence against women: A practical guide for researchers and activists.* Washington DC, United States: World Health Organization, PATH.

English, D.J., Upadhyaya, M.P., Litrownik, A.J., Marshall,J.M., Runyan, D.K., Graham, J., & Dubowitz, H. (2005). Maltreatment's wake: The relationship of maltreatment dimensions to child outcomes. *Child Abuse & Neglect, 29*, 597-619.

Karl, D. (2004). Behavioral state organization: Breastfeeding. *MCN: The American Journal of Maternal/Child Nursing, 29*, 293-298.

Kendall-Tackett, K. (Ed.). (2005). *Handbook of women, stress and trauma.* New York: Brunner-Routledge.

Lau, Y., & Chan, K.S. (2007). Influence of intimate partner violence during pregnancy and early postpartum depressive symptoms on breastfeeding among Chinese women in Hong Kong. *Journal of Midwifery & Women's Health, 52*(5), e15-e20.

Perkins, C., Klaus, P., Bastian, L., & Cohen, R. (1996). *Criminal victimization in the United States, 1993: A National Crime Victimization Survey Report.* The U.S. Department of Justice Bureau of Justice Statistics. Washington, DC: USGPO. Retrieved from http://www.bjs.gov/content/pub/pdf/cvus93.pdf.

Russell, D.E.A. (1986). *The secret trauma incest in the lives of girls and women.* New York: Basic Books.

Silberg, J., Waters, F., Nemzer, E., McIntee, J., Wieland, S., Grimminck, E., Nordquist, L., & Emsond, E. (2003). *Guidelines for the evaluation and treatment of dissociative symptoms in children and adolescents-2003-ISSD Task Force on Children and Adolescents.* Retrieved from http://www.isst-d.org/default.asp?contentID=50.

Stevens, L. (2001). *A practice approach to gender-based violence: Aa programme guide for health care providers and managers.* New York: United Nations Fund for Population Activities.

CHAPTER 6

The Changing Definition of Family: Issues in Lactation Consulting Related to Same Sex

Ellen Chetwynd

Feminism is about choice. Our life partners, and the families we create with them, are some of the most important choices we make in our lives. Breastfeeding advocates need to be fully cognizant of the options open to parents, whether gestational or non-gestational, regardless of sex or gender, in order to provide supportive care to all families. It is not enough to be open to the unfamiliar; we must also be knowledgeable in the way we counsel parents, whether we are providing lactation support as a peer or professional.

The landscape of marriage is rapidly changing around the world. In the United States, thirty-seven states currently accept marriages between same-sex couples (Freedom to Marry, 2015). [Same-sex marriage is now legal in all 50 states in the U.S.] According to the 2010 American Community Survey (ACS) results, 1% of coupled households (including married and unmarried domestic partnerships) are same-sex households, and 20% of same-sex households reported having children (Loquis, 2011). Of all the same-sex couple households with children,

21% were either step children or adopted children (Loquis, 2011). Open adoptions provide creative and cooperative options for all individuals choosing to be parents, but particularly for same-sex couples who might find policies and protocols within state institutions to be restrictive.

Overall, as social acceptance of same-sex relationships increases, the proportion of same-sex adoptions in the United States is also growing. Between 2000 and 2009, the number of same-sex adoptions in the United States doubled, and lesbian and bisexual women are considering and pursuing adoption at rates higher than heterosexual couples (Gates, Badgett, Macomber, & Chambers, 2001). The increasing number of adoptions combined with a growing emphasis on breastfeeding will likely accelerate the numbers of women in same-sex relationships who consider inducing lactation to feed an adoptive baby. Health care providers advising women who are inducing lactation should remain open and attentive to the myriad arrangements that may present themselves during counseling.

The literature on the success of non-puerperal lactation (nursing without pregnancy) is mixed and true prevalence trends are difficult to ascertain (Bryant, 2006). Research on lactation induction, whether it is re-lactation, or induction without previous breastfeeding experience, typically follows three types of protocols: (1) only breast stimulation, either once the baby is present, or beginning with pumping prior to the arrival of the child (Abejide, 1997; Auerbach & Avert, 1981; Thearle & Weissenberger, 1984); (2) use of breast stimulation and galactogogues, such as herbs or medications that can increase lactation (Banapurmath, 1993); or (3) use of hormones in combination with galactogogues and breast stimulation to simulate a hormonal milieu similar to pregnancy, along with the galactogogues and breast stimulation (Nemba, 1994; Szucs, Axline, & Rosenman, 2010; Thearle & Weissenberger, 1984). While herbs are commonly used as galactogogues in current standard clinical care, the most common galactogogue studied for lactation induction is metoclopramide, sometimes combined with a single shot of medroxyprogesterone (Nemba, 1994).

Method

We followed the lactation induction and breastfeeding experience of a lesbian couple from their decision to induce lactation to their postpartum experience with nursing and milk sharing. In this case, the families had agreed that all three mothers would nurse their child for the first ten days after the birth while they stayed together at the birth mothers' home, and the birth mother would continue to pump and share her milk as long as she was able.

Results

The adoptive mothers (ages 38[participant A] and 46[participant B]) were both in good health, and neither had ever been pregnant or lactated previously. With the help of their International Board Certified Lactation Consultant and their primary care doctors, they decided to use hormonal birth control pills for approximately 3 months. They then stopped the birth control pills and began domperidone, fenugreek, herbal lactation tea, and breast stimulation (breast pumping) 4-6 times a day one month prior to their baby's due date. Both mothers successfully produced milk. For participant B, milk production began on day 2, and on day 12 for participant A. The milk was thin, white, and had the appearance of mature milk rather than colostrum. By the time the baby was born, each mother was producing 1-2 oz a day (Figure 1).

The baby was born at term via a spontaneous vaginal home delivery and weighed 3.8 kg (70th percentile). The adoptive mothers stayed with the birth family for the first 10 days. During this time, both adoptive mothers, as well as the birth mother, nursed the baby. Both adoptive mothers continued their galactogogues, but found it difficult to maintain their pumping regimen. Each adoptive mother was able to pump once a day. While the baby nursed with all three mothers, he had a preference for A's left breast over her right and either of Bs breasts. As a result, it was this breast that received the most stimulation. Once home, both mothers nursed using a supplemental feeder made by the midwife out of a bottle with a neonatal nasogastric tube inserted through the nipple. Supplements were a combination of cows' milk formula, breastmilk pumped by the birth mother and shipped for several months after the birth, and breastmilk donated by friends. Neither mother pumped. Each mother put her son to breast equally, trading the feedings back and forth between them. The largest measured feeding he received from the breast, measured using pre- and post-weights on a breastfeeding scale, was 14 mL.

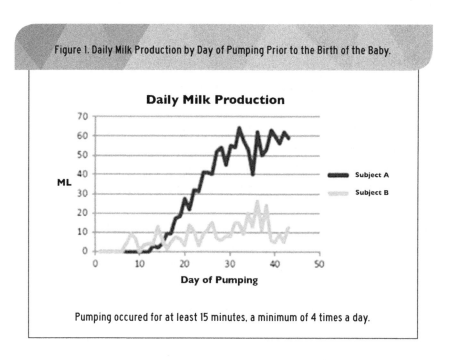

Figure 1. Daily Milk Production by Day of Pumping Prior to the Birth of the Baby.

Pumping occured for at least 15 minutes, a minimum of 4 times a day.

Although both women felt that breastfeeding was good for bonding, producing milk was more important to A than to B. The couple discussed having A do the majority of the feedings in order to maximize their overall potential milk production; however, they eventually decided against this due to the disequilibrium it would introduce into their shared feeding responsibilities. In addition, B enjoyed using the supplemental nurser for bonding and comforting the baby. The adoptive moms nursed their son for 7 months.

It is the exception rather than the norm among female-only couples for both mothers to want to lactate; in this instance, both felt that although they had not produced as much milk as they had hoped, but the experience of nursing their infant had been worthwhile.

Discussion and Conclusion

For same-sex couples inducing lactation, the duplication of biologically defined roles intrinsic to nursing shared between multiple mothers introduces unique physical consideration, including lack of full breast stimulation, and negotiation around variation of production between partners. For the health care provider advising women inducing lactation, it is important to remain open and attentive to the myriad arrangements that may present themselves during counseling. In this case, the dynamic of three nursing mothers during the first weeks postpartum likely contributed to the decreased milk production for both adoptive mothers after the birth of their baby.

When counseling same-sex parents, it is important to additionally consider the adoption process itself, as it may introduce unique demands and anxieties because of continued discriminatory practices and policies that exist in some states or agencies. Women should be counseled in the nutritive and non-nutritive benefits of breastfeeding, as well as being open to varying personal feelings about breasts, as not all women identify with the female gender, and thus not all women would consider lactation as a choice for themselves. The personal priorities of each parent should be addressed individually and respected.

This chapter is a summary of one of two pilot studies published based on the experience of these two mothers. Here, we focus on the qualitative research; however, we also collected and analyzed the mothers' non-puerperal milk composition over the course of their induction, which is, to our knowledge, the first study of the composition of induced non-puerperal human milk in the literature. To fully understand induced lactation in this context, further work is needed on appropriate means of induction, the composition of induced milk, and the social implications of adoptive nursing within non-traditional family settings.

Full articles about the two pilot studies briefly described in this article can be found at:

Perrin M.T., Wilson E., Chetwynd E., & Fogleman A (2015). A pilot study on the protein composition of induced non-puerperal human milk. *Journal of Human Lactation, 31*(1), 166-171.

Wilson E., Perrin M.T., Fogleman A., & Chetwynd E (2015). The intricacies of induced lactation for same-sex mothers of an adopted child. *Journal of Human Lactation, 31*(1), 64-67.

References

Abdjide, O.R., Tadese, M.A., Babajide, D.E., Torimiro, S.E., Davies-Adetugbo, A.A., & Makanjuola R.O. (1997). Non-puerperal induced lactation in a Nigerian community: case reports. *Annals of Tropical Paediatrics, 17*(2), 109-114.

Auerbach, K.G., & Avery, J.L. (1981). Induced lactation. A study of adoptive nursing by 240 women. *American Journal of Diseases in Childhood, 135*(4), 340-343.

Banapumath, C.R., Banapurmath S., & Desaree N. (1993). Successful induced non-puerperal lactation in surrogate mothers. *Indian Journal of Pediatrics, 60*(5), 639-643.

Bryant C.A. (2006). Nursing the adopted infant. *Journal of American Board of Family Medicine,* 19(4), 374-379.

Gates G.J., Badgett M.V.L., Macomber J.E., & Chambers K. (2001). *Adoption and foster care by gay and lesbian parents in the United States.* Washington, DC: The Williams Institute and Urban Institute.

Lofquis, D. (2011) *Same sex couple housing.* American Community Survey Briefs. Retrieved from https://www.census.gov/prod/2011pubs/acsbr10-03.pdf.

Nemba, K. (1994). Induced lactation: A study of 37 non-puerperal mothers. *Journal of Tropical Pediatrics, 40*(4), 240-242.

States | Freedom to Marry. (2015). *States.* Retrieved from http://www.freedomtomarry.org/states on June 11, 2015.

Szucs K.A., Axline S.E., & Rosenman M.B. (2010). Induced lactation and exclusive breastmilk feeding of adopted premature twins. *Journal of Human Lactation, 26*(3), 309-313.

Thearle, M.J., & Weissenberger R. (1984) Induced lactation in adoptive mothers. *Australian and New Zealand Journal of Obstretrics & Gyneaecology, 24*(4), 283-286.

Section 2
**Increasing
Racial Equity**

CHAPTER 7

Moving Mothers of Color from the "Margins to the Center" of the Breastfeeding Movement: 10 Key Principles for Applying Black Feminist Theory in Public Health

Quinn M. Gentry

The purpose of this paper is to introduce 10 principles of how public health professionals can apply black feminist theory in the breastfeeding movement in their work as researchers, intervention developers, frontline health educators and program implementers, and social and health equity advocates. In general, Black feminism is an interpretative framework for understanding the meaning of research findings on multiple levels with close attention to social, political, and economic dynamics that explains how Black women are impacted by social and health issues in particular. When thinking about how to apply Black feminism in public health, and more specifically, in breastfeeding, Black feminism is a valuable framework on at least three broad levels (Collins, 2000):

1. **Interpretive framework**: Black feminist theory provides an interpretive framework for examining how social, political, and economic issues that impact Black women, in particular.

2. **Examination of repeat patterns of power and control:** Black feminism is generally defined as a pattern of thought that recognizes how systems of power are configured around and maintain socially constructed categories of race, class, and gender.

3. **Action-oriented:** The larger premise is grounded in a "politics of empowerment" that demands action at the individual (agency) and systematic levels.

The core of this paper focuses on how to move from theory to action by examining 10 themes or principles in Black feminism with special attention on how to apply them in breastfeeding advocacy.

Theme No.1: Respect Individual's Right to Self-Definition and Self-Valuation

In conducting my research on black women in general and Black mothers, in particular, the resounding theme is that mothers on the margin want to be recognized as "more than mothers." The following are a few of the diverse/within groups of mothers who are on the margins of the breastfeeding movement because of the multiple roles and status set they have in society: (1) adolescent and young mothers between the ages of 15-21(Shanok & Miller, 2007; Zachry, 2005); (2) "mothers" between the ages of 11-14 years old (Boyer & Fine, 1992); (3) minimum-wage/hourly wage job working mothers (Baker & Milligan, 2008); (4) mothers with rapid repeat pregnancy (Boardman, Allsworth, Phipps, & Lapane, 2006); (5) single, working moms who have "2nd shifts" (Johnston & Esposito, 2007); (6) mothers with alcohol and drug dependency problems (Gentry, 2004); (7) collegiate mothers (Flam,

2014); (8) unwanted pregnancies carried to full term (Finer at al., 200); and (9) the "dysfunctional," "distant," and/or "deviant" (Schur, 1984) mom as defined by society standards of motherhood.

One way to fully understand the unmet needs of mothers on the margin is to examine their lives through the theory of Maslow's Hierarchy of Needs where health educators take into account the competing needs of mothers on the margin as it relates to her needs for (1) basic necessities, (2) safety, (3) belongingness and love, (4) self-esteem, and (5) self-actualization (Maslow, 1943).

Theme No. 2: Controlling Images

The theme of controlling images suggests that health educators pay close attention to the words, socialization processes, and symbols used to objectify a group of people in ways that justify continued economic and social disenfranchisement. For breastfeeding, it requires that we acknowledge the historical beginning of Black women serving as nursemaids for White mothers. The controlling images of Black mothers being forced to give their breastmilk to White babies continue to surface as historical barriers as to why Black women in today's time do not breastfeed.

One of the many ways to addressing the lingering impact of controlling images is to replace the "public health" model of building rapport to one of building a relationship. I developed the RELATE model as a way to engage clients as subjects and not public health objects. The "RELATE" Model is comprised of six core elements as follows: (1) reality, (2) empathy, (3) listening, (4) action, (5) touch-base, and (6) empower (Gentry, 2015).

Theme No. 3: Race, Class, and Gender

When it comes to marginalized mothers, health educators must understand the interconnectedness of race, class, and gender as a way to detect "who" and "what" is influencing and informing breastfeeding choices. From a Black feminist standpoint, this is done by examining how race, class, and gender intersect to inform individual factors and choices, the social context within which breastfeeding, and the social constraints that are beyond control of the individual mother.

Theme No. 4: Unique Experiences

A thorough understanding of unique experiences among diverse groups of mothers on the margins of breastfeeding will result in breastfeeding advocates being more committed to multiple levels of intervention. For example, at the community level, interventions need to address the lingering impact of racism, stigma, and shame associated with breastfeeding among poor mothers, in particular. At the small group intervention level, health educators can create opportunities for support systems to continue beyond the group level engagement. Individual sessions are needed as well to unpack those barriers that may be more personal and embarrassing, or even dangerous to discuss in a community or group-level setting.

Theme No. 5: Matrix of Domination

The theme on the matrix of domination represents the overall organization of power relationships, rules, and regulations associated with systems in our society. For breastfeeding, that means that we must immerse ourselves in deeper understanding of how the following systems impact breastfeeding decisions before we "blame the victim" for her choice to not breastfeed: (1) family, (2) social and health services, (3) political/governing, (4) educational, and (5) business/economics.

Theme No. 6: Structure and Agency

Organizations and individuals must change in order to create opportunities for optimum-levels of health and well-being. First, Black feminism is compatible with public health theories on behavioral change. In the case of breastfeed, behavioral change theory represents the "agency" of individual mothers to make changes in her decision and action to breastfeed (Gentry, Elifson, & Sterk, 2005; Prochaska, Redding, & Evers, 2008).

At the structural level, public health professionals need to be more politicized to the changes needed in the "taken-for-granted" rules and regulations governing home, school, work, and community-based programs that conflict with mothers' willingness and ability to breastfeed.

Theme No. 7: Reality, Roles, Relationships, and Risk-taking

Closely related to the "Relate" model discussed earlier, breastfeeding advocates must be more sensitive to the everyday reality of mothers on the margin. As an example, the doula model typically associated with middle- and upper-class, primarily White mothers was adapted and tailored for adolescent mothers of color. The overall conclusion of the program was that doulas had to go beyond the call of her traditional "doula duties" to really reach and engage this group of marginalized mothers (Gentry, Nolte, Gonzalez, Pearson, & Ivey, 2010).

Theme No. 8: Rigorous Research, Responsible Application

This theme suggests that a Black feminist approach is very much grounded in examining the empirical research on breastfeeding among adolescent mothers. For this project, a cursory review of existing findings on breastfeeding among mothers on the margin revealed the following reasons as to why these mothers choose not to breastfeed: (1) embarrassment, (2) no visible milk production, (3) increased breast size, (4) breast soreness, (5) pain, (6) lack of interest, (7) family choice, (8) father's choice, (9) poor maternal nutrition, (10) inconvenience, (11) leaking milk, and (12) return to school/work (Dykes, Moran, Burt, & Edwards, 2003; Dyson, Green, Renfrew, McMillan, & Woolridge, 2010; Earle, 2000; Feldman-Winter & Shaikh, 2007; Hannon, Willis, Bishop-Townsend, Martinez, & Scrimshaw, 2000; Ineichen, Pierce, & Lawrenson, 1997).

Black feminist action-oriented stance, however, suggests that researchers unraveling these barriers have a responsibility to continue the work needed to develop theory-based and/or data-informed solutions for removing these constraints.

Theme No. 9: Problem-Solution Paradigm

In looking at ways to solve problems associated with mothers on the margin and breastfeeding, my model for advancing Black feminism offers a dynamic framework for examining the problems and related solutions. The problem-solution paradigm includes deeper discussions about the following "Ps" as a way to comprehensively address any and all problems associated with a particular public health issue: (1) problem-definition, (2) p-values, (3) personal experiences, (4) person(s)-impacted (partners, parents, peers, professionals), (5) places of risk and protection, (6) practices, (7) programs, (8) partnerships, and (9) policy.

Theme No. 10: Empowerment, Activism, and Social Justice

As we conclude this 10th anniversary of this conference, I want to leave you with a final message of empowerment as grounded in the 10th theme that focuses on Empowerment, Activism, and Social Justice. This is where we talk about the links between knowledge and action at the most radical extreme if necessary, much like the "ACT-UP" movement in New York when gay males took to the streets in New York to demand social justice for those impacted by HIV/AIDS. So too must those of us fighting in the breastfeeding movement be willing to act-up for the inclusion of marginalized mothers. We must all commit to bring our A-game! I want to end my thoughts on advancing Black feminism in breastfeeding with "7 As" that remind us to bring our "A" game

1. Bring comprehensive *assessment* tools that examine issues commonly raised among mothers on the margin of breastfeeding.
2. Bring *analytic skills* that are sensitive to the unique experiences of Black women and girls in breastfeeding.
3. Bring the courage to *address* health risks with relevant interventions and appropriate implementation settings that are more effective from marginalized and disenfranchised mothers.
4. Bring a spirit of *advocacy* for challenging and changing individuals, organizations, and systems that perpetuate health threats that result in mothers on the margins not breastfeeding.
5. Bring your positive *affirmations* to the field to help build up those who frontline staff who get beat up, broken down, and take unfair hits in advocating for breastfeeding among mothers on the margin.
6. Bring your willingness to *aggravate* people, politicians, and policies that work against positive health outcomes for women.
7. Bring your willingness to *act-up,* disrupt, and dismantle the matrix of domination.

Act up, disrupt, and dismantle, because, as Audrey Lorde reminds us, the master's tools will never dismantle a system that works for the powerful minority; that responsibility belongs to the mothers and daughters of the breastfeeding movement. So, I need you to awaken, arise, and work in unity, share the knowledge, and love those who are unlovable until they can love themselves and their children.

Thank you!

References

Baker, M., & Milligan, K. (2008). Maternal employment, breastfeeding, and health: Evidence from maternity leave mandates. *Journal of Health Economics, 27*(4), 871-887.

Boardman, L. A., Allsworth, J., Phipps, M. G., & Lapane, K. L. (2006). Risk factors for unintended versus intended rapid repeat pregnancies among adolescents. *Journal of Adolescent Health, 39*(4), 597-e1.

Boyer, D., & Fine, D. (1992). Sexual abuse as a factor in adolescent pregnancy and child maltreatment. *Family Planning Perspectives,* 4-19.

Collins, P. H. (2000). *Black feminist thought: Knowledge, consciousness, and the politics of empowerment.* New York: Routledge.

Dykes, F., Moran, V. H., Burt, S., & Edwards, J. (2003). Adolescent mothers and breastfeeding: Experiences and support needs—an exploratory study. *Journal of Human Lactation, 19*(4), 391-401.

Dyson, L., Green, J. M., Renfrew, M. J., McMillan, B., & Woolridge, M. (2010). Factors influencing the infant feeding decision for socioeconomically deprived pregnant teenagers: The moral dimension. *Birth, 37*(2), 141-149.

Earle, S. (2000). Why some women do not breast feed: Bottle feeding and fathers' role. *Midwifery, 16*(4), 323-330.

Feldman-Winter, L., & Shaikh, U. (2007). Optimizing breastfeeding promotion and support in adolescent mothers. *Journal of Human Lactation, 23*(4), 362-367.

Finer, L. B., & Henshaw, S. K. (2006). Disparities in rates of unintended pregnancy in the United States, 1994 and 2001. *Perspectives on Sexual and Reproductive Health,* 90-96.

Flam, L. (2014) *Breast-feeding mom's college graduation photo stirs controversy.* TODAY. Retrieved from http://www.today.com/parents/breast-feeding-moms-college-graduation-photo-stirs-controversy-2D79780389.

Gentry, Q. (2004). A Black feminist critique of the social construction of crack cocaine along race, class, and gender lines. In R.D. Coates (Ed.), *Race and ethnicity: Across time, space, and discipline.* (pp. 239-253). The Netherlands: Brill Academic Publishers.

Gentry, Q. M., Elifson, K., & Sterk, C. (2005). Aiming for more relevant HIV risk reduction: A Black feminist perspective for enhancing HIV intervention for low-income African American women. *AIDS Education & Prevention, 17*(3), 238-252.

Gentry, Q. M., Nolte, K. M., Gonzalez, A., Pearson, M., & Ivey, S. (2010). "Going beyond the call of doula": A grounded-theory analysis of the diverse roles community-based doulas play in the lives of pregnant and parenting adolescent mothers. *Journal of Perinatal Education, 19*(4), 24.

Gentry, Q.M. (2015). *Cultivating our gems: Strategies for raising, mentoring, and modeling the way for adolescent girls.* Atlanta, GA: Messages of Empowerment Productions Publication.

Gentry, Q.M., Elifson, K., & Sterk, C. (2005). Aiming for more relevant HIV risk reduction: A Black feminist perspective for enhancing HIV intervention for low-income African American women. *AIDS Education and Prevention, 17*(3), 238-252.

Hannon, P. R., Willis, S. K., Bishop-Townsend, V., Martinez, I. M., & Scrimshaw, S. C. (2000). African-American and Latina adolescent mothers' infant feeding decisions and breastfeeding practices: a qualitative study. *Journal of Adolescent Health, 26*(6), 399-407.

Ineichen, B., Pierce, M., & Lawrenson, R. (1997). Teenage mothers as breastfeeders: Attitudes and behaviour. *Journal of Adolescence, 20*(5), 505-509.

Johnston, M. L., & Esposito, N. (2007). Barriers and facilitators for breastfeeding among working women in the United States. *Journal of Obstetric, Gynecologic, & Neonatal Nursing, 36*(1), 9-20.

Maslow, A. H. (1943). A theory of human motivation. *Psychological Review, 50*(4), 370.

Prochaska, J. O., Redding, C. A., & Evers, K. E. (2008). The Transtheoretical Model and stages of change. In K. Glanz, B. K. Rimer, & K. Viswanath (Eds.), *Health behavior and health education: Theory, research, and practice, 4th Ed.* (pp. 97-121). San Francisco: Jossey-Bass.

Schur, E. M. (1984). *Labeling women deviant: Gender, stigma, and social control.* New York: McGraw-Hill.

Shanok, A. F., & Miller, L. (2007). Stepping up to motherhood among inner-city teens. *Psychology of Women Quarterly, 31*(3), 252-261.

Zachry, E. (2005). Getting my education: Teen mothers' experiences in school before and after motherhood. *The Teachers College Record, 107*(12), 2566-2598.

CHAPTER 8

Breastfeeding Disparities and Implications for the Life Course

Sarah Verbiest,
Amanda Zabala, and Elizabeth Thomas

Disparities in maternal and infant outcomes remain a prevalent and significant issue in the United States. The U.S. is one of only 17 countries worldwide, and the only high-income country, where the rate of maternal mortality is increasing. Between 1990 and 2013, the maternal mortality ratio in the U.S. increased from 12 to 28 maternal deaths for every 100,000 live births (World Health Organization [WHO], 2014). In addition, severe maternal morbidity currently affects more than 50,000 women in the U.S. every year, with the rate of hospitalizations due to severe delivery complications more than doubling between 1998 and 2010 (Centers for Disease Control and Prevention [CDC], 2014a). Disparities in these rates of maternal mortality and morbidity are particularly evident, with Black women being three-to-four times more likely to die from pregnancy-related causes than White women (Tucker, Berg, Callaghan, & Hsia, 2007). Black women are also two times more likely to suffer from severe maternal morbidity than their White counterparts (Creanga, Bateman, Kuklina, & Callaghan, 2014).

In terms of infant outcomes, rates of preterm birth, low birth weight, and infant mortality continue to be significantly greater for Blacks than they are for Whites. In 2013, the overall preterm birth rate was 11.4%; however, 16.3% of Black infants were born preterm, compared to just 10.2% of White infants (Martin, Hamilton, Osterman, Curtin, & Mathews, 2015). Even after accounting for known risk factors (e.g., income, education, chronic conditions, risky health behaviors), this disparity in preterm birth persists (Lu & Halfon, 2003). Similarly, the rate of low birth weight in 2013 was 8.0%; though, the rate for Black infants (13.1%) was nearly twice that of White infants (7.0%) (Martin et al., 2015).

In addition to these adverse birth outcomes for Black Americans, disparities in infant feeding practices also exist, and have persisted over time. Among all infants born in 2000, 70.3% had ever breastfed, 34.5% breastfed for 6 months, and 16.0% breastfed for 12 months. Among infants born in 2008, these percentages increased to 74.6%, 44.4%, and 23.4%, respectively (CDC, 2013). Among Black women, the prevalence of breastfeeding initiation in 2000 was 47.4%, increasing to 58.9% by 2008. Comparatively, the prevalence of breastfeeding initiation among White women increased from 71.8% to 75.2% in this timeframe. From 2000 to 2008, breastfeeding at 6 and 12 months increased significantly among both populations (CDC, 2013). Data from the 2011 National Immunization Survey (NIS) indicate that rates of breastfeeding initiation have continued to increase, with 61.6% of Black and 81.1% of White women initiating breastfeeding practices (CDC, 2014b). Still, while the gap between Black and White breastfeeding initiation has narrowed, Black infants maintain the lowest prevalence of breastfeeding initiation and duration (CDC, 2014b).

Life Course Theory

The causes of the racial disparities in birth outcomes and breastfeeding practices are still not fully understood. However, since Lu and Halfon (2003) developed the life course perspective in 2003, maternal and child health professionals have expanded their views of health determination (Lu & Halfon, 2003). Life course theory is a conceptual framework that aims to provide an explanation for health, disease, and disparities patterns among differing populations and over time (Fine & Kotelchuck, 2010). The life course perspective synthesizes two longitudinal models—an early programming model and a cumulative pathways model—ultimately pointing to broad social, economic, and environmental factors as underlying causes of persistent inequalities in health for a wide range of diseases and conditions across population groups (Fine & Kotelchuck, 2010; Lu et al., 2010). The life course theory ultimately conceptualizes birth outcomes as the product of a lifetime of exposures, and the early programming model, in particular, provides a rationale for supporting breastfeeding practices.

The early programming component of the life course perspective posits that early life exposures influence future health outcomes. Breastfeeding, therefore, provides a number of benefits for infants and children, including nutritionally balanced meals, protection against common childhood illnesses and infections, better survival during the first year of life, and a lower chance of developing certain allergies or Type 1 diabetes (American Academy of Pediatrics [AAP], 2012; National Institute of Child Health & Human Development [NICHD], 2009). There are also demonstrated physical and emotional benefits of breastfeeding from infants' skin-to-skin contact with their mother (UNICEF, n.d). In addition to these proximal benefits, indirect evidence also suggests that overweight and obesity occur less often among children who were breastfed (Yamakawa, Yorifuji, Inoue, Kato, & Doi, 2013). Research has also shown a connection between breastfeeding and better cognitive development in children through school age (Quigley et al., 2012).

Though the benefits of breastfeeding are often focused on the infant, there are known benefits for mothers as well. Short term, mothers experience less blood loss following childbirth and improved healing; improved postpartum weight loss; emotional benefits from close interaction with their infant; lower likelihood of experiencing postpartum depression; and the same physical and emotional benefits associated with skin-to-skin contact with their infants. In a more long-term sense, breastfeeding mothers have a lesser chance of developing certain health conditions, including rheumatoid arthritis, cardio-vascular disease, and certain cancers (AAP, 2012; NICHD, 2009; UNICEF, n.d.).

In 2010, Lu et al. used the aforementioned life course approach to propose a 12-point plan to reduce the Black-White disparities in birth outcomes (Lu et al., 2010). Recognizing that early life disadvantages and cumulative allostatic load over the life course are significant factors to be addressed, North Carolina adapted this original plan to specifically improve the health of mothers, children, and communities within the state.

North Carolina Perinatal Health Strategic Plan

The 12 points suggested by Lu et al., and which form the framework of North Carolina's plan are summarized in Table 1. The North Carolina plan is comprehensive, and will be described elsewhere upon final publication by the NC Division of Public Health. Certainly, the accumulation of these points suggests a multifaceted approach to addressing disparities in birth outcomes; however, a specific focus on breastfeeding practices and promotion is woven throughout. Many aspects of the plan respond to needs that are universal to all mothers, such as the creation of breastfeeding-friendly policies and designations, and promoting the role of fathers in changing culture. Recognizing that eliminating disparities in breastfeeding will also require targeted actions, the plan includes a number of strategies that address concerns specific to, or disproportionately experienced by, minority women.

Providing culturally competent care is a crucial component in addressing disparities. While the U.S. population is 63.4% White and 12.3% Black, 87% of International Board Certified Lactation Consultants (IBCLCs) are White, and just 1.6% are Black (Mojab, 2015). The disproportionately small number of minority IBCLCs reflects the barriers in access to the specialized education, financial investment, and contact hours required for certification. The North Carolina plan includes increased access to the numbers of IBCLCs per live birth, especially those of color, and calls for increased educational and financial support for these professionals. Others who work with breastfeeding mothers, such as home visitors, can benefit from training to focus on community building and empowering families. Listening sessions with women, families, and communities will enhance the systems that support breastfeeding and speak directly to the needs voiced by the populations served. Enhancing home visiting and other health care services, along with diversifying the breastfeeding support workforce, will be powerful tools in providing culturally competent care.

Table 1

A 12-Point Plan to Close the Black-White Gap in Birth Outcomes (Lu et al., 2010)

Goal 1: Improving Health Care for Women
● Point 1. Provide interconception care to women with prior adverse pregnancy outcomes
● Point 2. Increase access to preconception health and health care to women and men
● Point 3. Improve the quality of maternal care
● Point 4. Expand health care access over the life course for women and men
Goal 2: Strengthening Families and Communities
● Point 5. Strengthen father involvement in families
● Point 6. Enhance coordination and integration of family support services

- Point 7. Create reproductive social capital in all communities
- Point 8. Invest in community building

Goal 3: Addressing Social and Economic Inequities

- Point 9. Close the education gap
- Point 10. Reduce poverty among families
- Point 11. Support working mothers and families
- Point 12. Undo racism

The plan includes expansion of the breastfeeding peer support program to all counties in North Carolina. Peer support is an acknowledged strategy for increased breastfeeding initiation and duration, and can be an important component in reducing disparities (Johnson, Kirk, Rosenblum, & Muzik, 2015). Peer counseling also increases partner support for breastfeeding and strengthens the father's role in the family (Johnson et al., 2015).

Support for working families is another critical component in reducing racial disparities in breastfeeding. Black mothers working outside the home are disproportionately affected by barriers to breastfeeding and milk expression, such as short maternity leaves and inflexible work conditions (Johnson et al., 2015). Expanding paid leave, making high-quality childcare more accessible, and improving business support for breastfeeding will be of particular benefit to Black mothers.

While we celebrate the progress that has been made in increasing breastfeeding rates among mothers, multiple, coordinated efforts are needed to accelerate the pace of this change, especially for Black mothers. To close the gaps in birth and breastfeeding outcomes, statewide initiatives must reach women throughout their reproductive lives. Addressing disparities in breastfeeding from a life course perspective provides insight into the generational effects of these inequities, and highlights opportunities to redress them at the policy, community, and individual levels.

References

American Academy of Pediatrics (AAP). (2012). Breastfeeding and the use of human milk. *Pediatrics, 129*(3), e827–e841. Retrieved from http://pediatrics.aappublications.org/content/129/3/e827.full.pdf+html.

Centers for Disease Control and Prevention (CDC). (2013). *Progress in increasing breastfeeding and reducing racial/ethnic differences — United States, 2000–2008 births. MMWR, 62*(5), 77-80. Retrieved from http://www.cdc.gov/mmwr/preview/mmwrhtml/mm6205a1.htm.

Centers for Disease Control and Prevention (CDC). (2014a). *Severe maternal morbidity in the United States.* Retrieved from http://www.cdc.gov/reproductivehealth/MaternalInfantHealth/SevereMaternalMorbidity.html.

Centers for Disease Control and Prevention (CDC). (2014b). *Rates of any and exclusive breastfeeding by socio-demographics among children born in 2011.* http://www.cdc.gov/breastfeeding/data/nis_data/rates-any-exclusive-bf-socio-dem-2011.htm.

Creanga, A. A., Bateman, B. T., Kuklina, E. V., & Callaghan, W. M. (2014). Racial and ethnic disparities in severe maternal morbidity: A multistate analysis, 2008-2010. *American Journal of Obstetrics and Gynecology, 210*(5), 435-e1-8.

Fine, A., & Kotelchuck, M. (2010). *Rethinking MCH: The life course model as an organizing framework.* Retrieved from http://mchb.hrsa.gov/lifecourse/rethinkingmchlifecourse.pdf.

Johnson, A., Kirk, R., Rosenblum, K.L., & Muzik, M. (2015). Enhancing breastfeeding rates among African American women: A systematic review of current psychosocial interventions. *Breastfeeding Medicine, 10*(1), 45-62.

Lu, M. C., & Halfon, N. (2003). Racial and ethnic disparities in birth outcomes: A life course perspective. *Maternal and Child Health Journal, 7*(1), 13-30.

Lu, M. C., Kotelchuck, M., Hogan, V., Jones, L., Wright, K., & Halfon, N. (2010). Closing the Black-White gap in birth outcomes: A life-course approach. *Ethnicity & Disease, 20*(1 Suppl 2), S2-62-76.

Martin, J. A., Hamilton, B. E., Osterman, M. J. K., Curtin, S. C., & Mathews, T. (2015). Births: Final data for 2013, *National Vital*

Statistics Reports, 64(1); Hyattsville, MD: National Center for Health Statistics.

Mojab, C. G. (2015). Pandora's Box is already open: Answering the ongoing call to dismantle institutional oppression in the field of breastfeeding. *Journal of Human Lactation, 31*(1), 32-35.

National Institute of Child Health & Human Development (NICHD). (2009). *Breastfeeding.* Retrieved from http://www.nichd.nih.gov/health/topics/Breastfeeding/.

Quigley, M. A., Hockley, C., Carson, C., Kelly, Y., Renfrew, M. J., & Sacker, M. (2012). Breastfeeding is associated with improved child cognitive development: A population-based cohort study. *Journal of Pediatrics, 160*(1), 25-32.

Tucker, M. J., Berg, C. J., Callaghan, W.M., & Hsia, J. (2007). The black-white disparity in pregnancy-related mortality from 5 conditions: Differences in prevalence and case-fatality rates. *American Journal of Public Health, 97*(2), 247–251.

UNICEF. (n.d.). *Skin-to-skin contact.* Retrieved from http://www.unicef.org.uk/BabyFriendly/News-and-Research/Research/Skin-to-skin-contact/.

Yamakawa, M., Yorifuji, T., Inoue, S., Kato, T., & Doi, H. (2013). Breastfeeding and obesity among schoolchildren: A nationwide longitudinal survey in Japan. *JAMA Pediatrics, 167*(10), 919–925.

World Health Organization (WHO). (2014). *Trends in maternal mortality: 1990 to 2013.* Retrieved from http://apps.who.int/iris/bitstream/10665/112682/2/9789241507226_eng.pdf?ua=1.

CHAPTER 9

Reflections on the Concept of General Self-Efficacy in Breastfeeding Research and Practice

Cecilia E. Barbosa, Kellie E. Carlyle, and Saba W. Masho

The influence of self-efficacy on breastfeeding initiation and duration has been widely reported in the breastfeeding literature (Dennis, 2002; Meedya, Fahy, & Kable, 2010; Spencer & Grassley, 2013). Bandura (1984) described perceived self-efficacy as a person's confidence in their ability to perform a given task, or at a given level of performance, and affects how barriers and facilitators are perceived (Bandura, 2004). For example, a person with low self-efficacy could perceive breastfeeding barriers as insurmountable, whereas someone with high self-efficacy may pay scant attention to barriers. As Bandura (1977) stated,

> People fear and tend to avoid threatening situations they believe exceed their coping skills, whereas they get involved in activities and behave assuredly when they judge themselves capable of handling situations that would otherwise be intimidating (p. 194).

Although self-efficacy is typically described as domain-specific, some researchers have conceptualized a broader form called general self-efficacy (GSE) (Sherer & Maddux, 1982), or "a broad and stable sense of personal competency to deal effectively with a variety of stressful situations" (Luszczynska, Scholz & Schwarzer, 2005, p. 440). The level of GSE is a reflection of an accumulation of experiences over a lifetime and can influence the level of self-efficacy toward a newly-learned behavior (Imam, 2007). Both types of self-efficacy can be developed through personal or vicarious experiences, verbal persuasion, or physiological arousal (Bandura, 1977; Imam, 2007).

The periods of pregnancy, childbirth, and breastfeeding present unique circumstances for differentiating both conceptualizations of self-efficacy. When a woman becomes pregnant, she has already experienced, during her lifetime, successes and failures in multiple domains that influence her level of GSE. A first birth brings multiple new stresses and demands on mothers—those with high GSE would be expected to adapt to, and cope with, these demands and stresses better than someone with low GSE. Similarly, someone with low GSE would be expected to need greater support during pregnancy to withstand and prepare for these new demands and stresses.

The behavior of breastfeeding illustrates the difference between GSE and domain-specific self-efficacy. A first-time expectant woman has no personal experience with breastfeeding, and, unless she has had a high level of exposure vicariously through close family or friends, would be expected, in early pregnancy, to have low breastfeeding self-efficacy (BSE). However, this same expectant woman could, based on previous experiences, enter pregnancy with either high or low GSE. With a high GSE, she would be expected to be more adept at quickly learning and mastering this new skill than a woman with low GSE. This study explores this idea by identifying and describing qualitative differences and similarities in general self-efficacy among low-income African American women who engage in different infant feeding practices.

Method

Data from this study originated from a larger study aimed at understanding the barriers and facilitators faced by low-income African American women who have different infant feeding practices (Barbosa, 2014). Focus groups and interviews were conducted in Richmond, Virginia from November 2012 through May 2013 with 28 adult non-Hispanic/Latina African American mothers of children who were recipients of public assistance. Mothers whose oldest child was less than 2 years old were included in the study. Women were grouped according to their infant- feeding practice, as follows: only formula-fed their babies ($n = 9$); breastfed for 3 months or less ($n = 13$); and breastfed for at least 4 months ($n = 6$). Further details on the methods are described elsewhere (Barbosa, 2014).

The present study focuses on data segments in the intrapersonal category identified as either breastfeeding incentives or disincentives. [These are the intrapersonal, interpersonal, institutional, community levels from McLeroy's ecological model (McLeroy, K., Bibeau, D., Steckler, A., & Glanz, K.,1988).] Specifically, the analysis examined three areas of GSE as identified by Sherer and Maddux (1982): determination to initiate behavior; persistent effort to complete the behavior; and persistence under adversity. Once identified, differences and similarities in GSE among the three infant feeding groups were analyzed.

Results

All women who breastfed for at least four months had intended to breastfeed; the majority expressed a strong commitment to breastfeeding. One woman's strong commitment led her to pump her milk while driving.

> I try to train my body. I never wore breast pads or nothing like that ... I went and I bought that car charger—one where you just plug it into the little cigarette lighter, and even driving to work, I pumped.

Another woman valued planning:

> ... you have to kind of learn yourself and ... you have
> to kind of be a planner ... I think it's just making sure
> you plan ahead for when you're not gonna be around
> your baby, and you're not gonna nurse.

A high level of persistence in the face of adversity was also a common theme. One woman persisted in spite of pain: "It's painful for a few days, but you'll get over it and it'll become a lot easier." Others withstood the negative influence of family members.

> My family... they have a strange view of it [breastfeeding]. I told them I was supposed to breastfeed and ...
> they were like "Ew," my sister and my mother. I'm like,
> "Okay, I mean, that's what it's there for," and my aunts,
> like, all of them ... they think it's nasty or something.

The women who breastfed for less than 3 months varied in their prenatal infant feeding intentions, including women who had intended to formula-feed, who were ambivalent, or who intended to do so for an unspecified long time. The mothers also varied in their level of commitment to breastfeeding. For example, one woman had directed hospital staff to follow her breastfeeding-friendly birthing plan, while another was dissuaded by her grandmother's painful breastfeeding experience, and yet another stated: "I planned to breastfeed [when I was pregnant], but when I tried it I didn't like it." Their accounts of weaning illustrate how they dealt with adverse situations. One working woman said: "This is my first child, and the breastfeeding came pretty easy to me, but it just got difficult with—as far as working—and trying to do that at the same time for me." Another one stopped breastfeeding when she started feeling soreness: "I ate my regular food and he was doing good, until I started getting sore, so I was like, you going on the bottle." She does not mention seeking help or information for her sore breasts.

Seven of the 9 women who only formula-fed their babies had intended to do so while they were pregnant. Several women expressed fear and insecurity around breastfeeding. One woman feared the unknown ("Being insecure and scared ... I fear change. I didn't want to do something that I knew was different"). Another woman expressed fear of her baby's hunger ("And I agree with her, like with the fear ... I didn't know if the baby was gonna latch. I didn't know if I had enough"). In contrast, they viewed formula-feeding as more convenient, familiar, and compatible with their lifestyles.

Discussion

This pilot study illustrated examples of strong GSE among women who breastfed for at least 4 months, and weaker GSE among women who breastfed for shorter periods, or who did not breastfeed. The women's approaches to adverse situations highlighted these differences. However, it is possible that those who breastfed for shorter periods may have faced more challenging circumstances, for example, at work. According to social cognitive theory, human behavior is a product of the individual, behavioral, and environmental influences.

Three studies (Dennis & Faux, 1999; Hernandez, 2014; Ystrom, Niegel, Klepp, & Vollrath, 2008) examined the relationship between GSE and breastfeeding, using a GSE Scale (Luszczynska et al., 2005). Reporting on a Norwegian prospective cohort study, Ystrom et al. (2008) concluded that a higher GSE score, when adjusted for negative affect, predicted predominant breastfeeding compared to bottle-feeding. Dennis and Faux (1999) found a negative correlation between the BSE scale and a 24-item GSE scale ($r=-.20$, $p=.03$) when measured postpartum in the hospital, and Hernandez reported no significant correlation between a 10-item GSE scale and intensity of breastfeeding at 6 weeks in a sample of Hispanic women ($r=.07$, $p>.05$). While these study results appear inconsistent, the study methods differed and the results are not comparable.

The cited examples, and the focus group results, suggest that further study, on the reciprocal influence of GSE upon BSE and, in turn, on breastfeeding initiation and duration, could lead better tailoring of interventions to increase breastfeeding. If a relationship exists between GSE and breastfeeding, an assessment of GSE could be combined with a BSE assessment during an early prenatal visit to inform the level of support an expectant mother might need, prenatally through postpartum, to breastfeed successfully. In addition, placing attention on increasing girls' or women's GSE prior to or during pregnancy may be as important as imparting specific breastfeeding skills.

References

Bandura, A. (1977). Self-efficacy: Toward a unifying theory of behavioral change. *Psychological Review, 84*(2), 191-215.

Bandura, A. (1984). Recycling misconceptions of perceived self-efficacy. *Cognitive Therapy and Research, 8*(3), 231-255.

Bandura, A. (2004). Health promotion by social cognitive means. *Health Education & Behavior, 31*, 143-164.

Barbosa, C. (2014). *Barriers and facilitators to infant feeding among low-income African American women.* Retrieved from Scholars Compass. Paper 3610.

Dennis, C. (2002). Breastfeeding initiation and duration: A 1990-2000 literature review. *Journal of Obstetric, Gynecologic, & Neonatal Nursing, 31*(1), 12-32.

Dennis, C., & Faux, S. (1999). Development and psychometric testing of the Breastfeeding Self-Efficacy Scale. *Research in Nursing and Health, 22*(5), 399-409.

Hernandez, I. (2014). *Acculturation, self-efficacy and breastfeeding behavior in a sample of Hispanic women.* Retrieved from: http://scholarcommons.usf.edu/etd/5239.

Imam, S. (2007). Sherer et al. General Self-efficacy scale: Dimensionality, internal consistency, and temporal stability. Proceedings from the *Redesigning Pedagogy: Culture, Knowledge and understanding Conference*, Singapore. Retrieved from: http://kaputzan.free.fr/outilsdupsy/index.php/doc-riasec/doc_download/80-sherer-general-self-efficacy-scale-sgses.

Luszczynska, A., Scholz, U., & Schwarzer, R. (2005). The General Self-Efficacy Scale: Multicultural validation studies. *Journal of Psychology, 139*(5), 439-457.

McLeroy, K., Bibeau, D., Steckler, A., & Glanz, K. (1988). An ecological perspective on health promotion programs. *Health Education Quarterly, 15*(4), 351-377.

Meedya, S., Fahy, K., & Kable, A. (2010). Factors that positively influence breastfeeding duration to 6 months: A literature review. *Women and Birth, 23*, 135-145.

Sherer, M., & Maddux, J. (1982). The Self-Efficacy Scale: Construction and validation. *Psychological Reports, 51*, 663-671.

Spencer, B., & Grassley, J. (2013). African American women and breastfeeding: An integrative literature review. *Health Care for Women International, 34*(7), 607-625.

Ystrom, E., Niegel, S., Klepp, K., & Vollrath, M. (2008). The impact of maternal negative affectivity and general self-efficacy on breastfeeding: The Norwegian Mother and Child Cohort Study. *Journal of Pediatrics, 152*, 68-72.

CHAPTER 10

Breastfeeding Beliefs and Attitudes Among Black Americans

Kelly McGlothen and Sara Gill

Substantial evidence exists, documenting the superiority of breastfeeding and breastmilk for mothers, babies, and society. In 2011, the Surgeon General identified improving breastfeeding rates as a priority for the nation, and particularly those with disparate rates (U.S. Department of Health and Human Services, 2011). The Healthy People 2020 Breastfeeding Objectives call for an increase in the proportion of infants that are ever breastfed to 81.9%, and for 60.6% to continue to breastfed for 6 months (Healthy People, 2013). Only 58.9% of Black American mothers initiate breastfeeding, and 30.1% continue for 6 months (Healthy People, 2013). Persistently a disparity, African American breastfeeding rates might be deemed one causal factor for the high morbidity and mortality rates for this population (Cottrell & Detman, 2013). African Americans consistently have some of the highest rates of diabetes, breast cancer, asthma, and obesity (Adler et al., 1994).

Black mothers face barriers to breastfeeding that are both complex and multi-dimensional. Whether a mother breastfeeds or not is influenced by intersectional factors, including cultural beliefs related to infant feeding practices. In order to increase breastfeeding initiation and continuation rates in this population, cultural beliefs must first be explored so that culturally appropriate interventions can be designed. Previous studies suggest that a woman's infant feeding decision is made based on factors, such as her perception of women's roles as a mother, her life experience, and perceptions of societal response and support (Bentley, Dee, & Jensen, 2002). The aim of this study was to describe low-income, Black Americans' beliefs and attitudes about breastfeeding.

Method

This was a qualitative descriptive study. Eight focus groups, each consisting of 4 to 7 participants were conducted: five focus groups consisted of pregnant and/or parenting women, two groups with grandmothers, and one group with fathers (Table 1 displays the demographics of the participants). Participants were recruited from the community, including a community outreach center, churches, beauty shops, and a barber shop. A semi-structured interview guide was used to elicit discussion. Participants were asked to discuss: 1) what they heard about breastfeeding, 2) what they thought about breastfeeding, 3) what made breastfeeding easy, 4) what made breastfeeding difficult, and 5) identify how and when they made feeding decisions, and who influenced their decision. Participants received a $20 gift card to compensate for their time. Audiotapes were transcribed and analyzed using qualitative content analysis. Demographic data was analyzed using descriptive statistics.

Table 1

Participant Demographics

	Number	Age	Marital Status	Level of Education	# of Children	# of Breastfed Children	Employment	Family Income
Mothers	15	X=32.2 Range: 22-44	7 married	Range: < H.S. to college graduate	Range: 1-7	Range: 0-7	14 Employed	Median: 30,000-39,999
Fathers	7	X= 26 Range: 19-30	4 married	Range: H.S. graduate to some college	Range: 1-3	Range: 0-3	7 Employed	Median: 20,000-29,999
Grandmothers	8	X= 55.8 Range: 42-76	4 married	Range: < H.S. to some college	Range: 2-12	Range: 1-10	1 Employed	Median: 10,000- 19,000

*Note: X = mean; H.S. = High School.

Results

Perceived Breastfeeding Benefits

There are numerous health benefits associated with breastfeeding, such as decreased risks of obesity for children who are breastfed, and reductions in rates of breast and ovarian cancer for a mother who breastfeeds (World Health Organization [WHO], 2013). All participants could describe the benefits of breastfeeding for both mothers and babies. All stated that breastfeeding was "the best way to feed your baby." In addition to the health benefits, mothers mentioned that breastfeeding allowed them to "be able to bond better with [their] child." Fathers included financial benefits, stating that "it beats paying for formula. Why get formula when you're getting something better and it's free?" All participants stated that they would recommend breastfeeding to everyone. Mothers and grandmothers noted that breastfeeding was more convenient than formula-feeding.

> You didn't have to wash a bottle. You didn't have them crying until you made the bottle. You have to wake up in the middle of the night but it's easier to lay them with you and nurse them.

Perceived Breastfeeding Difficulties

As aforementioned, Black women steadily have some of the lowest breastfeeding rates among all ethnicities and races, which may be attributed to several breastfeeding barriers (Beal, Kuhlthau, & Perrin, 2003). Mothers described a number of breastfeeding difficulties, including health issues (mother and/or infant), pain, insufficient milk, employment, additional family responsibilities, and infant temperament. Fathers identified similar difficulties as the mothers adding that lack of previous breastfeeding experience was problematic. Grandmothers added that breastfeeding "can be a lot of work." Grandmothers also believed that a nutritious diet could make breastfeeding difficult;

"So momma has to be careful, because if you like to eat, you know, certain things, you just have to watch it until you finish breastfeeding." Despite the perceived difficulties, all participants stated that they would recommend breastfeeding to everyone.

Breastfeeding Beliefs and Practices

Mothers described making the feeding decision in late pregnancy, or after their babies were born. All participants said that health care providers, both physicians and nurses, were most influential regarding infant feeding. Participants also mentioned that WIC classes and school health classes presented positive breastfeeding messages images; however, they were "few and far in between." Many mothers described receiving discouraging comments about breastfeeding from family members, usually the maternal grandmother. "My grandmother and my mother both told me not to breastfeed because I guess they don't do it; they bottle-fed."

Conclusions

The findings reported are consistent with past literature on Black breastfeeding beliefs and attitudes (Jefferson, 2013; Leigh 2010). Relationships between African American women's life experience, and their attitudes and perceptions of infant feeding exist. Findings from one study suggested that positive breastfeeding attitudes, and greater probability of breastfeeding intention, were observed among participants who knew someone who had a higher level of education and breastfed their infant, as well (Jefferson, 2013). Similarly, women in our study stated that they felt more likely to continue breastfeeding when they had the support of their family and peers, or knew someone who breastfed. Consistent with our findings, another study concluded that women also felt that their own community and society, including their environment and mass media, influenced their choice to breast-feed or bottle-feed (Leigh, 2010). According to Leigh, women felt that there were more frequent images of women bottle-feeding than breast-feeding. This, in turn, influenced the perception of infant feeding for the mother, regardless of whether the mother being portrayed in the media was feeding formula in the bottle, or if the bottle contained expressed breastmilk.

"Social support, infant health, bonding, and breastfeeding strategies are enabling factors along with mothers' personal commitments to continue breastfeeding beyond 6 months" (Gross, 2014, p. 70). Spouses and maternal grandmothers play a significant role in a mothers' infant feeding decisions. Infant feeding is a cultural mainstay in Black families; therefore, having an understanding of factors that enable mothers to find breastfeeding success would assist stakeholders and health care providers in giving support.

Breastfeeding peer support has also consistently been identified as aiding in breastfeeding success in low-income mothers (Anderson, Damio, Young, Chapman, & Perez- Escamilla, 2005; Chapman, Morel, Damio, & Perez- Escamilla, 2010; Gross, 2014; Raisler, 2000). Through the use of peer breastfeeding support persons, organizations, such as WIC, should continue to work to normalize breastfeeding, as well as provide clients with culturally familiar resources. Peer counselors can serve in churches, schools, and community health care centers. Media, such as local radio stations and billboard advertisements, could also promote breastfeeding in those communities. Businesses, such as beauty salons, and community spiritual centers, such as churches, could become "mother-friendly" establishments that promote their support of breastfeeding (Texas Mother-Friendly Work-Site, 2011).

In order to achieve WHO's (2013) aim to increase the global rate of exclusive breastfeeding at 6 months to at least 50% by 2025, comprehensive education and breastfeeding support must be afforded to all mothers. This includes African American mothers who experience greater breastfeeding disparities than other ethnicities. Implementing the Ten Steps from the WHO-UNICEF Baby-Friendly Hospital Initiative, particularly in hospitals that serve African American women, could support women's infant feeding choices in the prenatal, intra-partum, and postpartum periods (WHO, 2013). Researchers should work to gain a better understanding of both micro- and macro-level contextual factors that affect African American mothers. Having a greater knowledge of the complex experiences of breastfeeding among Black women will help to improve infant feeding disparities. This, in turn, will further advance the development and implementation of interventions that target the multifaceted ways in which African American women are successful with breastfeeding.

References

Adler, N., Boyce, T., Chesney, M., Folkman, S., Kahn, R., & Syme, S. (1994). Socioeconomic status and health: The challenge of the gradient. *American Psychological Association, 49*(1), 15-24.

Anderson, A. K., Damio, G., Young, S., Chapman, D. J., & Perez- Escamilla, R. (2005). A randomized trial assessing the efficacy of peer counseling on exclusive breastfeeding in a predominately Latina low-income community. *Archives of Pediatrics & Adolescent Medicine, 159, 9*(836-841), 836-841.

Beal, A. C., Kuhlthau, K., & Perrin, J. M. (2003). Breastfeeding advice given to African American and White women by physicians and WIC counselors. *Public Health Reports, 118,* 368-376.

Bentley, M. E., Dee, D. L., & Jensen, J. L. (2002). Breastfeeding among low income, African American women: Power, beliefs and decision making. *Journal of Nutrition, 133,* 305S-309S.

Berlin, L. J., Brady- Smith, C., & Brooks-Gunn, J. (2002). Links between childbearing age and observed maternal behaviors with 14-month olds in the Early Head Start Research and Evaluation Project. *Infant Mental Health Journal, 23*(1-2), 104-129.

Chapman, D. J., Morel, K., Damio, A. K., & Perez- Escamilla, R. (2010). Breastfeeding peer counseling: From efficacy through scale-up. *Journal of Human Lactation, 26*(3), 314-326.

Cottrell, B. H., & Detman, L. A. (2013). Breastfeeding concerns and experiences of African American mothers. *Maternal and Child Nursing, 38*(5), 297-304.

Gross, T. T. (2014). *"We've got to first learn that breastfeeding is for us"* *A positive deviance inquiry of the long-term breastfeeding experiences of African- American women in the WIC program* (p.70).

Healthy People. (2013). *Maternal and child health objectives.* Retrieved from http://www.healthypeople.gov/2020/topicsobjectives2020/objectiveslist.aspx?topicId=26.

Jefferson, U. T. (2013). Infant feeding attitudes and breastfeeding intentions of Black college students. *Western Journal of Nursing Research.* Retrieved from http://wjn.sagepub.com/content/early/2013/12/09/0193945913514638.

Leigh, J. L. (2010). *Breast is best but bottle is next: Mother's perception of the portrayals of breastfeeding in the media* (Doctoral dissertation, University of Houston). Retrieved from https://repositories.tdl.org/uh-ir/bitstream/handle/10657/183/LEIGH-.pdf?sequence=2.

Raisler, J. (2000). Against the odds: Breastfeeding experiences of low-income mothers. *Journal of Midwifery & Women's Health*, *45*(3), 253. http://dx.doi.org/.

Texas mother-friendly worksite. (2011). *Community.* Retrieved from http://texasmotherfriendly.org/community#all/page1.

U.S. Department of Health and Human Services (2011). *Executive Summary: The Surgeon General's Call to Action to Support Breastfeeding.* Retrieved from http://www.surgeongeneral.gov/library/calls/breastfeeding/executivesummary.pdf.

World Health Organization [WHO]. (2013). *WHO aims to increase global rate of breastfeeding for six months to 50% by 2025.* Retrieved from http://www.news-medical.net/news/20130730/WHO-aims-to-increase-global-rate-of-breastfeeding-for-six-months-to-5025-by-2025.aspx.

*Building Women's Experiences into
Practice, Promotion, and Support*

Constraints to Practicing Exclusive Breastfeeding for HIV Positive South African Women

Courtenay Sprague, Hannah Fraley, and Vivian Black

HIV in women and their children remains a considerable public health threat and major cause of mortality, contributing to 40% of total maternal and child deaths in high HIV prevalence countries, such as South Africa (Black et al., 2009; UNAIDS, 2012). Pregnancy, labor, delivery, and breastfeeding are modes of mother-to-child HIV transmission (MTCT) (UNAIDS, 1998). In 2001, the number of new HIV infections in children was 550,000, declining by 52% to 260,000 in 2012 (UNAIDS, 2013). Given that HIV is fully preventable, additional advances in averting new pediatric HIV infections must be made to reduce child mortality, in line with Millennium Development Goal 4 (UNAIDS, 2012). The key problem and question is, *"How do we prevent new HIV infections in children in high HIV prevalence, lower-resource settings, through effective prevention of mother-to-child HIV transmission (PMTCT) programs?"*

The goal of PMTCT programs is to reduce or eliminate risk of HIV transmission (WHO, 2010). Different approaches have been implemented to attain this goal. In order to achieve uptake and effectiveness, strategies must match sociocultural context and available resources, while recognizing women's rights and limitations in resource-limited contexts (Gable et al., 2008; Lazarus et al., 2013; Östlin et al., 2001). Recent approaches to safe infant feeding, like South Africa's, may be limited by a range of factors, which need to be overcome to protect and promote child and women's health (UNAIDS, 2012).

We highlight key differences in PMTCT approaches in low- and middle-income countries (LMICs), compared to high-income countries (HICs), such as the United States. Based on a review of recent published research, we then present challenges facing low-income Black South African women who seek to practice exclusive breastfeeding (EBF) in line with revised WHO guidelines (2010).

Two Approaches to Prevent Pediatric HIV through Safe Infant Feeding Guidelines

The historic approach to PMTCT has been risk elimination. This encompasses 6 months of exclusive formula-feeding (EFF) + lifelong combination antiretroviral therapy (cART) for the mother, with avoidance of breastfeeding: a successful strategy in reducing pediatric HIV to < 2% in HICs like the U.S (NIH, 2014; WHO, 2010). In contrast, new 2010 WHO guidelines are based on risk reduction. They recommend 6 months of EBF and cART for the life of the mother or the duration of breastfeeding, and pediatric antiretroviral prophylaxis. These recommendations are based on evidence of malnourishment, stunting, and other adverse effects on child health and survival when milk substitutes, e.g., formula milk, were used in PMTCT programs in poorer-resource settings in contexts of high HIV prevalence (Black et al., 2008; Coutsoudis et al., 2001; Iliff et al., 2005; Landes et al., 2012; Taha et al., 2006; Thior et al., 2006). For children, mixed feeding (breastfeeding combined with non-nutritive liquids and solids) continues to generate higher risk of both HIV and child malnourishment (Black et al., 2008).

South Africa Implements the WHO 2010 Revised EBF Guidelines

South Africa has the greatest number of people living with HIV in a single country (Government of South Africa, 2012a-b). Of a population of 54 million, 6.4 million are living with HIV (Shisana et al., 2014). HIV prevalence in Black South African women (of African descent) of reproductive age is exceptionally high, ranging from 23%-43% (Government of South Africa, 2012a; Shisana et al., 2014). From 2001-2011, South Africa followed the HIC approach of EFF, adopting the new EBF policy in mid-year 2011: a shift representing a major change and the implementation of new procedures that would be executed by health providers across the country (Ijumba et al., 2012, 2013).

Over 92% of women living with HIV in South Africa are poor, of lower social status, unemployed, dependent on a partner or parents, and with high school level education (Gauteng Provincial Department of Health, 2011; Government of South Africa, 2013). Rural women may not have access to safe water and/or electricity (Government of South Africa, 2013, 2012b). Corollary health threats linked to gender hierarchies include intimate partner violence, which ranges from 31% to 55% (Boonzaier, 2005; Dunkle et al., 2004; Gass et al., 2010; Sprague et al., 2015).

The majority of HIV-positive women are reliant on freely available HIV services in the public health system and guidance from health providers concerning safe infant feeding, generally nurses (Sprague, 2009). Under the previous EFF policy, we (Sprague and Black) conducted in-depth interviews with 83 South African women with HIV, 32 caregivers of children with HIV, and 38 key informants in 2009 (Sprague, Chersich, & Black, 2011). Our findings indicated that individual and health systems' factors hindered women's capacity to practice EFF, with poor feeding guidance by health personnel. Against this background, we conducted a literature review to identify South African women's feeding experiences, practices, and challenges to exclusively breastfeed in order to document women's lived experiences, and anticipate challenges as the new policy is implemented. These exploratory research questions guided the review: What are HIV positive South African women's attitudes and practices with regard to exclusive breastfeeding? What challenges, if any, do they face in practicing EBF?

Method

We employed an analytical framework to develop inclusion criteria based on three health determinants likely to influence women's EBF practices, encompassing individual-level factors, sociocultural determinants, and health care/health systems factors. We reviewed studies published from 2010-2014, extracting articles from PubMed and CINAHL databases, using search criteria that included: WHO, EBF, South Africa, policy, HIV positive women, and safe infant feeding. Of 91 articles reviewed, five met our inclusion criteria. These all focused on challenges facing HIV positive South African women seeking to practice EBF; included direct quotations representing women's experiences; and were published in the last several years, with attention to the latest evidence on EBF (Ijumba et al., 2013; Madiba & Letsoalo, 2013; Nor et al., 2011; Zulliger et al., 2013). Research on EBF under the new policy remains limited, however. Only one was published following the full implementation of South Africa's new EBF policy (Ijumba et al., 2013). Thus, the research reviewed serves to inform the implementation of the new policy, with attention to women's lived experiences.

Themes

Findings revealed women's struggles to elect and practice EBF. Individual-level factors included lack of empowerment to elect feeding methods; struggles with HIV disclosure and adherence to cART (leading to mixed-feeding); fear of MTCT; previous experience of infant feeding; and lack of knowledge of EBF benefits (Madiba & Letsoalo, 2013; Zulliger et al., 2013). Working women, women seeking work, and teen mothers expressed preferences to formula-feed for its greater autonomy, pointing to a lack of support within workplaces or by employers to encourage EBF. Consequently, women perceived EBF was not feasible (Zulliger et al., 2013).

Social-cultural factors encompassed use of substitute mothers to breastfeed infants; intergenerational power exerted (primarily over teenage mothers' feeding choices) (Ijumba et al., 2012); cultural practice of cleansing the baby's stomach with water; pressure by family to supplement breastmilk with food due to perceptions that breastmilk is insufficient for the baby's needs (Madiba & Letsoalo, 2013; Nor et al., 2013).

Health care/systems factors included: poor infant feeding counseling of women; inadequate breastfeeding guidance and support, e.g., latching (Ijumba et al., 2013; Zulliger et al., 2013), myths, and confusion about the reasons for dismantling the formula program (breastfeeding was perceived as sub-optimal and punitive); inadequate health personnel training in communicating EBF benefits (Ijumba et al., 2012, 2013).

Conclusion

While early in the implementation of the new EBF policy in South Africa, research indicates acceptability, feasibility, and uptake of EBF by HIV positive women have not yet been demonstrated (Ijumba et al., 2013, 2012; Lazarus et al., 2013). The opportunity to promote child health and prevent new HIV infections through EBF exists but will require concerted attention to multi-level interventions (UNAIDS,

2013), encompassing: (a) to advance women's education, employment, and economic participation, which underpin women's health behaviors, including support for EBF in workplaces; (b) *sociocultural interventions* that engage widely accepted cultural feeding practices, passed on from mother to daughter, such as cleansing; (c) *health systems' interventions* to train health providers in engaging with women; improving trust and communication between patients and providers; effective public health messaging in communities that explain EBF benefits; and (d) *policies and interventions* must involve HIV positive women as stakeholders in the policy-formulation process; attend to women's social, economic, and cultural constraints, expected norms, gender relations, while creating and promoting the enabling conditions for the health and well-being of HIV positive women and their children to be promoted and protected (Östlin et al., 2001).

References

Black, V., Brooke, S., & Chersich, M.F. (2009). Impact of HIV treatment on maternal mortality at a tertiary center in South Africa: a five-year audit. *Obstetrics & Gynecology, 114*, 292–299.

Black, RE, Allen, L.H., Bhutta, Z.A., Caulfield, L.E., de Onis, M., Ezzati, M., Mathers, C., & Rivera, J. (2008). Maternal and child undernutrition: Global and regional exposures and health consequences. *Lancet, 371* (9608), 243-260.

Boonzaier, F. (2005). Women abuse in South Africa: A brief contextual analysis. *Feminism and Psychology, 15*(1), 99-103.

Centers for Disease Control and Prevention (CDC). (2013). *Today's HIV/AIDS Epidemic*. Retrieved from http://www.cdc.gov/nchhstp/newsroom/docs/hivfactsheets/todaysepidemic-508.pdf.

Coutsoudis, A., Pillay, K., Kuhn, L. et al. (2001). Method of feeding and transmission of HIV-1 from mothers to children by 15 months of age: Prospective cohort study from Durban, *South Africa AIDS, 15*, 379–387.

Dunkle, K., & Decker, M. (2013). Gender-based violence and HIV: Reviewing the evidence for links and causal pathways in the general population and high-risk groups. *American Journal of Reproductive Immunology, 69*(suppl 1), 20-26.

Dunkle, K., Jewkes, R., Brown, H. et al. (2004). Gender-based violence, relationship power, and risk of HIV infection in women attending antenatal clinics in South Africa. *Lancet, 363*, 1415-1421.

Gable, L., Gostin, L., & Hodge, J. (2008). HIV/AIDS, reproductive and sexual health and the law. *American Journal of Public Health, 98*(10), 1779-1786.

Gass, J., Stein, D., Williams, D.P. et al. (2010). Intimate partner violence, health behaviours and chronic physical illness among South African women. *South African Medical Journal, 100*, 582-585.

Gauteng Provincial Department of Health and Social Development. (2011). *Annual performance plan.* Retrieved from http://www.health.gpg.gov. za/Documents/APP%202011_copy2.pdf.

Government of South Africa. (2013). *MDG Country Report.* Retrieved from http://www.za.undp.org/content/dam/south_africa/docs/ Reports/The_Report/MDGOctober-2013.pdf.

Government of South Africa (2012a). *The 2012 national antenatal sentinel HIV & herpes simplex type 2 prevalence survey in South Africa.* Retrieved from http://www.hst.org.za/publications/2012-national-antenatal-sentinel-hiv-herpes-simplex-type-2-prevalence-survey.

Government of South Africa. (2012b). *National strategic plan on HIV, STIs and TB 2012-2016.* Retrieved from http://www.gov.za/documents/ national-strategic-plan-hiv-stis-and-tb-2012-2016.

Ijumba, P., Doherty, T., Jackson, D., Tomlinson, M., Sanders, D., & Persson, L. (2013). Free formula milk in the prevention of mother-to-child transmission programme: Voices of a peri-urban community in South Africa on policy change. *Health Policy and Planning, 28*, 761-768.

Ijumba, P., Doherty, T., Jackson, D., Tomlinson, M., Sanders, D., & Persson, L. (2012). Social circumstances that drive early introduction of formula milk: an exploratory qualitative study in a peri-urban South African community. *Maternal and Child Nutrition, 10*, 102-111. doi: 10.1111/mcn.12012.

Iliff, P.J., Piwoz, E.G., Tavengwa, N.V. et al. (2005). Early exclusive breastfeeding reduces the risk of postnatal HIV-1 transmission and increases HIV-free survival. *AIDS, 19*, 699–708.

Landes, M., van Lettow, M., Chan, A.K., Mayuni I., Schouten E.J. et al. (2012) Mortality and health outcomes of HIV-exposed and unexposed children in a PMTCT cohort in Malawi. *PLoS ONE, 7*(10), e47337. doi:10.1371/journal.pone.0047337

Lazarus, R., Struthers, H., & Violari, A. (2013). Promoting safe infant feeding practices - the importance of structural, social and contextual factors in southern Africa. *Journal of International AIDS Society, 16*, 1-15.

Madiba, S., & Letsoalo, R. (2013). HIV disclosure to partners and family among women enrolled in prevention of mother to child transmission of HIV program: Implications for infant feeding in poor resourced communities in South Africa. *Global Journal of Health Science, 5*(4), 1-11.

National Institutes of Health (US). (2014). *Recommendations for use of antiretroviral drugs in pregnant HIV-1-infected women for maternal health and interventions to reduce perinatal HIV transmission in the United States.* Retrieved from http://aidsinfo.nih.gov/contentfiles/lvguidelines/PerinatalGL.pdf.

Nor, B., Ahlberg, B. M., Doherty, T., Zembe, Y., Jackson, D., & Ekstrom, E. (2011). Mother's perceptions and experiences of infant feeding within a community-based peer counseling intervention in South Africa. *Maternal and Child Nutrition, 8*, 448-458.

Östlin, P., Sen, G., & George, A. (2001). Gender, health and equity—the intersections. In T. Evans, M. Whitehead, F. Diderichsen, A. Bhuiya, & M. Wirth (Eds.) *Challenging inequities to health: From ethics to action.* Oxford, UK: Oxford University Press.

Shisana, O., Rehle, T., Simbayi L.C. et al (2014). *South African National HIV Prevalence, Incidence and Behaviour Survey, 2012.* Cape Town: Human Sciences Research Council.

Sprague, C., Woollett, N., Parpart, J., Hatcher, A., Sommers, T., Brown, S., & Black, V. (2015). When nurses are also patients: IPV and the health system as an enabler of women's health and institutional agency in Johannesburg. *Global Public Health, 1*(1), 1-15. http://dx.doi.org/10.1080/17441692.2015.1027248.

Sprague, C., Chersich, M., & Black, V. (2011). Health system weaknesses constrain access to PMTCT and maternal HIV services in South Africa: A qualitative enquiry. *AIDS Research and Therapy, 8*, 10-19.

Sprague, C. (2009). *Cui bono: A capabilities approach to understanding HIV prevention and treatment for pregnant women and children in South Africa* (PhD thesis). University of the Witwatersrand, South Africa. Retrieved from http://wiredspace.wits.ac.za/handle/10539/8234.

Taha, T.E., Kumwenda, N.I., Hoover, D.R. et al. (2006). The impact of breastfeeding on the health of HIV-positive mothers and their children in sub-Saharan Africa. *Bulletin of the World Health Organization, 84*, 546–554.

Thior, I., Lockman, S., Smeaton, L.M. et al. (2006). Breastfeeding plus infant zidovudine prophylaxis for 6 months vs formula-feeding plus infant zidovudine for 1 month to reduce mother-to-child HIV transmission in Botswana: A randomized trial: The Mashi Study. *Journal of the American Medical Association, 296,* 794–805.

UNAIDS. (2013). *2013 Progress report on the global plan towards the elimination of new HIV infections among children by 2015 and keeping their mothers alive. Geneva: UNAIDS.* Retrieved from http://www.unaids.org/ sites/default/files/en/media/unaids/contentassets/documents/ unaidspublication/2013/20130625_progress_global_plan_en.pdf.

UNAIDS. (2012). *Global Report: UNAIDS report on the global HIV epidemic.* Geneva: UNAIDS. Retrieved from: http://www.unaids.org/en/ media/unaids/contentassets/documents/epidemiology/2012/ gr2012/20121120_UNAIDS_Global_Report_2012_with_annexes_ en.pdf.

UNAIDS. (1998). *Mother to child transmission of HIV: UNAIDS technical update.* Geneva: UNAIDS. Retrieved from http://data.unaids.org/ Publications/IRC-pub03/meetingmarch98_en.pdf.

WHO. (2010). *Guidelines on HIV and infant feeding: Principles and recommendations for infant feeding in the context of HIV and a summary of evidence.* Geneva: WHO. Retrieved from http://whqlibdoc.who. int/publications/2010/9789241599535_eng.pdf.

Zulliger, R., Abrams, E., & Myer, L (2013). Diversity of influences on infant feeding strategies in women living with HIV in Cape Town, South Africa: A mixed-methods study. *Tropical Medicine and International Health, 18*(12), 1547-1554. doi: 10.11111/tmi.12212.

"But just the swelling didn't go good ... Just didn't. So, I just stopped": Factors in Initiation and Continuation of Breastfeeding and Pumping among Adolescent Mothers

Brittany D. Chambers and Paige Hall Smith

Despite the scientific evidence supporting the long-term benefits of breastfeeding for mother and child, 77% of women initiated breastfeeding while only 49% of women exclusively breastfeed their infants until 6 months in the United States (U.S.) in 2013 (Center for Disease Control and Prevention [CDC], 2014). Among women who breastfeed in the U.S., adolescent mothers are less likely to initiate and continue breastfeeding (Gartner et al., 2005; Peterson & Da Vanzo, 1992; Smith, Avery, & Gizlice, 2004). In fact, approximately 43% of adolescent mothers' initiated breastfeeding in the hospital and 21% continued to breastfeed until their infants were 6 months old (Ryan, 1997). Adolescent mothers often fall into multiple groups that are less likely to initiate and continue breastfeeding (CDC, 2010). For example, minority adolescents and those residing in high poverty neighborhoods are more likely to become parents during adolescence compared to White adolescents and those living in more affluent neighborhoods (CDC, 2012). In 2011, 57% of adolescent births were to African American and Latino adolescents (CDC, 2012). Research has shown that adult and adolescent women who are African American, and have a low socioeconomic status, are less likely to initiate and continue breastfeeding (Apostolakis-Kyrus, Valentine, & DeFranco, 2013; Dykes, & Williams 1999).

The purpose of this study was to examine factors across the social ecology that influence adolescent mothers' infant feeding practices.

Method

Study Population and Enrollment

Participants in this study were 18 pregnant adolescents participating in a 7-week childbirth education class offered by the Teen Parent Mentoring Program (TPMP) of a Young Women's Christian Association (YWCA)'s located in a large urban city in the U.S. The childbirth education curriculum included a weekly breastfeeding education component that was currently being evaluated. Staff from TPMP described the nature of the study to adolescents, and received signed assent from adolescents and consent from their guardian. The institutional review board at the University of North Carolina, Greensboro approved this study.

Data Collection

Two semi-structured interviews were conducted in-person with participants by a trained graduate research assistant. The baseline interview, conducted before 7-week program began, included questions regarding expectations and concerns for motherhood; how motherhood would alter their lives; infant feeding expectations; social and community knowledge and norms surrounding infant feeding, future goals, and aspirations; and their living situation and support network.

The second semi-structured interview took place two weeks after the participant had stopped breastfeeding. During the follow-up interview, participants were asked questions about their day-to-day interactions with family, friends, and the baby's father, as well as new responsibilities; their living situation including a support network, challenges and joys of motherhood, infant feeding decisions including challenges with breastfeeding, and goals and aspirations for themselves and their children. Infant feeding practices were tracked weekly by telephone interview.

Data Analysis

The interviews were transcribed verbatim by a professional transcriptionist. We used the social ecological model as a framework for the analysis reported here (McLeroy, Bibeau, Steckler, & Glanz, 1988). Data was coded into five categories that corresponded with research questions asked during interviews: rationale for breastfeeding, breastfeeding practice, breastfeeding messages and support from others, breastfeeding experiences, and breastfeeding cessation. For each of these categories, we identified that factors at three levels of the social ecology were influential in shaping the women's decisions and experiences: structural, interpersonal, and intrapersonal. Collaborative coding and analysis took place, coding each transcript multiple times for accuracy.

Definitions

In this study, breastfeeding is defined as providing babies with human milk directly from the breast, and pumping is defined as expressing milk from the breast, and feeding babies human milk from a bottle.

Results

Three of the 18 participants were lost to follow-up. As a result, only 15 adolescent mothers were included in this study. Most (89%) were in high school at the time of the study, although one adolescent mother was in middle school, one was in college, and three were not in school at baseline. The majority (77.8%) of the participants reported African American as their race/ethnicity, followed by Hispanic/Latino (11.1%). One participant reported White as their race/ ethnicity, and another as mixed race.

At baseline, 83.3% of participants intended to exclusively breast-feed or mix-feed their infants, while one participant was undecided about infant feeding. After birth, 87.5% of participants initiated breast-feeding. Among participants who initiated breastfeeding, the majority (83.3%) of participants did not breastfeed past 3 weeks; however, one participant continued to mix-feed her infant by providing formula and human milk by pumping up to 5 weeks postpartum. Two participants exclusively breastfed: one for 3 months, and one for 6 months.

Barriers Associated with Breastfeeding

Adolescent mothers revealed structural, interpersonal, and intrapersonal level factors that impacted their infant-feeding experiences.

Structural Factors

Adolescent mothers discussed interactions with three institutions: school, health care clinics and offices, and the Women's Infant and Children's (WIC) program. However, they only discussed barriers related to school and with health care clinics. The majority of participants did not associate school with breastfeeding, and many stated that they would stop breastfeeding once they returned to school. Specifically, one participant reported receiving no support for her needs as a mother from school personnel: "Yeah, because they [school personnel] was probably like, 'Why is this 12-year-old pregnant? I just don't understand.'" Adolescent mothers reported similar interactions in hospital and clinical settings. Another adolescent expressed, "I had to stop [breastfeeding] because the birth control that my doctor put me on. I found out later on that it had steroids in it." These experiences suggest that institutions may have difficulty recognizing adolescents as mothers, preferring to continue to interact with in them in their more familiar role as teenagers in need of education and contraception, not as teenage mothers in need of education and contraception.

Two adolescent mothers attempted to breastfeed and attend school; however, one was able to take online GED courses from home and continued to breastfeed for 6 months. The adolescent mother who attempted to breastfeed in a traditional high school setting found that the need for her to pump led to an insufficient milk supply (an intrapersonal level factor): "I tried pumping [at school]. And I pumped [at school] for a while, but I wasn't pumping enough. Like, I was only pumping out one [breast]. I was trying to pump out of both [breasts]. But milk was only coming out of one [breast]." This experience indicates an interaction between adolescent mothers' personal aspirations to breastfeed, and lack of support to breastfeed in institutions such as schools.

Interpersonal Factors

Adolescent mothers reported hearing many negative attitudes about breastfeeding from these in their social networks. For example, one participant stated:

> My friends thought it was pretty nasty. They asked a lot of very weird questions as far as breastfeeding. Like, um, one friend, I don't know why she asked this. But she was like, "Do you feel weird, you being a girl, and your daughter being a girl, feeding her by your breast?" I was like, "No, not really."

Additionally, adolescents discussed a lack of support from family members and spouses. Lack of support from family members that seemed to come from both their own lack of experience with breastfeeding, as well as myths, such as "you want to get up in the middle of the night and breastfeed? You know, you're tired and stuff."

Adolescent mothers also discussed an intersection between institutions and social constraints, where many participants mentioned that they stopped breastfeeding as recommended by their mother and doctor. For example, the mother of one young women [who participated in her follow-up interview] mentioned, "I think the formula was a little bit more convenient as far as going back to school, being so young. You know? You know, so that transition, too, and not only [that], but the pain. But, you know, that played a part in it, too. What's she going to do when she go to school?" While another adolescent mother expressed similar decisions made for her by a doctor:

> Un, just that he—well, he first—when he first came out, I fed him, and he latched on good. He was on for 30 minutes. But, then, after that he would just—he wouldn't latch on no more. He would just sleep. But they said that was usual. But, then, he still wouldn't latch on. Like, I'd be, like, 3 hours. So, the doctors gave him a bottle. And I just kept giving him the bottle, so.

Intrapersonal Factors

Although all adolescent mothers were aware of the health benefits of breastfeeding for both mother and child, the majority of them expressed negative attitudes towards breastfeeding. For example, some adolescents viewed breastfeeding as a "gross" process that should be done in private.

> Because I'm the kind of person, I'm shy. I don't want to be in public doing that. I think—I mean, I see other

ladies doing it. But I think that's not ladylike. I think
it's gross.

A few adolescent mothers also discussed unpleasant experiences with
breastfeeding, which caused them to discontinue breastfeeding early
on. For example, "I don't know. I didn't like the feeling. I didn't like
it. It hurt."

Success Stories: Factors Associated with Breastfeeding

Two adolescent mothers exclusively breastfeed for 3 and 6 months,
respectively. These young women identified factors across the social
ecology that helped them navigate some of the challenges they experienced with breastfeeding. Organizational support from WIC staff and
lactation consultants at the hospital played integral roles in adolescent
mothers successfully initiating breastfeeding, and having adequate
resources to pump.

> Like, at first my milk wasn't coming down. Like, she
> wasn't getting anything out. And it was making my
> nipples really swollen and sore. So, it, like, made me
> not want to [breastfeed]. But just, basically, they [lacta-
> tion consultants] would come in and show me different
> ways that I could do it, you know, that would relieve
> the pain and make her latch on better. And, then, you
> know they gave me a hand-held pump. So, before I
> would try to breastfeed her, you know, to try to pull
> the milk down. They [lactation consultants] gave me
> the pump to try to pump it for a little. And that actu-
> ally worked pretty well. My milk came down before I
> actually got out of the hospital, so.

These mothers also expressed that they received support and advice
from a family member who had previously breastfeed. This made
their transition to being a breastfeeding mother easier. Lastly, these
two adolescent mothers discussed the benefits of participating in the

TPMP infant feeding course to learn about the health benefits of breastfeeding for mother and baby, which assisted them in making an informed decision about their infant-feeding choices.

Conclusion

Factors associated with initiation and continuation of breastfeeding among adolescent mothers were identified on all levels of the social ecology. The majority ($n = 12$) of participants initiated breastfeeding. However, all but two adolescent mothers discontinued breastfeeding at 5 weeks postpartum or before. These findings are similar to other studies (Apostolakis-Kyrus et al., 2013; Bica & Giugliani, 2014; Smith et al., 2012). Studies have shown that there are many factors that contribute to adolescent mothers' early cessation of breastfeeding, including return to school, dependency on family members, negative physical experiences, and lack of support (Bica & Giugliani, 2014; Smith et al., 2012). Findings from this study, as well as others, suggest that policies and training regarding breastfeeding and adolescent pregnancy be incorporated in school settings to better support adolescent mothers' infant-feeding decisions (Handa & Schanler, 2013). This may include trainings for school personnel on destigmatizing adolescent pregnancy, as well as a space and support group for adolescent mothers. It is important for organizations that interact with adolescent mothers attend to their needs, both as adolescents and as mothers. Institutional failure to recognize and support these young mothers in all their multiple roles may undermine them all.

This study also indicated the need for the incorporation of sexuality in infant-feeding education curricula tailored towards adolescent mothers and, specifically, the functioning of the breast, and acceptability of breastfeeding in public. Future studies should further explore the support adolescent mothers need, given the multiple roles they play in society (e.g., adolescent, mother, daughter, and student) to successfully initiate and continue breastfeeding if that is their desire.

References

Apostolakis-Kyrus, K., Valentine, C., & DeFranco, E. (2013). Factors associated with breastfeeding initiation in adolescent mothers. *Journal of Pediatrics, 163*(5), 1489-1494.

Bica, O. C., & Giugliani, E. R. J. (2014). Influence of counseling sessions on the prevalence of breastfeeding in the first year of life: A randomized clinical trial with adolescent mothers and grandmothers. *Birth, 41*(1), 39-45.

Center for Disease Control and Prevention [CDC]. (2010). *Provisional breastfeeding rates by socio-demographic factors, among children born in 2007.* Retrieved from http://www.cdc.gov/breastfeeding/data/NIS_data/2007/socio-demographic_any.htm.

Center for Disease Control and Prevention [CDC]. (2012). *About teen pregnancy.* Retrieved from http://www.cdc.gov/teenpregnancy/aboutteenpreg.htm.

Center for Disease Control and Prevention [CDC]. (2014). *Breastfeeding report card, United States /2013.* Retrieved from http://www.cdc.gov/breastfeeding/pdf/2013breastfeedingreportcard.pdf.

Chin, N., & Dozier, A. (2012). The dangers of baring the breast: Structural violence and formula-feeding among low-income women. In P.H. Smith, B.L. Hausman, & M.H. Labbok (Eds.). *Beyond health, beyond choice: Breastfeeding constraints and realities.* New Brunswick, NJ: Rutgers University Press.

Dykes, F., & Williams, C. (1999). Falling by the wayside: A phenomenological exploration of perceived breast-milk inadequacy in lactating women. *Midwifery, 15*(4), 232-246.

Gartner, L. M., Morton, J., Lawrence, R. A., Naylor, A. J., O'Hare, D., Schanler, R. J., & Eidelman, A. I. (2005). Breastfeeding and the use of human milk. *Pediatrics, 115*(2), 496-506.

Handa, D., & Schanler, R. J. (2013). Role of the pediatrician in breastfeeding management. *Pediatric Clinics of North America, 60*(1), 1-10.

McLeroy, K. R., Bibeau, D., Steckler, A., & Glanz, K. (1988). An ecological perspective on health promotion programs. *Health Education & Behavior, 15*(4), 351-377.

Peterson, C. E., & DaVanzo, J. (1992). Why are teenagers in the United States less likely to breast-feed than older women? *Demography, 29*(3), 431-450.

Ryan, A. S. (1997). The resurgence of breastfeeding in the United States. *Pediatrics*, *99*(4), e12.

Smith, P. H., Avery, M., & Gizlice, Z. (2004). SCHS Studies. *North Carolina State Center for Health Statistics*, 1997-2001. Retrieved from http://www.schs.state.nc.us/SCHS/pdf/SCHS142.pdf.

Smith, P. H., Coley, S. L., Labbok, M. H., Cupito, S., & Nwokah, E. (2012). Early breastfeeding experiences of adolescent mothers: A qualitative prospective study. *International breastfeeding journal*, *7*(1), 13.

CHAPTER 13

Biopsychosocial Vulnerability, Lactation, and Postpartum Depression

Alison Stuebe

C onventional wisdom holds that breastfeeding prevents post-partum depression and increases bonding between the mother and infant. Some authors have gone so far as to suggest that not breastfeeding triggers depression because it mimics conditions associated with the death of the infant (Gallup, Nathan Pipitone, Carrone, & Leadholm, 2009). However, emerging evidence suggests that the relationship between lactation and maternal mood is complex. For example, in a recent study, women who achieved their breastfeeding intentions were less likely to be depressed that women who did not breastfeed; however, women who were not able to achieve their intentions were more likely to be depressed than those who neither intended to breastfeed nor initiated (Borra, Iacovou, & Sevilla, 2014). Moreover, women who did not plan to breastfeed, but did so, were *more* likely to be depressed at 18 months postpartum than women who formula-fed. These results suggest that intended, successful breast-feeding is protective, but the data raise questions about the impact of promoting breastfeeding among women who are reluctant to initiate, or who are at risk for early weaning. Furthermore, this work underscores the need to provide psychological support for women who are unable to achieve their infant feeding intentions. This paper will explore what is known about the relationship between breastfeeding and depression, discuss neuroendocrine mechanisms that may link these two disorders, and consider implications for supporting mothers who are experiencing depression and anxiety symptoms.

Relationship between Breastfeeding and Depression

Several authors have found evidence that maternal anxiety and depression precede early weaning. Paul et al. (Paul, Downs, Schaefer, Beiler, & Weisman, 2013) measured state anxiety during the post-partum stay, and found that high anxiety (indexed by Spielberger State Anxiety Inventory $\geq$ 40) was associated with reduced breastfeeding duration (p=0.003). Hahn-Holbrook et al. found higher rates of prenatal depression, indexed by CES-D score, among women who were not breastfeeding at 3 months (33%), compared with women who were breastfeeding at all (22%), or exclusively breastfeeding (17%).

There is also evidence to suggest that breastfeeding difficulties predict postpartum depression. In a longitudinal study conducted in Norway, low breastfeeding self-efficacy was also associated with postpartum depression symptoms (Haga et al., 2012). In analyses of the Infant Feeding Practices Study II, we found that severe breast-feeding-associated pain the first 2 weeks after birth was associated with depression symptoms at 2 months postpartum (Watkins, Melt-zer-Brody, Zolnoun, & Stuebe, 2011). In the same cohort, 19% of women with depression symptoms experienced disrupted lactation, defined as early, undesired weaning due to problems with pain, latch, and/or low milk supply, compared with 11% of women without depression symptoms (Stuebe et al., 2014). A recent systematic review confirmed that depression during pregnancy predicts shorter breastfeeding dura-tion, and postpartum depressive symptoms predict earlier weaning (Dias & Figueiredo, 2014). Taken together, the literature suggests that there is considerable overlap between breastfeeding difficulties and depressive symptoms, underscoring the need to screen and treat for both conditions.

Associations between breastfeeding difficulties and depression may reflect both decreased self-efficacy in the setting of depression symptoms, and perturbation of neuroendocrine mechanisms implicated in maternal mood and lactation physiology (Stuebe, Grewen, Pedersen, Propper, & Meltzer-Brody, 2012). For example, the neurosteroid allopregnanolone has been implicated in early postpartum mood symptoms. This progesterone metabolite is a potent GABA agonist, and levels rise rapidly during pregnancy, with concomitant down-regulation of the GABA receptor. Progesterone and allopregnanolone levels fall precipitously after birth, and maternal GABA receptors must upregulate to compensate. In an animal model, Maguire et al. (Maguire & Mody, 2008) studied maternal behavior in a knockout mouse model, and found loss of the GABA(R) delta gene prevented postpartum recruitment of GABA receptors, resulting in aberrant mothering behavior and decreased pup survival. The rapid fall in progesterone levels coincides with secretory activation in the breast, such that women who are sensitive to fluctuating allopregnanolone levels face greater challenges when navigating engorgement and onset of milk production.

Neuroendocrine Mechanisms

Oxytocin has also been implicated in the pathophysiology of depression and early weaning. The hormone oxytocin is essential for lactation physiology, because it stimulates let down, which is the contraction of myoepithelial cells and transfer of milk from individual alveolar lumens through the ductal system to the areola, where it is accessible to the infant. Oxytocin also plays a central role in pair bonding and maternal behavior, and is thought to down-regulate the hypothalamic pituitary adrenal axis and modulate responses to stress. In a pilot study ($N=47$), we compared oxytocin levels during breastfeeding among women with and without anxiety symptoms, and we found that higher levels of anxiety were associated with lower oxytocin area under the curve during feeding at 2 months postpartum (Stuebe, Grewen, & Meltzer-Brody, 2013). We further found that, among women with symptoms, oxytocin during feeding was associated with higher, rather than lower, maternal cortisol response during a standardized social stressor (Cox et al., 2015). These results suggest that oxytocin signaling during lactation is dysregulated in women with symptoms of depression and anxiety.

Emerging evidence suggests a complex relationship between oxytocin and postpartum depression. In a small crossover design study enrolling 25 women with postpartum depression, Mah et al. tested inhaled oxytocin vs. placebo (Mah, Van Ijzendoorn, Smith, & Bakermans-Kranenburg, 2012). The authors found that oxytocin made mothers sadder ($p=0.01$), and they were more likely to describe their infants as difficult ($p=0.04$), but they rated their relationship quality more positively ($p=0.04$). Jonas et al. have explored genetic variants in oxytocin and found that early life adversity, indexed by Childhood Trauma Questionnaire, moderates the relationship between oxytocin genotype, and both postpartum depression score and breastfeeding duration (Jonas et al., 2013). For women with the high-risk genotype (rs2740210 CC), early life adversity markedly reduced breastfeeding duration and increased depression scores, whereas for women with the lower risk genotype (AA/CA), early life adversity did not affect breastfeeding duration, and more modestly increased depression scores.

Emerging evidence regarding oxytocin and postpartum depression suggests that exogenous oxytocin may be a useful treatment for women experiencing postpartum depression and/or breastfeeding difficulties. However, as Kim et al. have reviewed (Kim et al., 2014), more research is needed to determine individual differences among patients that may moderate the effect of oxytocin, as well as evaluate the dosage, timing, side-effects, and safety with long-term adminstration.

In our ongoing NIH-funded study, "Mood, Mother, and Infant: The psychobiology of impaired dyadic development" (R01 HD073220), we are quantifying the role of oxytocin in maternal mood disorders and insecure attachment. At study enrollment, we used validated instruments to measure maternal childhood experiences, relationship style, and antenatal attachment (Parental Bonding Instrument, Experiences in Close Relationship Scale-Short Form (ECR-S), Maternal Antenatal Attachment Scale). At 2 months postpartum, mothers rated their emotions during infant feeding over the past week with the Modified Differential Emotions Scale (mDES). We found that more negative paternal bonding and more avoidant or anxious relationship style were associated with more negative emotions during infant feeding, whereas greater antenatal attachment was associated with more possitive emotions. We similarly found that higher trait anxiety and greater depression symptoms were correlated with negative emotions during feeding. Ongoing analyses will measure asociations between these psychometric measures and oxytocin during feeding.

Discussion and Conclusion

These findings suggest that the biological and psychological experience of breastfeeding may differ among women with and without depression, anxiety, or adverse early life experiences. Women with depression and anxiety require additional support to enable them to achieve their infant feeding goals, and appopriate support depends on the individual woman's specific psychobiological vulnerabilities. Such specific needs have important implications for the care and support of mothers and infants. Before conception, and during pregnancy, approaches are needed that explore each woman's risk factors for depression, anxiety, and parenting difficulties, and engage her in supportive interventions. Realistic anticipatory guidance regarding breastfeeding and early parenting, together with plans for coping with setbacks, may help vulnerable women to navigate early lactation.

After birth, providers need to ask women how breastfeeding is going—and listen for, and address, both emotional and technical challenges. In the setting of clinical depression, anxiety, or extensive breastfeeding difficulties, the provider should ask the mother what is going well with her and her baby. Using this information, the provider, mother, and other caregivers can craft a feeding approach that increases the activities that are going well, and reduces those that are not. Assuring families that "Breastfeeding is a part of motherhood – it's not the point of motherhood," may help families to integrate their lived experience with their infant feeding goals. Further resesarch is needed to develop and test strategies that value a woman's experience of breastfeeding and that are tailored to her individual psychobiological strengths and vulnerablilities. Ultimately, such work will enable more women to achieve their infant feeding goals.

References

Borra, C., Iacovou, M., & Sevilla, A. (2014). New evidence on breastfeeding and postpartum depression: The importance of understanding women's intentions. *Maternal and Child Health Journal, 19*(4), 897-907. doi: 10.1007/s10995-014-1591-z.

Cox, E. Q., Stuebe, A., Pearson, B., Grewen, K., Rubinow, D., & Meltzer-Brody, S. (2015). Oxytocin and HPA stress axis reactivity in postpartum women. *Psychoneuroendocrinology, 55*, 164-172. doi: 10.1016/j.psyneuen.2015.02.009

Dias, C. C., & Figueiredo, B. (2014). Breastfeeding and depression: A systematic review of the literature. *Journal of Affective Disorders, 171C*, 142-154. doi: 10.1016/j.jad.2014.09.022.

Gallup, G. G., Jr., Nathan Pipitone, R., Carrone, K. J., & Leadholm, K. L. (2009). Bottle feeding simulates child loss: Postpartum depression and evolutionary medicine. *Medical Hypotheses.* doi: S0306-9877(09)00507-6 [pii]10.1016/j.mehy.2009.07.016.

Haga, S. M., Ulleberg, P., Slinning, K., Kraft, P., Steen, T. B., & Staff, A. (2012). A longitudinal study of postpartum depressive symptoms: Multilevel growth curve analyses of emotion regulation strategies, breastfeeding self-efficacy, and social support. *Archives of Women's Mental Health, 15*(3), 175-184. doi: 10.1007/s00737-012-0274-2.

Jonas, W., Mileva-Seitz, V., Webb Girard, A., Bisceglia, R., Kennedy, J. L., Sokolowski, M., . . . Steiner, M. (2013). Genetic variation in oxytocin rs2740210 and early adversity associated with postpartum depression and breastfeeding duration. *Genes, Brain, and Behavior, 12*(7), 681-694. doi: 10.1111/gbb.12069.

Kim, S., Soeken, T. A., Cromer, S. J., Martinez, S. R., Hardy, L. R., & Strathearn, L. (2014). Oxytocin and postpartum depression: Delivering on what's known and what's not. *Brain Research, 1580*, 219-232. doi: 10.1016/j.brainres.2013.11.009.

Maguire, J., & Mody, I. (2008). GABA(A)R plasticity during pregnancy: Relevance to postpartum depression. *Neuron, 59*(2), 207-213. doi: S0896-6273(08)00537-0 [pii]10.1016/j.neuron.2008.06.019.

Mah, B. L., Van Ijzendoorn, M. H., Smith, R., & Bakermans-Kranenburg, M. J. (2012). Oxytocin in postnatally depressed mothers: Its influence on mood and expressed emotion. *Progress in Neuro-psychopharmacology & Biological Psychiatry, 40C*, 267-272. doi: 10.1016/j.pnpbp.2012.10.005.

Paul, I. M., Downs, D. S., Schaefer, E. W., Beiler, J. S., & Weisman, C. S. (2013). Postpartum anxiety and maternal-infant health outcomes. *Pediatrics, 131*(4), e1218-1224. doi: 10.1542/peds.2012-2147.

Stuebe, A. M., Grewen, K., & Meltzer-Brody, S. (2013). Association between maternal mood and oxytocin response to breastfeeding. *Journal of Women's Health, 22*(4), 352-361. doi: 10.1089/jwh.2012.3768.

Stuebe, A. M., Grewen, K., Pedersen, C. A., Propper, C., & Meltzer-Brody, S. (2012). Failed lactation and perinatal depression: Common problems with shared neuroendocrine mechanisms? *Journal of Women's Health (Larchmt), 21*(3), 264-272. doi: 10.1089/jwh.2011.3083.

Stuebe, A. M., Horton, B. J., Chetwynd, E., Watkins, S., Grewen, K., & Meltzer-Brody, S. (2014). Prevalence and risk factors for early, undesired weaning attributed to lactation dysfunction. *Journal of Women's Health (Larchmt), 23*(5), 404-412. doi: 10.1089/jwh.2013.4506.

Watkins, S., Meltzer-Brody, S., Zolnoun, D., & Stuebe, A. (2011). Early breastfeeding experiences and postpartum depression. *Obstetrics & Gynecology, 118*(2 Pt 1), 214-221. doi: 10.1097/AOG.0b013e3182260a2d.

Mothers, Recommendations for Improving Breastfeeding Support in Health Care Settings

Marie Dietrich Leurer and Eunice Misskey

In an effort to explore factors behind low exclusive breastfeeding rates, this research sought the experiential wisdom of mothers regarding the characteristics of effective breastfeeding support. While exclusive breastfeeding for the first 6 months is recognized as optimal for infant and maternal health (Horta, Bahl, Martines, & Victoria, 2007), only 1-17% follow this recommendation in the United States, United Kingdom, and Australia despite initiation rates of between 77 % to 96% (Australian Institute of Health & Welfare, 2013; McAndrew et al., 2012). Up to 60% of mothers discontinue breastfeeding earlier than desired (Odom, Li, Scanlon, Perrine, & Grummer-Strawn, 2013), highlighting the need for effective breastfeeding support.

Method

To investigate the issues behind those statistics, an infant nutrition survey was distributed by public health nurses in a Canadian health region to mothers who had initiated breastfeeding, and whose infants were 6 up to 12 months of age. Two open-ended questions asked mothers how the health care system could provide better support to help mothers feed their babies, and what could be done to help make women's breastfeeding experiences positive. Qualitative interpretive description (Thorne, 2008) was used in analyzing the narrative responses. A total of 191 women completed the survey (35 % response rate), with respondents having a higher education and income than the general population.

Findings

The respondents provided thoughtful feedback on how they felt the health care system could improve the breastfeeding support offered, with the following categories evident.

Happy with Current Level of Support

A significant number of mothers (85/191) wrote of their satisfaction with the current level of breastfeeding support, although some who were satisfied also provided suggestions for how services could be improved:

> My public health nurse helped me a lot, visiting me, getting the weight and measurement of my baby, the information she gave me. Especially in my case, a new mom and have no family here, I felt good, someone caring, sense of belonging, encouragement and support (M49).

> Everyone was great and knew what they were talking about, so very helpful answering new mom's endless questions (M124).

Quality of Breastfeeding Advice

Mothers commonly expressed concerns regarding the quality of the breastfeeding information received from health care professionals

(HCPs). They reported receiving inadequate or conflicting advice, and recommended strategies to ensure HCPs: (a) provide consistent information; and (b) have sufficient lactation knowledge.

> I found that every nurse, and every shift change, brought in new staff, and each one told you how to feed your baby, and everyone's advice was different. And then, the public health nurse had her advice. It may be easier if you have less information, and more trust in the mother and baby relationship, or more of a relationship between the health care staff, so they know what has been told or taught to the mother (M74).

> I think it should be routine for a lactation consultant to visit you in the hospital when you are there starting to breastfeed your baby. The nurse that I had was younger than me, had no children, and while she had knowledge about breastfeeding, she was not able to help me as much as I would've liked (E27)

> The nurses on the mother-baby unit were not well educated or helpful. They kept trying to give formula so the babies "would sleep better." The public health nurse and maternity visiting program nurses were good, but not well educated about breastfeeding twins (M137).

Nature of the Interpersonal Interactions

While some mothers were very happy with their interpersonal interactions with HCPs, others felt support should be more respectful and caring. Mothers sought: (a) encouragement, support and empathy; (b) respect for their preferences and knowledge; and (c) respect for decision to use formula (21% of respondents were no longer breastfeeding).

> By listening to the mom's needs and frustration. We need help, and not somebody to scold us for not do-

ing things right. It is a learning experience and we need guidance. We are very sensitive after childbirth (M89).

I have heard lots of moms having a negative experience with breastfeeding their babies because of a nurse who thinks she knows better, and instead of listening to the mother, pushes and decides what is best for [the] baby. New moms are exhausted and vulnerable and I think some of the nurses take advantage of that (M10).

Everyone pushes breastfeeding so much now that when you can't breastfeed your baby, or choose not to for another reason, then as a mother, you feel bad because the books, and nurses, and everyone are pushing it so much in our society. The health district and maternity center at the hospital should let mothers know that if they can't breastfeed, that doesn't mean they are failing as a mom, that there are other alternatives which are still healthy for your baby (E42).

Timely and Accessible Breastfeeding Support

Access to timely breastfeeding support was an issue for some mothers. The first 24 hours after birth, in particular, was a critical time, although some also desired improved access, and at other times, prenatally and during the lactation period.

During my hospital day, I received a quick demonstration on breastfeeding at 3:30 a.m., after having given birth at 11 p.m. I was absolutely exhausted, and there was no follow-up from the nurses after the original demonstration. The demonstration was helpful. However, the timing could have been better (M85).

I really think getting a good support system right away in the hospital is super important … The maternity visiting only helps you for a couple weeks, and then if you have trouble, you have to go seek it out elsewhere, but when you're exhausted the last thing you want to do is seek someone out, and find out where to get help. It's a lot easier to get a bottle (E21).

Breastfeeding Promotion

A diversity of views was apparent regarding breastfeeding promotion efforts. Some mothers expressed displeasure with the current emphasis on breastfeeding, while others expressed the desire for even more breast-feeding promotion. Mothers also sought increased societal level support for breastfeeding, and greater acceptance for breastfeeding in public.

They should just continue to discuss the benefits of breastfeeding, and also how much it saves you cost wise if you don't use formula (E2).

Stop being so pushy about breastfeeding, and making a new mom feel badly for not wanting to/having trouble. The pressure that a new mom feels to breastfeed can really turn them off of it (E30).

To somehow make the public more aware of breastfeeding and its benefits, not to be so judgmental of those who do choose to nurse. Also for it to be mandatory for all public places to have a private spot for mother to nurse, or at least a chair (M120).

Community Resources

Awareness of breastfeeding resources beyond the health care system was an issue, as some mothers sought access to peer support systems, and more information about other community-based resources. Comments suggested HCPs should play a role in providing information about existing community supports, and in establishing informal support groups.

> Design a website where instructional videos can be seen, maybe a chat forum for mothers, and more support groups to attend (M9).

> Off-site (out of hospital) feeding clinics could be increased. Perhaps a peer group option as well (i.e., one public health staff leads a group of interested moms, babies around the same age) could be helpful (M4).

> As a new mom, it helps to listen to other new moms who successfully breastfed their babies. It is important to recognize that it is not always an easy process, but with patience and determination, and the right support and tools, it is achievable. It is easy to give up without guidance and support (M89).

Discussion

HCPs offering breastfeeding support need to have the necessary skills and competencies to provide consistent and accurate information in a respectful and empathetic manner. Health care organizations could facilitate this goal by reviewing the adequacy of orientation and continuing education for HCPs. They could enhance awareness between HCPs regarding advice given to mothers by improving communications strategies. Breastfeeding support programs should also be timely and accessible from prenatal throughout the lactation period.

Given evidence that all forms of extra breastfeeding support increase the duration of exclusive breastfeeding (Renfrew, McCormick, Wade, Quinn, & Dowswell, 2012), improving the breadth and accessibility of such supports could help address the gap between initiation and exclusive 6-month breastfeeding rates. Commonly cited reasons for early cessation, such as perceived insufficient milk supply, infant latch/suck difficulties, maternal discomfort and pain, concern that the baby is not satisfied, and maternal psychological responses (Hauck,

Fenwick, Dhaliwal, & Butt, 2011; Li, Fein, Chen, & Grummer-Strawn, 2008) could be mitigated with high quality, timely support.

Health care organizations could also play an expanded role by encouraging breastfeeding-friendly public policies and education to the wider community, and by creating and/or providing linkages to community-based resources. Future research could further investigate outcome measures of the quality, accessibility, and timeliness of breastfeeding supports. Given evidence that support positively impacts breastfeeding duration rates, we hope the insights of mothers in this research provide the guidance needed to increase effectiveness of breastfeeding support programs.

References

Australian Institute of Health and Welfare. (2012). *Australia's Health 2012* (Australia's Health series no. 13 Cat. No. AUS 156). Canberra, Australia: Author. Retrieved from http://www.aihw.gov.au/WorkArea/DownloadAsset.aspx?id=10737422169.

Center for Disease Control and Prevention & Health Promotion. (2013). *Breastfeeding Report Card United States 2013.* Retrieved from http://www.cdc.gov/breastfeeding/pdf/2013breastfeedingreportcard.pdf.

Hauck, Y. L., Fenwick, J., Dhaliwal, S. S., & Butt, J. (2011). A Western Australian survey of breastfeeding initiation, prevalence, and early cessation patterns. *Maternal and Child Health Journal, 15*(2), 260-268. doi:10.1007/s10995-009-0554-2.

Horta, B., Bahl, R., Martines, J., & Victora, C. (2007). *Evidence on the long-term effects of breastfeeding: Systematic reviews and meta-analyses.* Geneva: World Health Organization. Retrieved from http://whqlibdoc.who.int/publications/2007/9789241595230_eng.pdf.

Li, R., Fein, S. B., Chen, J., & Grummer-Strawn, L. M. (2008). Why mothers stop breastfeeding: mothers' self-reported reasons for stopping during the first year. *Pediatrics, 122*(Suppl 2), S69-S76. doi: 10.1542/peds.2008-1315i.

McAndrew, F., Thompson, J., Fellows, L., Large, A., Speed, M., & Renfrew, M. (2012). *Infant feeding survey 2010: Summary.* Leeds, UK: Health & Social Care Information Centre.

Retrieved from http://www.hscic.gov.uk/catalogue/PUB08694/Infant-Feeding-Survey-2010-Consolidated-Report.pdf.

Odom, E.C., Li, R., Scanlon, K. S., Perrine, C. G., & Grummer-Strawn, L. (2013). Reasons for earlier than desired cessation of breastfeeding. *Pediatrics, 131*(3), 726-732. doi: 10.1542/peds.2012-1295.

Renfrew, M.J., McCormick, F.M., Wade, A., Quinn, B., & Dowswell, T. (2012). Support for healthy breastfeeding mothers with healthy term babies. *Cochrane Database of Systematic Reviews,* 2012(5), 1-207. doi: 10.1002/14651858.CD001141.pub4.

Thorne, S. (2008). *Interpretive description.* Walnut Creek, CA: Left Coast Press Inc.

CHAPTER 15

The Risks of
Risk-Based Language

Alison Stuebe

In her 1996 essay, "Watch Your Language," Diane Wiessinger challenged health professionals to reframe the way we talk about breastfeeding in comparison with formula- feeding:

> When we fail to describe the hazards of artificial feeding, we deprive mothers of crucial decision-making information. The mother having difficulty with breastfeeding may not seek help just to achieve a "special bonus"; but she may clamor for help if she knows how much she and her baby stand to lose (p. 1).

The essay argues that by presenting the "benefits of breastfeeding," we imply that formula feeding is normal, and breastfeeding is an optional bonus (Wiessinger, 1996). Conversely, when we recognize breastfeeding as the biological norm, and present the risks of formula, breastfeeding becomes an imperative.

Wiessinger's argument is powerful, and in many venues, the frame has shifted from "benefits of breastfeeding" to "risks of formula-feeding." However, framing formula-feeding as a risky activity may have unintended consequences. Central to Wiessinger's argument is that risk-based language provides a woman with information so that she will "clamor for help if she knows how much she and her baby stand to lose" (p. 1). This argument presumes that a woman has access to resources that will allow her to overcome breastfeeding challenges. In the absence of such resources, there may be risks to risk-based language.

Evidence from other fields of health promotion suggests that the effect of fear appeals depends on the target individual's perceived threat and efficacy. A threat is defined as a "danger of harm, characterized by the degree of severity, and the degree to which one is susceptible to this threat (and a threatening communication is a message conveying one or both of these elements)" (p. S9) (Peters, Ruiter, & Kok, 2013). Efficacy is defined as "One's ability to negate the harm, a function of the effectiveness of a potential response in negating the harm (response efficacy), and one's capability to enact that response (self-efficacy)" (p. S9). The evidence suggests that fear appeals are most effective in individuals with high-efficacy and low- perceived threat. Faced with information about risk, these individuals are proactive, and they can change their behavior to avoid risk. Arguably, when Wiessinger was writing in the mid-1990s, these proactive individuals were considering breastfeeding. These women were highly educated, and they had sufficient resources to seek out and pay—out-of-pocket, if needed—for professional lactation support. In this high-efficacy population, risk-based language was highly effective.

Among women with low self-efficacy, however, the psychology literature suggests that fear appeals may trigger a defensive response, reducing, rather than increasing, the target behavior. Individuals with low-efficacy, who perceive high threat become avoidant—they recognize that a threat exists, but they are unable to change their behavior, and become defensive, in some cases increasing the adverse behavior. In a recent meta-analysis, Peters et al. (2013) concluded that fear appeals should be used only in the context of an intervention that has been shown to increase efficacy. These findings are consistent with a central tenet of social-cognitive theory: in order for an individual to adapt a health behavior, the individual must believe the behavior is possible. "Unless people believe they can produce desired effects by their actions, they have little incentive to act or to persevere in the face of difficulties" (Bandura, 2004, p.144). This work suggests that risk-based language should be used with caution in populations that face personal, social, or systemic barriers to breastfeeding. Building efficacy, rather than emphasizing the risks of formula, may enable more mothers and infants to initiate and sustain breastfeeding.

This mismatch between fear appeals, and solutions for systemic barriers to breastfeeding, characterized public response to The National Breastfeeding Awareness Campaign ("Public Service Campaign to Promote Breastfeeding Awareness Launched," 2004). This campaign emphasized the risks of not breastfeeding through public service advertisements, including radio, television, print, and billboards. The campaign's video clips earned particular notoriety—in one clip, a pregnant woman rides a mechanical bull, with the caption, "You wouldn't take risks before your baby's born. Why start after? Breast-feed exclusively for 6 months." Another clip showed two pregnant women participating in a logrolling competition with the same caption. The implied message—that only thrill-seeking, reckless mothers would choose to formula-feed—was widely criticized (Bernier, 2011). A *New York Times* article about the campaign, titled "Breast-feed or else," generated more than 100 letters to the editor ("Letters: Breast-feed or Else," 2006). One mother, who was unable to establish a full milk supply, wrote,

> Why should I be made to feel like an irresponsible parent if that is my only option? The language of "risk" often implies a choice has been made. For a number of parents, that is not the case.

Others emphasized the importance of efficacy to breastfeeding messaging: "… to shame new mothers for using formula is the wrong approach. The burden must be on society, and in the workplace, to improve support for breastfeeding … New mothers need support, not admonitions."

Data on breastfeeding intention and outcomes supports the letter writer's contention that mothers need support; the majority of women initiate breastfeeding, yet two-thirds wean earlier than they had intended, and 45% report early, undesired weaning (Stuebe et al., 2014). For these women, the problem is not their desire to breastfeed, but their capacity to act on that desire and achieve their goals.

In addition to the mismatch between fear-appeals and self-efficacy, risk-based language may also adversely affect how women experience breastfeeding, motivating women to sustain breastfeeding due to fear of formula. Such motivation may foster an obsessive, rather than harmonious, passion for breastfeeding. These two types of passion are contrasted in Robert Vallerand's essay, "On the Psychology of Passion" (Vallerand, 2008). Obsessive passion arises when social acceptance or self-esteem is tied to an activity, whereas harmonious passion arises when an individual chooses the activity freely. Evidence suggests that obsessive passion may drive an individual to pursue a particular course of action with rigid persistence, with potential negative effects on health and wellbeing. For example, dancers with obsessive passion were more likely to ignore pain when injured, and continue to perform, whereas those with harmonious passion were more likely to seek information on the injury and its treatment. In the context of breastfeeding, an obsessive passion for avoiding formula might lead women to continue breastfeeding despite severe pain, or signs of infant dehydration, unnecessarily delaying treatment, and potentially leading to lasting harm for the mother, baby, or both.

Psychologist Barbara Fredrickson hypothesized that the obsessive patient is driven by negative emotions, which narrow cognition, whereas positive emotions broaden cognition and support harmonious passion (Fredrickson, 2001). My concern is that similar patterns may arise for breastfeeding women. When a mother breastfeeds because formula is risky, the associated negative emotions may derail breastfeeding. If her infant requires a supplement because lactogenesis is delayed, and she has learned that "just one bottle" devastates the infant gut for months, she may conclude that the damage has been done, and she might as well give up breastfeeding altogether. For the mothers who struggle with perinatal depression, obsessive passion may manifest with extreme statements such as, "Every time I feed my baby formula, I feel like I'm killing him because I am giving him poison" (Raines, 2012). Conversely, presenting breastfeeding as a nurturing connection between mother and child may foster harmonious passion for breastfeeding, ultimately sustaining a longer-lasting, and more positive, breastfeeding relationship.

Such nurturing relationships are addressed at the end of Wiessinger's (1996) essay. She writes:

> Easy, long-term breastfeeding involves forgetting about the "breast," and the "feeding" (and the duration, and the interval, and the transmission of the right nutrients in the right amounts, and the difference between nutritive and non-nutritive suckling needs, all of which form the focus of artificial milk pamphlets), and focusing instead on the relationship. Let's all tell mothers that we hope they won't "breastfeed"—that the real joys and satisfactions of the experience begin when they stop "breastfeeding," and start mothering at the breast (p. 4).

This notion of mothering at the breast, rather than avoiding the risks of formula, has the potential to foster more harmonious breastfeeding relationships. However, for many women, financial constraints require a return to the paid workforce. In the absence of widespread paid maternity leave, babies at work, or on-in onsite childcare, "mothering at the breast" is available to a privileged few.

The potential adverse effects of risk-based language raise important questions. As we search for ways to enable mothers to integrate their reproductive and productive work, how might risk-based language help engage families and stakeholders? How might it hurt? How might we embed efficacy building into our conversations and messaging? Nearly two decades after Wiessinger's essay, it may be time to reconsider what language to watch. It may be time to move beyond the risk-based frame, and focus on removing barriers, building efficacy, and cultivating nurturing relationships between mothers and babies.

References

Bandura, A. (2004). Health promotion by social cognitive means. *Health Education & Behavior, 31*(2), 143-164. doi: 10.1177/1090198104263660.

Bernier, R. (2011). *A critique of the National Breastfeeding Awareness Campaign: Three ways in which the campaign was flawed.* Retrieved from http://challengingdogma-fall2011.blogspot.com/2011/12/critique-of-national-breastfeeding.html.

Fredrickson, B. L. (2001). The role of positive emotions in positive psychology. The broaden-and-build theory of positive emotions. *American Psychologist, 56*(3), 218-226.

Letters: Breast-feed or Else. (2006). *The New York Times.* Retrieved from http://www.nytimes.com/2006/06/20/science/20webletters.html.

Peters, G.J., Ruiter, R.A., & Kok, G. (2013). Threatening communication: a critical re-analysis and a revised meta-analytic test of fear appeal theory. *Health Psychology Review, 7*(Suppl 1), S8-s31. doi: 10.1080/17437199.2012.703527.

Public Service Campaign to Promote Breastfeeding Awareness Launched. (2004). Retrieved from http://archive.hhs.gov/news/press/2004pres/20040604.html.

Raines, C. (2012). [Personal communication].

Stuebe, A. M., Horton, B. J., Chetwynd, E., Watkins, S., Grewen, K., & Meltzer-Brody, S. (2014). Prevalence and risk factors for early, undesired weaning attributed to lactation dysfunction. *Journal of Women's Health (Larchmt), 23*(5), 404-412. doi: 10.1089/jwh.2013.4506.

Vallerand, R. J. (2008). On the psychology of passion: In search of what makes people's lives most worth living. *Canadian Psychology/ Psychologie Canadienne, 49*(1), 1-13. doi: 10.1037/0708-5591.49.1.1.

Wiessinger, D. (1996). Watch Your Language! *Journal of Human Lactation, 12*(1), 1-4. doi: 10.1177/089033449601200102.

CHAPTER 16

Perceived Likeliness to Breastfeed and Current Infant Feeding Attitudes Among Japanese University Students

Manami Hongo and Miki Akiyama

Infant feeding attitudes among youth are important and are known to be formed long before pregnancy (Arora, McJunkin, Wehrer, & Kuhn, 2000; Howard et al., 2000). Young students' infant feeding attitudes, and their intentions to breastfeed, are related (Fairbrother & Stanger-Ross, 2010; Kavanagh, Lou, Nicklas, Habibi, & Murphy, 2012; Lou et al., 2014; Tarrant & Dodgson, 2007).

In Japan, many mothers do not breastfeed exclusively, even though they wish to breastfeed. Ninety-six percent (96%) of mothers intended to breastfeed prenatally in 2005 (The Ministry of Health, Labor, and Welfare [MOH], 2007). Moreover, while the rate of "any" breastfeeding at 1 to 2 months postpartum was 95% in 2010, 43.8% were mixed-feeding (MOH, 2011).

While maternal attitudes toward infant feeding are known to be associated with intention to breastfeed (De La Mora, Russell, Dungy,

Losch, & Dusdieker, 1999; Nanishi & Jimba, 2014), it remains unknown which attitude patterns are associated with intention among youth. In addition, infant feeding attitudes and intentions have been scarcely explored among youth in Japan (Yeo, Mulholland, Hirayama, & Breck, 1994). Therefore, the objective of this study was to identify current infant feeding attitude patterns associated with perceived likeliness to breastfeed, rather than mixed-feed, among university students in Japan.

Method

A cross-sectional study was conducted using a self-administered questionnaire at a private university in Kanagawa, Japan in July 2011. Participants were female and male university students who were attending one of the following official activities provided by the Faculty of Policy Management, and/or the Faculty of Environment and Information Studies at the university: 4 lecture classes, 5 circles (autonomous student activities officially approved by the university), and 6 seminars. Convenience sampling was performed. The approached activities were those with which the first researcher (then a senior student) had contact. The ethical principles of health research and codes of conduct provided by our institution were followed. The questionnaire was filled out anonymously. We considered a student's submission of the questionnaire as consent to participate.

Infant feeding attitudes were measured using the Japanese version of the Iowa Infant Feeding Attitude Scale (IIFAS-J) (Nanishi & Jimba, 2014) on a 5-point Likert scale. The IIFAS consists of 17 statements, among which 9 are written in favor of formula-feeding, and are reversed scored for the analyses (De La Mora et al., 1999). The Cronbach's alpha of the IIFAS-J was 0.66 (Nanishi & Jimba, 2014). The IIFAS-J excludes item 17 from the original IIFAS, "A mother who occasionally drinks alcohol should not breastfeed her baby," because of its low item-total correlation. Infant feeding attitude patterns were examined using principal components analysis.

Intention was measured as perceived likeliness to breastfeed. It was defined as perceiving a higher probability of breastfeeding than mixed-feeding (i.e., "My future partner and/or I will probably breast-feed rather than mixed-feed"). The probability of breastfeeding was rated on a 6-point Likert scale (0 = 0%, 1 = 1–20%, 2 = 21–40%, 3 = 41–60%, 4 = 61–80%, 5 = 81–100%) (Marrone, Vogeltanz-Holm, & Holm, 2008). The probability of mixed-feeding was rated accordingly. Participants who gave higher ratings on the former scale, compared to the latter scale, were identified as having a perceived likeliness to breastfeed, rather than mixed-feed.

Multiple logistic regression analysis was conducted to examine the association of attitude patterns with perceived likeliness to breastfeed, as opposed to mixed-feed. Possible confounders were age, gender, "had been mainly breastfed," and "had observed breastfeeding in public." Both "had been mainly breastfed" and "had observed breastfeeding in public" were measured as dichotomous variables. Models included these covariates in order to determine adjusted odds ratios.

Results

Of the 291 questionnaires that were distributed, 275 were returned (95%). None of the participants had children. Three participants were omitted from the analysis for answering none of the IIFAS-J questions. Seventy-seven participants who were unsure of their infant feeding history were also excluded from the analysis. Therefore, data from 177 university students (106 women, 71 men) who completed the questions required for the analysis were further analyzed (61%). Characteristics of participants are shown in Table 1.

Table 1. Characteristics of participants (*N* = 177).

Variable		n (%)
Gender	Male	71 (40.1)
	Female	106 (59.9)
Age	Mean ± SD = 20.5 ± 1.5 (Min 18, Max 25)	---
Main feeding method as a baby	Had not been mainly breastfed — Formula-fed	16 (9.0)
	Had not been mainly breastfed — Mixed-fed	93 (48.0)
	Had been mainly breastfed	76 (42.9)

*Note: Percentages may not add up to 100% due to rounding.

Table 2. Factor coefficients (based on varimax rotated factors).

	IIFAS-J Items	Factor 1	Factor 2	Factor 3	Factor 4	Factor 5
Q.1 (RS)	No lasting nutritional benefits	- 0.01	0.04	0.45	0.02	- 0.23
Q.2 (RS)	Less convenient	- 0.07	0.48	0.09	0.07	- 0.04
Q.3	Bonding	0.25	- 0.02	- 0.16	0.08	0.18
Q.4 (RS)	Lack of iron	0.03	- 0.13	0.44	- 0.15	0.01
Q.5	Overfeeding (formula)	- 0.03	- 0.04	- 0.01	0.56	- 0.10
Q.6 (RS)	Back to work	0.06	0.26	0.03	- 0.19	0.22
Q.7	Joy of motherhood	0.20	- 0.05	- 0.05	0.10	0.16
Q.8 (RS)	Should not breastfeed in public	0.01	0.00	- 0.04	0.12	0.45
Q.9	Baby's health (healthier)	0.24	0.03	0.02	- 0.04	- 0.11
Q.10 (RS)	Overfeeding (breastfeeding)	- 0.06	0.02	0.39	0.18	0.07
Q.11 (RS)	Father feeling left out	- 0.06	- 0.07	- 0.10	- 0.12	0.59
Q.12	Baby's ideal food	0.34	- 0.12	0.07	- 0.20	- 0.04
Q.13	More easily digested	0.27	- 0.00	0.11	- 0.10	- 0.21
Q.14 (RS)	Baby's health (no difference)	- 0.04	0.03	0.21	0.40	0.14
Q.15	More convenient	- 0.04	0.53	- 0.14	- 0.01	- 0.08
Q.16	Less expensive	0.15	- 0.01	- 0.10	0.22	0.04

*Note: (RS): Reversed scored; Bold: the highest coefficient score among the factors.
IIFAS-J items above are short forms of the questionnaire items.

Factor analysis identified five attitude patterns (Table 2): benefits of breastfeeding (Factor 1), perceived convenience of breastfeeding (including returning to work) (Factor 2), perceived disadvantages of breastfeeding (Factor 3), unsure and ambivalent about formula-feeding (Factor 4), and social perceptions (public breastfeeding/role of the father) (Factor 5) (see Table 2). The overall Cronbach's alpha was 0.64 (see Table 2).

An increase of one unit on the Factor 2 score corresponded to being more than twice as likely to perceive likeliness to breastfeed rather than to mixed-feed. After adjusting for gender, age, "had been mainly breastfed," and "had observed breastfeeding in public," perceived future likeliness to breastfeed was positively associated with Factor 2 (adjusted odds ratio (AOR): 2.03 [95% confidence interval (CI): 1.45–2.83], "had been mainly breastfed" (AOR: 3.29 [95% CI: 1.61–6.72]) and "had observed breastfeeding in public" (AOR: 2.26 [95% CI: 1.10–4.64]) (see Table 3).

Table 3. Association between infant feeding attitude patterns and perceived likeliness to breastfeed.

Variables	Perceived likeliness to breastfeed > mixed-feed ($N = 177$) AOR [95% CI]
Factor 1: Benefits of breastfeeding	1.24 [0.90–1.69]
Factor 2: Perceived convenience or inconvenience (including returning to work)	2.03 [1.45–2.83]
Factor 3: Perceived disadvantages of breastfeeding	1.24 [0.90–1.71]
Factor 4: Unsure or ambivalent about formula feeding	1.27 [0.92–1.75]
Factor 5: Social perceptions (public breastfeeding/role of the father)	1.25 [0.90–1.73]
Had been breastfed	3.29 [1.61–6.72]
Had observed breastfeeding in public	2.26 [1.10–4.64]
Age	1.06 [0.82–1.36]
Gender (Female)	0.59 [0.28–1.25]

Note: The factor variables categorize the predicted factor scores by quantiles. The highest quantile corresponds to 3 while the lowest quantile corresponds to 0. The adjusted odds ratio (AOR) indicates how many times the perceived likeliness to breastfeed is larger than that to mixed-feed, given a quantile increase in the attitude variable.

Discussion

Using principle component analysis, we found that perceived convenience of infant feeding methods, including returning to work, is associated with perceived likeliness to breastfeed. Students who thought breastfeeding was convenient perceived that they would be more likely to breastfeed than mixed-feed. Our findings are consistent with previous research that has shown positive associations of intention with attitude with different scales (Fairbrother & Stanger-Ross, 2010; Kavanagh et al., 2012; Lou et al., 2014; Tarrant & Dodgson, 2007).

In our study, having observed breastfeeding in public, and having been breastfed, were associated with perceived likeliness to breastfeed rather than to mixed-feed. Positive associations of breastfeeding intention with observation experience (Ebrahim et al., 2011), and having been breastfed have also been reported (Kavanagh et al., 2012; Lou et al., 2014; Tarrant & Dodgson, 2007). However, some studies did not find a significant association between observation experience and breastfeeding intention (Fairbrother & Stanger-Ross, 2010; Marrone et al., 2008; Tarrant & Dodgson, 2007). This may be due to differences in the definition of intention. In our study, perceived likeliness included personal efficacy for breastfeeding, whereas other studies asked participants' merely about preferences for different methods. When youth learn that breastfeeding is convenient, and that it can be combined with working, this may enhance their self-efficacy to breastfeed in the future. Research on the difference between preference and perceived likeliness to breastfeed may facilitate further understanding of the youth's intentions towards infant feeding.

This is the first study to explore the youth's attitude patterns associated with perceived likeliness to breastfeed in Japan. Since this research was completed at a private university, the results might not be generalizable to the general youth population. However, to our knowledge, this is the first study of its nature conducted among university students in Japan from non-health/childcare specialty courses (Tsutsumi, Takano, & Mihashi, 2004).

Conclusion

Perceived convenience or inconvenience of infant feeding (including returning to work) was significantly associated with increased perception of likeliness to breastfeed. Therefore, information about breastfeeding management and increasing convenience may positively affect the youth's future likeliness to breastfeed.

References

Arora, S., McJunkin, C., Wehrer, J., & Kuhn P. (2000). Major factors influencing breastfeeding rates: Mother's perception of father's attitude and milk supply. *Pediatrics, 106(5)*, E67. doi:10.1542/peds.106.5.e67.

De La Mora, A., Russell, D. W., Dungy, C. I., Losch, M., & Dusdieker, L. (1999). The Iowa Infant Feeding Attitude Scale: Analysis of reliability and validity. *Journal of Applied Social Psychology, 29(11)*, 2362–2380. doi:10.1111/j.1559-1816.1999.tb00115.x.

Ebrahim, B., Al-Enezi, H., Al-Turki, M., Al-Turki, A., Al-Rabah, F., Hammoud, M. S., & Al-Taiar, A. (2011). Knowledge, misconceptions, and future intentions towards breastfeeding among female university students in Kuwait. *Journal of Human Lactation, 27(4)*, 358–366. doi:10.1177/0890334411411163.

Fairbrother, N., & Stanger-Ross, I. (2010). Reproductive-aged women's knowledge and attitudes regarding infant-feeding practices: An experimental evaluation. *Journal of Human Lactation, 26(2)*, 157–167. doi:10.1177/0890334409352853.

Howard, C., Howard, F., Lawrence, R., Andresen, E., DeBlieck, E., & Weitzman, M. (2000). Office prenatal formula advertising and its effect on breast-feeding patterns. *Obstetrics and Gynecology, 95(2)*, 296–303. doi:10.1016/S0029-7844(99)00555-4.

Kavanagh, K. F., Lou, Z., Nicklas, J. C., Habibi, M. F., & Murphy, L. T. (2012). Breastfeeding knowledge, attitudes, prior exposure, and intent among undergraduate students. *Journal of Human Lactation, 28(4)*, 556–564. doi:10.1177/0890334412446798.

Lou, Z., Zeng, G., Orme, J. G., Huang, L., Liu, F., Pang, X., & Kavanagh, K. F. (2014). Breastfeeding knowledge, attitudes, and intention in a sample of undergraduate students in Mainland China. *Journal of Human Lactation, 30(3),* 331–339. doi:10.1177/0890334414526058.

Marrone, S., Vogeltanz-Holm, N., & Holm, J. (2008). Attitudes, knowledge, and intentions related to breastfeeding among university undergraduate women and men. *Journal of Human Lactation, 24(2),* 186–192. doi:10.1177/0890334408316072.

Nanishi, K., & Jimba, M. (2014). Reliability and validity of the Japanese version of the Iowa Infant Feeding Attitude Scale: A longitudinal study. *Journal of Human Lactation, 30(3),* 346–352. doi:10.1177/0890334414534321.

Tarrant, M., & Dodgson, J. E. (2007). Knowledge, attitudes, exposure, and future intentions of Hong Kong university students toward infant feeding. *Journal of Obstetric, Gynecologic, and Neonatal Nursing, 36*(3), 243–254. doi:10.1111/j.1552-6909.2007.00144.x.

The Ministry of Health, Labor, and Welfare. (2007). *Junyu-rinyuno-shien guide [Guide for infant feeding and weaning].* Tokyo, Japan: Equal Employment, Children and Families Bureau, Ministry of Health, Labor, and Welfare. (in Japanese). Retrieved from http://www.mhlw.go.jp/shingi/2007/03/dl/s0314-17.pdf.

The Ministry of Health, Labor, and Welfare. (2011). *Survey on the growth of infants and preschool children in Japan, 2010.* Tokyo, Japan: Equal Employment, Children and Families Bureau, Ministry of Health, Labor, and Welfare. (in Japanese). Retrieved from http://www.mhlw.go.jp/stf/houdou/2r9852000001t3so-att/2r9852000001t7dg.pdf.

Tsutsumi, C., Takano, Y., & Mihashi, F. (2004). University students' perception on breastfeeding (1): Students from nutritionist and/or child care educational courses [Bonyuikuji ni kansuru ishikichosakenkyu (1) eiyoshi hoikushi youseikatei no gakusei no ishiki nituite]. *Journal of the Japan Child and Family Research Institute, 41,* 203–217. (in Japanese)

Yeo, S., Mulholland, P. M., Hirayama, M., & Breck, S. (1994). Cultural views of breastfeeding among high-school female students in Japan and the United States: A survey. *Journal of Human Lactation, 10(1),* 25–30. doi:10.1177/089033449401000124.

Advancing Strategies Across the Social Ecology

This section examines women's experiences with and prevention strategies to address challenges with breastfeeding across the social ecology.

Section 1

Advancing Supportive Public Policy

CHAPTER 17

A History of the
Infant Mortality Rate:
The Role of Milk

Jacqueline H. Wolf

During the first months of life, exclusive breastfeeding is a social equalizer. Exclusively breastfed babies enjoy the same start in life, whether they are from developing or developed countries, and whether their families are poor or rich. James Grant, the former Executive Director of UNICEF, described this phenomenon eloquently:

> Breastfeeding is a natural "safety net" against the worst
> effects of poverty... exclusive breastfeeding goes a long
> way toward canceling out the health difference between
> being born into poverty and being born into affluence
> ... It is almost as if breastfeeding takes the infant out of
> poverty for those first few months in order to give the
> child a fairer start in life and compensate for th injustice
> of the world into which it was born (Edwards & Byrom,
> 2007).

The many late 19th- and early 20th-century mothers whose infants died of "summer complaint," one of many names used at the time to describe

141

infant diarrhea, learned this lesson all too well. In that era, infants died of diarrhea by the tens of thousands each summer throughout North America, particularly in urban areas, where cows' milk traveled from rural dairy farmer to urban consumer for up to 72 hours in unrefrigerated railroad cars (Wolf, 2001). The high infant death rate spurred women's activism. "Save the babies" became a rallying cry (Meckel, 1990). One of the most influential women in this arena was Adelaide Hunter Hoodless, a Canadian mother whose fourth child died of diarrhea in 1889 due to tainted cows' milk. Hoodless went on to co-found the Women's Institute, the YWCA, the National Council of Women, and the Victorian Order of Nurses in order to put supports in place to help women safeguard their children (Adelaide Hunter Hoodless Homestead, 2015).

Physicians' activism also played a vital role in lowering infant mortality. Late 19th- and early 20th-century American doctors knew the dire consequences for babies who were not breastfed. As one pediatrician observed in 1909, cows' milk might be a second-best infant food but, he added, "I say 'best,' but in this connection the word is almost meaningless, for the difference between mother's milk and cows' milk is abysmal. The first is at once a perfect food and an efficient medicine, while the second is a very unsatisfactory food and no medicine at all" (Hirshberg, 1909).

In condemning the use of cows' milk as an infant food, some doctors conducted experiments to prove its dangers. Renowned pediatrician, Henry L. Coit, for example, fed human milk to puppies, and found that the puppies "remained alive, but were in a very miserable condition." Like the human infants with runny noses and stomach troubles that Coit attempted to treat, the pups were "inferior to the breast-fed animals, both at the time of the experiment and afterwards" (Coit, 1912).

Nineteenth- and early 20th-century pediatricians understood that mammals' milk is species-specific. They saw firsthand that one type of mammal cannot thrive on the milk of another. The high infant mortality rate from diarrhea was the most tangible proof of the importance of human milk to human health. The history of the infant mortality rate in the United States, however, is as much a story about cows' milk as about human milk.

Today, the leading causes of death in the United States are heart disease and cancer (Centers for Disease Control and Prevention [CDC], 2015). A century earlier, however, the country's leading killers were infectious diseases: #3 was pneumonia, #2 was tuberculosis, and the #1 killer was diarrhea. In 1900, 13 percent of infants died before their first birthday; more than half the dead died of diarrhea (Preston & Haines, 1991). When infant diarrhea struck, it killed almost 100 percent of its victims, and did so swiftly. Compared to adults, babies have meager water reserves and dehydrate quickly. In an era before rehydration therapy and antibiotics, infant diarrhea was untreatable. Doctors described the course of the illness: debilitating bouts of "violent" diarrhea were followed by a feeble pulse; shriveled, cold skin; sunken eyes; stupor; and coma. Death usually occurred within three to four days, but often within 24 hours of the first symptoms (Yale, 1885).

The most striking aspect of the contrast in the leading causes of death in early 20th- versus early 21st-century developed countries is the steep decline in killer infectious diseases. Most people associate this epidemiological shift with the medical knowledge accumulated in the last 100 years, and with the effective medical therapies, especially antibiotics and immunizations, that came with that knowledge. Yet, the eradication of deadly infectious disease was well under way before there were any effective therapies developed to treat those diseases. Prevention, not cure, was the solution.

One way that public health authorities thwarted infectious disease was to outlaw livestock in urban areas. Despite the benefits conferred by those animals as ready food and transportation sources, the domestication of animals also posed grave dangers, particularly in heavily populated areas. Diseases jumped the species barrier. Tuberculosis and smallpox, for example, came from cattle; influenza came from pigs and chickens (Diamond, 1997).

In addition to outlawing livestock in urban areas to diminish the spread of infectious disease, cities and towns built public health infrastructure to sanitize the environment. Municipal, county, and state governments built sewers to separate human waste from drinking water. Governments paid for filtering and chemically treating drinking water. State legislatures and city councils ordered milk be pasteurized and kept cold during shipping. These public health efforts led to changes in infection and mortality patterns (Tomes, 1998).

The #1 killer in the U.S., infant diarrhea, disappeared slowly over roughly four decades. In Chicago, infant deaths from diarrhea ebbed as municipalities passed laws governing the gathering, shipping, and sale of milk. In 1897, diarrhea caused 53.7% of 5,735 infant deaths in that city. In 1912, when the city's population was larger, diarrhea caused 39.4% of 6,689 infant deaths. In 1924, diarrhea caused 16.9% of 4,528 infant deaths. And in 1939, before there were any effective therapies to treat infant diarrhea—antibiotics, for example, were not available to the public until after WWII—only 1.4% of the 1,533 babies who died in Chicago that year died of diarrhea (Wolf, 2001).

As the leading cause of death in the United States, the eradication of infant diarrhea became a top public health priority. One of the first lessons the public needed to learn was that infant death is preventable. At the time, the medical community and public alike thought of infants as naturally weak, and thus, susceptible to a host of deadly ailments. Even public health workers had long dismissed infant deaths, particularly from diarrhea, as unavoidable; "We calmly accepted the annual harvest of death as if it were as inevitable as the weather; as if indeed a part of the weather. 'Hot weather, babies die' was our unconscious thought" (Infant Welfare Service, 1911, p. 177). Few associated the lack of refrigeration, and resulting spoiled food fed to infants during the summer, with the ailment that was killing so many.

Once the association was understood, public health posters explained that most infant deaths were "avoidable." Placards described the "preventable perils" threatening infants, including dirty cows' milk, bovine tuberculosis, and diarrheal disease (Bulletin Chicago School of Sanitary Instruction [BCSSI], n.d.). In other words, the food so many mothers fed their babies was killing them.

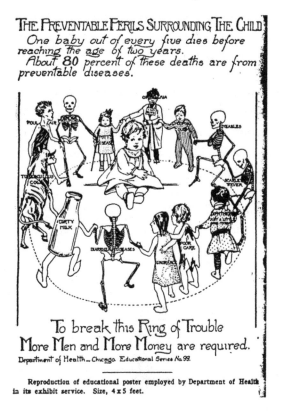

Reproduction of educational poster employed by Department of Health in its exhibit service. Size, 4 x 5 feet.

In this era before pure food laws, cows' milk could be deadly. Dairy cattle were often housed under filthy conditions and milked by dirty hands. Some of the milk sold was popularly known as "swill milk," produced by dairy cattle that were fed the cheap, fermented grain that was a byproduct of urban distilleries. Milk traveled for days in unrefrigerated railroad cars. Shipped in 8-gallon open vats, the milk was particularly easy for farmers, shippers, and merchants to adulterate. To stretch the commodity, water was often added to milk. Powered chalk was added as well to whiten milk as it grew dirty in its open vat. After the farmer or shipper skimmed cream from the top to sell separately at a higher price, he often replaced the cream with plaster to make the skim milk that remained appear whole again and rich with cream (Wolf, 2001). Merchants placed communal dippers in the milk vats so wary customers could sample the milk before purchase. Thus diphtheria, typhoid, scarlet fever, tuberculosis, and diarrhea all became milk-borne diseases.

In order to pinpoint the mothers most in need of education about the importance of breastfeeding, and the dangers of cows' milk, public health departments mapped every infant death from diarrhea in their jurisdictions. In the neighborhoods with the highest death rates, visiting nurses blanketed the community.

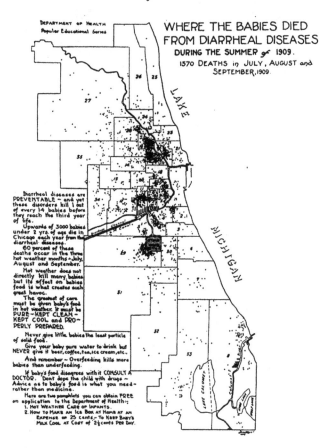

The health department hung posters. First and foremost, the posters urged mothers to breastfeed. One poster described the perilous path cows' milk followed as it made its way to the urban consumer. The poster depicted a long tube with one end attached to a cow's udder and the other end placed in the mouth of an emaciated infant. Between the cow and the baby, the tube snaked through a dairy barn, a railroad station, a railroad car, a milk depot, and a milkman's cart, ultimately landing on the steps of a home, in an uncapped bottle, baking in the sun, flies buzzing around the mouth of the bottle. The poster's narrative explained: "And Yet Some People Wonder Why So Many Babies Die! On the other hand, the mother-fed baby gets its milk fresh, pure and healthful—no germs can get into it. To Lessen Baby Deaths Let Us Have More Mother-Fed Babies" (BCSSI, 1911).

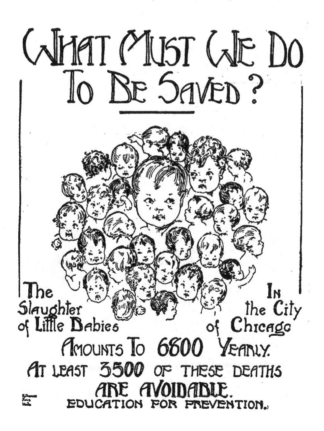

147

Most posters, however, focused solely on cows' milk. One depicted a mother cradling her infant, juxtaposed with a dairyman in his filthy workplace. The "healthman" appeared between the two. The poster read: "Bye Baby Bunting. Healthman's gone a hunting. To get the dirty milkman's skin/And save the Baby's life for him. Is your milkman a friend or an enemy of your baby? If you don't know ask the health department" (BCSSI, 1914). Another placard was headlined "Give the Bottle-Fed Baby a Chance for Its Life" and advised, "Buy only fresh milk in bottles [as opposed to treacherous 8-gallon open-vats]. Pasteurize milk at home. Keep milk on ice. Keep it away from flies. If flies beat the baby to it, let the flies have it. SAFE MILK¾SAVES SICKNESS" (BCSSI, 1912). Unfortunately, the relentless public health focus on cows' milk implied that cows' milk could be made safe for babies, negating the message of the other posters that instructed mothers to breastfeed.

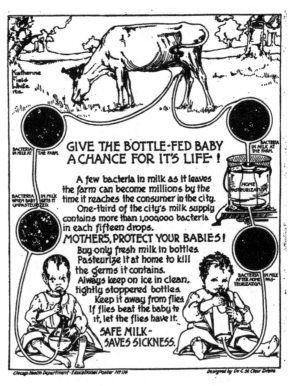

Cleaning up cows' milk became a crusade of urban newspapers. Newspapers ran headlines vilifying the dairy industry, and imploring legislators to regulate it. In Chicago, its clean-milk campaign began in 1892, and ended in 1926. Infant diarrhea there ebbed with every piece of legislation. That city ordered milk vats sealed in 1904, ordered milk be shipped in individual bottles in 1912, pasteurized in 1916, kept cold during shipping in 1920, and tested for bovine tuberculosis in 1926. By the early 1930s, due to almost 40 years of legislation, infant diarrhea as a cause of infant death had largely been eradicated (Wolf, 2001).

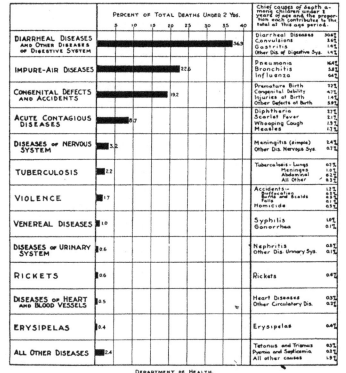

WHAT KILLS THE BABIES

This Diagram Shows the Chief Causes of Death Among Children Under Two Years of Age and the Ratio of Each Cause to the Total Deaths In This Age Division.

Department of Health, Chicago. Popular Education Series No.5

Public health workers lowered infant mortality largely by cleaning up the dairy industry despite a simultaneous campaign telling mothers, "The Proper Food for Babies is Mother's Milk—No sensible mother needs advice on this point" (BCSSI, 1910). In other words, the crusade to sanitize cows' milk had a far greater impact on public perception and behavior than the campaign to breastfeed. Far more visible than the breastfeeding campaign, the ubiquitous crusade to clean up cows' milk implied that cows' milk was more important than human milk to infants' health. And with the much-ballyhooed success of the cows' milk crusade came another implied message—that the problem of feeding cows' milk to human babies had finally been solved. The cow was now celebrated as "the foster mother of the human race" (Bonnie Mohr Studio, 1997-2013). The campaign to clean up the dairy industry gave enormous credence to the efficacy of cows' milk as a food for human babies. Breastfeeding no longer seemed vital to human health.

References

Adelaide Hunter Hoodless Homestead. (2015). *Adelaide's Story*. Retrieved from http://www.adelaidehoodless.ca/history/adelaides-story/.

Bonnie Mohr Studio. (1997-2013). *Foster mothers of the human race*. Retrieved from http://www.bonniemohr.com/store/foster-mothers-of-the-human-race.html.

Bulletin Chicago School of Sanitary Instruction. (2 July 1910). 13, 3.

Bulletin Chicago School of Sanitary Instruction. (25 April 1914).

Bulletin Chicago School of Sanitary Instruction. (3 June 1911).

Bulletin Chicago School of Sanitary Instruction. (31 August 1912).

Bulletin Chicago School of Sanitary Instruction. Chicago Department of Health Educational Poster 99. (Early 20th Century, exact date unknown.).

Centers for Disease Control and Prevention. (2015). *Leading causes of death*. Retrieved from http://www.cdc.gov/nchs/fastats/leading-causes-of-death.htm.

Coit, H.L. (1912). The effects of heated and superheated milk on the infant's nutrition (Recent Investigations). *Transactions of the American Pediatric Society*, 24, 128-138.

Diamond, J. (1997). *Guns, germs, and steel: The fates of human societies.* New York: W. W. Norton and Company.

Edwards, G., & Byrom, S. (Eds.). (2008). *Essential midwifery practice: Public health.* John Wiley & Sons. Malden, MA: Blackwell Publishers, Ltd.

Hirshberg, L. K. (1909). What you ought to know about your baby. *The Delineator,* 73, 262.

Infant Welfare Service, 1909-1910. (1911). *Report of the Department of Health of the City of Chicago for the Years 1907, 1908, 1909, 1910.* (Chicago), 177.

Meckel, R. A. (1990). *Save the babies: American public health reform and the prevention of infant mortality, 1850-1929.* Baltimore, MD: John Hopkins Press.

Preston, S.H., & Michael, R.H. (1991). *Fatal years: Child mortality in late Nineteenth-Century America.* Princeton: Princeton University Press.

Tomes, N. (1998). *The gospel of germs: Men, women, and the microbe in American life.* Cambridge: Harvard University Press.

Wolf, J. H. (2001). *Don't kill your baby: Public health and the decline of breastfeeding in the nineteenth and twentieth centuries.* Columbus, OH: Ohio State University Press.

Yale, L.M. (1885). Summer Complaint. *Babyhood,* 1, 203.

CHAPTER 18

Consideration for Environmental Contaminants in Breastmilk

Virginia T. Guidry

A mother's body is the environment for her children throughout pregnancy and during breastfeeding (Nickerson, 2006). Exposures in utero typically are much lower than exposures during breastfeeding. However, it is hard to distinguish the effects of exposure in utero from those that occur during breastfeeding because the developing fetus is more sensitive to these exposures than the breastfeeding infant. Additionally, some exposures are greater during breastfeeding due to the high fat content of breastmilk, and the lipophilic nature of many environmental chemicals (Anderson & Wolf, 2000; Nickerson, 2006). Increased detection of contaminants in breastmilk has resulted from improved sensitivity of laboratory testing, as well as increased efforts to conduct biomonitoring.

At background exposure levels typical of the United States, the many known health benefits of breastfeeding outweigh the potential harms from chemical exposures (Anderson & Wolf, 2000). It is important to acknowledge that contaminants can be measured in breastmilk, and understand that these exposures are a function of our surroundings. This information must be carefully presented to breast-feeding women in order to avoid the possibility of premature weaning due to fear of detrimental health effects (Brody, Morello-Frosch, Brown, & Rudel, 2009; Geraghty, Khoury, Morrow, & Lanphear, 2008).

Exposure Pathways

Chemicals mainly enter breastmilk via passive transfer from the mother's blood plasma (Anderson & Wolf, 2000). This transfer depends on a number of factors, including maternal body-burden, milk composition, length of breastfeeding, chemical transfer kinetics, chemical metabolism, and chemical characteristics, such as solubility and lipophilicity (Anderson & Wolf, 2000).

Maternal exposures to chemicals found in breastmilk mainly occur via food (Anderson & Wolf, 2000). Emissions from pollution sources, such as power plants, industrial facilities, and vehicular sources are deposited in air, water, and soil. Human exposures to pollutants can occur immediately, or over time, as contaminants are slowly released from environmental reservoirs, like soil and sediments under bodies of water. Pollutants enter the food chain and make their way into plants, meat, and fish that humans consume (Anderson & Wolf, 2000). This process can vary greatly by chemical.

In general, as maternal exposure to environmental chemicals decreases (e.g., due to the phasing out of sale and use of specific chemicals), so do breastmilk concentrations (Anderson, 2000). As background levels drop, however, exposures via breastmilk may comprise a greater proportion of a child's lifetime exposure (Anderson & Wolf, 2000). Some environmental chemicals that persist in the environment are exceptions to this pattern (Nickerson, 2006).

Contaminants of Concern

Persistent organic pollutants (POPs) are chemicals that do not break down in the environment, and thus, human exposures continue, even after production and use have ceased (Nickerson, 2006). After deposition and entering the food chain, which is the main source of exposure to these chemicals, POPs bioaccumulate so that animals at the top of the food chain have the highest body burdens (Nickerson, 2006). The recognition of their persistent nature often leads to bans on usage. However, many banned POPs are now ubiquitous. Many POPs are also lipophilic, which enhances transmission to breastmilk (Anderson & Wolf, 2000).

There are several prominent POPs. Polychlorinated biphenyls (PCBs) are the most widespread and concerning of human milk contaminants. Although banned in the United States (U.S.) since the 1970s, PCBs are still in production elsewhere. Dioxins are byproducts of the production and combustion of chlorinated compounds (e.g., for paper bleaching, waste incineration, and the manufacture of pesticides; Nickerson, 2006). Polybrominated diphenyl ethers (PBDEs) are flame retardants used in home furnishings that are still unrestricted in the U.S. Accordingly, U.S. breastmilk levels of PBDEs are 10 to 100 times higher than levels in Europe, where use is limited (Nickerson, 2006). Organochlorines are pesticides (e.g., DDT) that are banned in the U.S., but are still produced and used in other countries, especially for mosquito control. Organochlorine exposures have declined as chemicals are banned (Nickerson, 2006).

Heavy metals are another class of concerning contaminants, although less is known about the pharmacokinetics of heavy metals compared to POPs (American Academy of Pediatrics, 2001; Anderson & Wolf, 2000). Lead has been detected in breastmilk, and is a known neurotoxicant, but breastmilk is not a major source of exposure, in part because lead in breastmilk may not be completely absorbed (American Academy of Pediatrics, 2001). Mercury is also a contaminant of concern because of potential impacts on neurodevelopment (American

Academy of Pediatrics, 2001). Because they are in elemental form, heavy metals can't break down into other less harmful forms in the environment.

Possible Action

We need a better understanding of the relationship between a lifetime of environmental exposures for women, and the resulting exposures passed on to their children via breastmilk. We know that these chemicals can be harmful at some levels, but we don't know whether typical exposure levels via breastfeeding cause harm. A U.S. or global breastmilk biomonitoring program would provide data on contaminant levels in breastmilk over time, and alert public health officials if alarming increases in exposures were measured (Solomon, Weiss, Owen, & Citron, 2005).

Based on current knowledge, we should continue to encourage breastfeeding among women with typical background environmental exposures. Extreme circumstances, such as chemical disasters, may result in very high exposures that warrant an exception to this rule. An excellent resource for concerned mothers is the National Resources Defense Council's *Healthy Milk, Healthy Baby* report, which describes sources of exposure, summarizes the benefits of breastfeeding, and gives suggestions for moms to maintain a healthy environment (Solomon et al., 2005). Finally, we should follow the precautionary principle, and advocate for better public health policies that protect environmental quality for all. This is the most effective way to minimize exposures to mothers and their children, and thus, maximize the benefits of breastfeeding.

References

Anderson, H.A., & Wolff, M.S. (2000). Environmental contaminants in human milk. *Journal of Exposure Science and Environmental Epidemiology, 10,* 755-760.

American Academy of Pediatrics Committee on Drugs. (2001). The transfer of drugs and other chemicals into human milk. *Pediatrics, 108(3), 776-789.*

Brody, J.G., Morello-Frosch, R., Brown, P., & Rudel, R.A. (2009). Reporting individual results for environmental chemicals in breastmilk in a context that supports breastfeeding. *Breastfeeding Medicine, 4(2), 121.*

Geraghty, S.R., Khoury, J.C., Morrow, A.L., & Lanphear, B.P. (2008). Reporting individual test results of environmental chemicals in breastmilk: Potential for premature weaning. *Breastfeeding Medicine, 3(4), 207-213.*

Nickerson, K. (2006). Environmental contaminants in breastmilk. *Journal of Midwifery & Women's Health, 51(1), 26-34.*

Solomon, G., Weiss, P., Owen, B., & Citron, A. (2005). *Healthy milk, healthy baby: Chemical pollution and mother's milk.* Natural Resources Defense Council. Retrieved from http://www.nrdc.org/breastmilk/.

CHAPTER 19

Infant-feeding after Disasters: Wet-Nursing as Improvised Behavior and Formula Donations as Material Convergence

Sarah E. DeYoung

Disasters often exacerbate pre-existing inequities that exist in communities. These inequities have direct impacts on the health and well-being of nursing mothers and their infants. During emergencies, hospital staff and other public health facilities may need to re-route their normal daily initiatives and routines, which may affect infant-feeding practices (Bengin, Hormann, & Wang, 2010). Furthermore, ethics and logistical considerations surrounding the distribution of feeding supplies, such as formula or bottles following disasters, add to the complexity of infant nutrition immediately following a disaster (Callaghan et al., 2007; Carothers & Gribble, 2014; Dörnemann & Kelly, 2013; Gribble, 2014; Gribble, McGrath, MacLaine, & Lhotska, 2011; Hipgrave, Assefa, Winoto, & Sukotjo, 2011). The main rationale for restrictions on distribution of breastmilk substitutes following disasters is to avoid steering mothers away from breastfeeding their infants. Breastfeeding reduces the likelihood of diarrhea, an illness which can lead to increased rates of infant mortality (Gribble et al., 2011; WHO, 1997). Support for breastfeeding as a public health interventions can be a challenge for health workers after disasters, especially in developing areas, where bottle-feeding may be seen as a Western, and privileged, activity (Campbell, 2008; Gribble et al., 2011). This summary focuses on wet nursing and formula donations from the perspective of two subareas of disaster research: improvised behavior and material convergence, with wet nursing and formula donations as the respective issues viewed through the lens of theoretical and empirical findings of these subfields.

Wet Nursing as Improvisation

Community improvisation in disasters usually includes instances of self-organizing during a disaster in order to engage in protective action, relief activities, or evacuation (Quarantelli, 1985). For example, after the September 11th attacks on the World Trade Center, over 5,000 people were successfully evacuated across the Hudson River by private ferry owners without centralized command (Wachtendorf & Quarantelli, 2003). Another example of this would be of the Vietnamese community members using personal boats for evacuation during Hurricane Katrina (Airriess et al., 2008). Although these activities usually involve evacuation for protective action, another form of previously uncategorized improvised protective action that takes place is human milk sharing, or instances of wet nursing, during and after hazard events (e.g., Binns et al., 2012). This is a topic that warrants additional exploration in conjunction with existing research on community improvisation and emergent behaviors following disasters (Kendra & Wachtendorf, 2004), as well as with regards to the technical health protocols that may be related to spontaneous wet nursing.

Wet nursing after disasters is often retold in sensationalist narratives, and focuses on the wet nursing mother (Gribble, 2013). The framing may be problematic in these anecdotal narratives for several reasons. First, these heroic retellings of the wet nursing during, or after, a hazard event often fail to acknowledge the existence, plight, or complexities associated with the biological mother of the infant. In many cases, the mother has been killed in the hazard event, but it is unclear how or if, in many cases, the mother has survived, but is either missing, or unable to nurse her baby. Second, although narratives of wet nursing are valuable, they are often retold without an explanation for how the decision was made that wet nursing would occur. In some settings, it has been explained how family members may decide to nurse an infant, but not in the time immediately following the hazard. For example, in a study by Dörnemann and Kelly (2012), data were collected on nursing mothers more than one year after the 2010 Haiti earthquake. Nonetheless, the authors explain, "If a mother could not breastfeed, it was preferable that a close or extended family member should act as a wet nurse, rather than another woman who happened to have a baby of the same age" (p. 80). More clarification on how such decisions are made are both theoretically important, and important for public health workers in the post-disaster setting. For example, if the process of wet nurse-decision making has a general pattern within certain populations, that may facilitate organized milk sharing or wet nursing in the response and recovery phase of a disaster in which mass mortality has impacted many families. Knowing more about the process and occurrence of wet nursing after hazards might mean that aid and health workers could provide additional support (e.g., emotional and technical) for both the biological mothers, as well as the women who are acting as wet nurses.

Formula as Material Convergence

Supplies, volunteers, and machines flowing into a disaster-affected area can cause many problems in response, rescue, and recovery (Destro & Holguín-Veras, 2011; Holguín-Veras et al., 2014; Kendra & Wachtendorf, 2001; Perry & Lindell, 2003). In disaster research, material convergence is most studied within the subfield of humanitarian logistics (HL). Holguín-Veras et al. (2014), aptly describes material convergence in the following statement:

> Fundamentally, material convergence is a complex problem, with multifaceted logistical challenges: a huge quantity of items, an extremely heterogeneous flow, arriving within a short timespan to an area with limited space, resources, and personnel to process and distribute them to their intended recipients, and people in great need (p. 2).

Not only does the occurrence of material convergence potentially act as barriers for first responders engaging in search and rescue, but continued convergence in the form of donated supplies during the longer-term recovery phase can also be extremely problematic. For example, food intended for relief can rot if it is exposed to heat or water, supplies can take up space that might otherwise be used for daily activities in organizations, and human resources are needed to deal with these issues. Donations that are unneeded, or culturally inappropriate, are not uncommon, but of the possible kinds of donations, arguably one of the most dangerous is breast- milk substitute supplies. Material convergence of formula is an area of hazard research that has not been specifically applied is infant feeding *outside* of the context of: 1) general donations after hazards, and 2) public health research about formula distribution in vulnerable regions. Developing nations experiencing complex humanitarian emergencies or disasters are especially vulnerable to disruptions in infant feeding supplies, inadequate preparation of infant feeding supplies (e.g., water not adequately boiled), and stress on both the mother and the child due to the hazard event (Callaghan et al., 2007; Gribble et al., 2011). It should also be noted that formula distribution, when necessary and complying with the International Code of Marketing of Breastmilk Substitutes, must be strategic and targeted. As Gribble et al. (2011) describe,

> Although it is the breastfed babies who suffer most harm through inappropriate distributions, poor man-

agement of breast-milk substitutes also harms babies who cannot be breastfed. This is because those involved in such distributions are invariably unaware of the dangers of artificial feeding, and so do not provide the care-ers with the practical and educational support necessary to decrease risk, insofar as it can be reduced (p. 726).

Although the International Code of Marketing of Breastmilk Substitutes (Gribble et al., 2011) is acknowledged and reinforced across many governments and nongovernmental entities, it is unclear to what extent there is variation in adherence to Code standards after a disaster, especially by small emergent groups and individual actors. At the time that this summary is being composed, the author of this paper recently returned from field work deployment to Nepal after the April 2015 earthquake. Instances of formula distribution, although formally discouraged, were common among smaller emergent groups who may not have been familiar with the Code, or the implications for formula distribution (forthcoming, DeYoung & Suji).

Individual donors, and small emergent groups, and least likely to be subject to evaluation and restriction. Aside from public health implications, sociological and ethnographic assessment of these two issues, and under what circumstances they occur (wet nursing after disasters and formula donation distribution, respectively), is important because it sets an important theoretical framework for the processes of decision-making regarding infant feeding in a hazard and post-hazard setting. The most important reason for expanding research on infant feeding after disasters is, as stated succinctly by Gribble et al. (2011), "The importance of protecting the breastfeeding rights of women in emergencies relates to both infant and maternal outcomes" (p. 722). Not only is breastfeeding objectively healthy, but it is also more likely and sustainable in a resource low context, such as a developing region or post-disaster setting.

Summary

Although research is growing on the subject on infant feeding after disasters, continued work is required for several reasons: 1) formula donations continue to occur after disasters, despite the International Code of Marketing of Breastmilk Substitutes (Gribble et al., 2011). Wet nursing has also been documented, although barely beyond the level of sensationalism or anecdotal retelling (Gribble, 2013). To further explore the reasons and processes for how both of these processes occur goes beyond assigning valence of beneficiality or malevolence (for wet nursing and formula donation, respectively). The field studies, and ongoing data collection surrounding these two issues, can be foundational in informing health policy and community interventions. Without understanding how the processes unfold, and the how the various worldviews influence infant-feeding behavior, the implementation and sustainability of addressing these issues may be limited. By incorporating perspectives and research from disaster research, the ongoing research in these areas may be understood more fully.

References

Airriess, C. A., Li, W., Leong, K. J., Chen, A. C. C., & Keith, V. M. (2008). Church-based social capital, networks and geographical scale: Katrina evacuation, relocation, and recovery in a New Orleans Vietnamese American community. *Geoforum, 39*(3), 1333-1346.

Bengin H.G., Scherbaum V., Hormann, E, & Wang, Q. (2010). Breastfeeding after earthquakes. *Birth, 37*(3), 264-265.

Binns, C.W., Lee, M.K., Tang, L., Yu, C., Hokama, T., & Lee, A. (2012). Ethical issues in infant feeding after disasters. *Asia-Pacific Journal of Public Health, 24*(4), 672-680.

Callaghan, W. M., Rasmussen, S. A., Jamieson, D. J., Ventura, S. J., Farr, S. L., Sutton, P. D., & Posner, S. F. (2007). Health concerns of women and infants in times of natural disasters: Lessons learned from Hurricane Katrina. *Maternal and Child Health Journal, 11*(4), 307-311.

Campbell, S. (2008). Global challenges in protecting and promoting breastfeeding. *Primary Health Care, 18*(1), 41-48.

Carothers, C., & Gribble, K. (2014). Infant and young child feeding in emergencies. *Journal of Human Lactation, 30*(3), 272-275.

Destro, L., & Holguín-Veras, J. (2011). Material convergence and its determinants: case of hurricane Katrina. *Transportation Research Record: Journal of the Transportation Research Board*, (2234), 14-21.

DeYoung, S., & Suji, M. (in progress). Infant feeding and maternal well-being after the 2015 Nepal earthquake. *Field Exchange* (Emergency Nutrition Network).

Dörnemann, J., & Kelly, A. H. (2013). 'It is me who eats, to nourish him': A mixed-method study of breastfeeding in post-earthquake Haiti. *Maternal & Child Nutrition, 9*(1), 74-89.

Gribble, K.D. (2013). Media messages and the needs of infants and young children after Cyclone Nargis and the WenChuan Earthquake. *Disasters, 37*(1), 80-100.

Gribble, K.D. (2014). Formula-feeding in emergencies. In V.R. Preedy, R.R. Watson, & S. Zibadi (Eds.) *Handbook of dietary and nutritional aspects of bottle-feeding.* Human Health Handbooks no. 8. (pp. 143-161). Wageningen Academic Publishers.

Gribble, K.D., McGrath, M., MacLaine, A., & Lhotak, L. (2011). Supporting breastfeeding in emergencies: Protecting women's reproductive rights and maternal and infant health. *Disasters, 35*(4), 720-738.

Holguín-Veras, J., Jaller, M., Van Wassenhove, L. N., Perez, N., & Wachtendorf, T. (2014). Material convergence: Important and understudied disaster phenomenon. *Natural Hazards Review, 15*(1), 1-12. doi:10.1061/(ASCE)NH.1527-6996.0000113

Hipgrave, D. B., Assefa, F., Winoto, A., & Sukotjo, S. (2012). Donated breastmilk substitutes and incidence of diarrhoea among infants and young children after the May 2006 earthquake in Yogyakarta and Central Java. *Public Health Nutrition, 15*(02), 307-315.

Kendra, J. M., & Wachtendorf, T. (2001). Rebel food ... renegade supplies: Convergence after the World Trade Center attack.

Perry, R.W., & Lindell, M.K. (2003). Understanding citizen response to disasters with implications for terrorism. *Journal of Contingencies and Crisis Management, 11*(2), 49-60.

Quarantelli, E. L. (1985). Organizational behavior in disasters and implications for disaster planning. *Disaster Research Center*, Research Notes (Report 1).

Wachtendorf, T., & Kendra, J.M. (2005). Improvising disaster in the City of Jazz: Organizational response to Hurricane Katrina, Understanding Katrina: Perspectives from the Social Sciences. *Social Science Research Council.*

Wachtendorf, K.T., & Quarantelli, E.L. (2003). The evacuation of Lower Manhattan by water transport on September 11: An unplanned 'success.' *Joint Commission Journal on Quality and Patient Safety, 29*(6), 316-318.

CHAPTER 20

Policy Before Pressure: Iceland as a Model for Improving Postpartum Policies in the United States

Rachel Newhouse

The United States is underperforming in its duty to care for the newest generation of Americans, and those who give them life. While attempting to apply best health practices to infant feeding by promoting breastfeeding, there is very little practical support that exists in the form of specific postpartum policies that enhance breastfeeding. The policies that exist offer limited support to breastfeeding mothers, predispose her to conditions, like postpartum depression, and likely contribute to the skyrocketing infant and maternal mortality rates in the U.S. (Central Intelligence Agency, 2010, Central Intelligence Agency 2014a; Dagher, McGovern, & Dowd, 2014). Before public health officials, and the general public, put undue pressure on mothers to breastfeed, they need to look at the factors inhibiting breastfeeding that also inhibit the general health and well-being of the mom, infant, and family.

While the U.S. is struggling in this area, Iceland is leading much of the world in women's health policies, infant mortality, and maternal mortality. This paper will establish evidence that Iceland has a history of valuing its female citizens, demonstrate how government and policies impact the ability of a mother and infant to be healthy in the postpartum period, and suggest Iceland as a potential framework for the U.S. to consider in future development of postpartum policies.

Infant and Maternal Mortality

Much attention has been given to prenatal care and birth, which are undoubtedly influential to infant and maternal mortality rates, but infant mortality and maternal mortality statistics do not cease to be tabulated at birth. By definition, infant mortality is the death of an infant less than one-year-old, and maternal mortality is defined as death during pregnancy or within 6 weeks following the end of a pregnancy (Central Intelligence Agency, 2014b; World Health Organization, 2004).

With 21 deaths per 100,000 live births, the U.S. is ranked behind Iran and Croatia in the world for maternal mortality (Central Intelligence Agency, 2010). For infant mortality, the U.S. ranks directly below Serbia and Lithuania with 6.17 deaths per 1,000 live births (Central Intelligence Agency, 2010; Central Intelligence Agency, 2014b). In contrast, Iceland's infant mortality rate is nearly half the U.S. rate, and Iceland's maternal mortality is one fourth of the U.S. maternal mortality rate (Central Intelligence Agency, 2010; Central Intelligence Agency, 2014b). There is a comparison in Table 1 of the birth rates, maternal mortality rates, and infant mortality rates between Iceland and the U.S.

Table 1. Comparison of Birth Rates, Maternal Mortality Rates, and Infant Mortality Rates.

	Iceland	United States
Birth rate (per 1,000 population)	13.09	13.42
Maternal mortality (deaths per 100,000 live births)	5	21
Infant mortality (deaths per 1,000 live births)	3.15	6.17

Note. Data retrieved from the World Factbook from the Central Intelligence Agency (2010; 2014a; 2014b).

Key Historical Events in Iceland in the Women's Movement

The World Economic Forum (2013) recently published a report that featured Iceland as the country with the smallest gender gap in the world. The report uses ratios of women to men on a variety of indicators including health and survival, economic participation, and political empowerment to define the size of the gender gap. It is impossible to capture a country's history related to gender in a few paragraphs, but some key political highlights will be detailed to demonstrate the strength and longevity of support for women in Iceland.

Political Power

Coinciding with the international women's movement toward suffrage, Icelandic women won suffrage in 1915 for women (Styrkársdóttir, n.d.). The vote was key to Icelandic women gaining political footing, and provided fertile ground for the growing changes in the next century.

The Strike

One outstanding manifestation of women's use of political power in Iceland was the strike of 1975. It is estimated that on October 24, 1975, 90% of women in Iceland went on strike to demonstrate their importance to their country (Iceland: Women strike.1975; *The Guardian,* 2009). The strike put telephone communications at a standstill, closed newspapers, shut down theaters, cancelled flights due to lack of flight attendants, and closed nursery schools (Iceland: Women strike, 1975).

President Vigdís

Five years later, in 1980, Vigdís Finnbogadóttir became the first nationally elected female head of state in the world (The Vigdís Finnbogadóttir Institute of Foreign Languages, n.d.). President Vigdís served as president of Iceland for four consecutive terms, totaling 16 years in office.

Women continue to have a strong presence in Iceland at all levels of government. Table 2 provides a side-by-side comparison of women's political presence in both the United States and Iceland. While the labor force participation only differs by 9% between U.S. and Iceland, the difference in rates of female participation in government are marked.

Table 2. Gender Ratios: Labor Force Participation and Political Positions in Iceland and the United States

	Iceland	United States
Female-to-male ratio labor force participation	0.95	0.86
Female-to-male ratio of heads of state (in the last 50 years)	0.68	0
Female-to-male ratio in parliament	0.66	0.22
Female-to-male ratio in ministerial positions	0.60	0.47

*Note. Data retrieved from the Global Gender Gap Report by the World Economic Forum (2014).

Government and Policies

Government and Welfare

Icelandic welfare programs protect vulnerable populations in Iceland, including the elderly and single parents (Olafsdottir, 2007). Olafsdottir (2007) wrote,

> … female-friendly family policies of the Icelandic welfare state appear to eliminate the negative link between parenthood, especially single parenthood, and poor health outcomes. This indicates that the welfare

state may be successful in eliminating vulnerabilities related to gender and family as a negative impact on health (p. 249).

Health Care Policy

In Iceland, home nursing care, primary care maternity services, and maternity care (including hospitalization, medication, home birth, and multiple in-home postpartum follow-up visits) are provided free of charge under the national health care system in Iceland (The Commonwealth Fund, 2012).

The quality of health care a pregnant woman might receive in the U.S. depends upon the type of health care plan she has. Ideally, the majority of pregnant women would obtain health care insurance through the workplace. Nonetheless, Medicaid is a health care program funded jointly by the states and federal government to low-income pregnant and parenting women, who cannot receive insurance through the workplace, providing coverage for most health care services including prenatal, labor, delivery, and postpartum care (Medicaid.gov, n.d.). If a woman does not qualify for Medicaid, and otherwise has no coverage, the 2010 Affordable Care Act now requires individuals to have a private health plan to cover her maternity expenses, offering additional subsidy programs for people who do not qualify for Medicaid services. If a woman does not qualify for any of the aforementioned health care insurance options, she will have to pay for the services out-of-pocket. In addition, the normalized obstetric practice in the U.S. is to see women 6 weeks post-delivery for the first postpartum visit. This was established based on traditional cultural systems of care that took place for the 6 weeks postpartum, and remains in place, even though these traditions are no longer the norm (Gabbe et al., 2012).

Postpartum Leave Policies

As of 2013, the Icelandic government paid 90 days of maternity and paternity leave at 80% of full wages, with an additional 90 days to be shared between the parents (Eydal, 2012). This policy has been approved by the Icelandic parliament to be expanded to 5 months of paid leave per parent, and 2 months shared following the birth of a child still at 80% of full wages by 2016 (Eydal, 2012).

The U.S., Lesotho, and Papua New Guinea are the only countries in the world with no requirement for paid parental leave (International Labour Organization, 2012). The U.S. offers 12 weeks of unpaid job-protected leave through the Family Medical Leave Act, which protects a woman's job if she has a child, and takes time off postpartum. An individual is only provided this limited, unpaid leave if she or he qualifies. In the U.S., 41% of employees do not meet the conditions to be eligible for FMLA, and therefore, have no federal-level job protection if they take time off following the birth (Abt. Associates, 2012). Individual employers may have their own specific maternity/parental levels policies and procedures.

Workplace Breastfeeding Policies

Workplace breastfeeding policies in the U.S. vary from state to state, but typically require a private room that is not a bathroom with a locked door and a reasonable amount of time for employees to express breastmilk. Even these protections are not required if the company has less than 50 employees, and the time taken to express breastmilk is not required to be compensated (U.S. Department of Labor, 2010).

While the U.S. lacks specificity and universality of policies for breastfeeding at work, Iceland lacks them completely. How could this country, with such a narrow gender gap, and such excellent maternal and infant health statistics, not formally support breastfeeding? The key there is most likely formal support. While there are not workplace breastfeeding policies in place, Iceland, as a culture, has embraced, and seen the value in caring for postpartum women by providing paid maternity and paternity leave, and universal maternity health care (World Economic Forum, 2014). It is not a far leap to imagine that the reason for the lack of formal policies is due to a greater social acceptance of, and respect for, the needs of new mothers. Therefore, there has not been the necessity for such policies to this point in time.

Impact of Leave and Workplace Policies on Breastfeeding

With no required paid maternity leave, and typical 6-week follow up, it is no surprise to see U.S. breastfeeding rates lower at all periods than Iceland, with 80% paid parental leave, and paid-for home visits in the postpartum period (see Table 3) (Directorate of Health, 2008). When breastfeeding is touted as a way to improve infant health, policy makers and health care providers must consider the impact of lack of paid parental leave on the ability to breastfeed. Unfortunately, even though women are not granted leave, and many must, therefore, return to work quickly after giving birth, they are not even guaranteed protections for expressing breastmilk in the workplace. This conflict of systems and interests makes it very difficult for women to be able to breastfeed for the recommended first 12 months of an infant's life.

Table 3. Breastfeeding Rates: Iceland and the United States.

	Iceland	United States
Exclusively or partially breastfed	@ 1 week: 97.9%	Ever: 79.2%
Exclusively or partially breastfed @ 3 months	86.1%	49.4%
Exclusively or partially breastfed @ 12 months	29.1%	26.7%

*Note. Data retrieved from Directorate of Health (2008) and the Centers for Disease Control and Prevention (2014).

Conclusion

I hope that through reading this paper, the reader will have gained an understanding of how establishing policies and procedures supporting postpartum women are essential, as we expect women to be able to breastfeed for any duration. As has been demonstrated through Iceland and many other countries, breastfeeding rates increase as women receive more political support in the postpartum period. The U.S. will continue to fall behind in infant mortality, maternal mortality, and breastfeeding rates so long as the nation does not acknowledge the importance of supporting maternal and infant health in the postpartum period with adequate policies and health care practices. Luckily for the U.S., countries like Iceland have blazed the trail, and left an excellent framework behind that could be modified and adapted for the American people.

References

Abt. Associates. (2012). *Family and Medical Leave in 2012: Technical report.* Washington, D.C.: U.S. Department of Labor.

Centers for Disease Control and Prevention. (2014*). Breastfeeding Report Card: United States.* Retrieved from http://www.cdc.gov/breastfeeding/pdf/2014breastfeeding reportcard.pdf.

Central Intelligence Agency. (2010). Maternal mortality rate. In *The World Factbook.* Retrieved from https://www.cia.gov/1 ibrary/publications/the-world-factbook/rankorder/2223rank.html.

Central Intelligence Agency. (2014a). Infant mortality rate. In *The World Factbook.* Retrieved from https://www.cia.gov/library/publications/the-world-factbook/rankorder/2091rank.html.

Central Intelligence Agency. (2014b). Birth rate. In *The World Fact Book.* Retrieved from https://www.cia.gov/library/publications/the-world-factbook/rankorder/2054 rank.html.

Dagher, R. K., McGovern, P. M., & Dowd, B. E. (2014). Maternity leave duration and postpartum mental and physical health: Implications for leave policies. *Journal of Health Politics, Policy and Law, 39*(2), 369-416.

Directorate of Health. (2008). *Næring: Embætti landlæknis.* Retrieved from http://www.landlaeknir.is/tolfraedi-og-rannsoknir/tolfraedi/heilsa-og-lidan/naering/.

Eydal, G. B. (2012). Iceland 2012: *Revised law on paid parental leave.* Unpublished manuscript, University of Iceland, Reykjavík, Iceland.

Gabbe, S. G. (2012). *Obstetrics: Normal and problem pregnancies.* Philadelphia: Elsevier/Saunders.
Iceland: Women strike. (1975, Oct 25). *New York Times (1923-Current File)* Retrieved January 25, 2015, from ProQuest Historical Newspapers The New York Times (1851 - 2006). International Labour Organization. (2012). *Working conditions laws database.* Retrieved from http://www.ilo.org/dyn/travail/travmain.home.

Medicaid.gov. (n.d.). *Medicaid.* Retrieved from http://www.medicaid.gov/medicaid-chip-program-information/medicaid-and-chip-program-information.html.

Olafsdottir, S. (2007). Fundamental causes of health disparities: stratification, the welfare state, and health in the United States and Iceland. *Journal of Health and Social Behavior, 48*(3), 239-253. doi: 10.1177/002214650704800303

Styrkársdóttir, A. (n.d.). *Women's suffrage in Iceland.* Retrieved from http://kvennaso gusafn.is/index.php?page=womens-suffrage.

The Commonwealth Fund. (2012). *International Profiles of Health Care Systems.* Retrieved from http://www.commonwealthfund.org/~/media/Files/Publications /Fund%20Report/2012/Nov/1645_Squires_intl_profiles_hlt_care_systems_2012.pdf.

The day women went on strike. (2005, October 18). *The Guardian.* Retrieved from http://www.theguardian.com/world/2005/oct/18/gender.uk.

The Vigdís Finnbogadóttir Institute of Foreign Languages. (n.d.). *Vigdís Finnbogadóttir.* Retrieved from http://vigdis.hi.is/en/vigdis_finnbogadottir_0.

U.S. Department of Labor. (2010). *Fair Labor Standards Act: Break time for nursing mothers provision.* Retrieved from http://www.dol.gov/whd/nursing mothers/.

World Economic Forum. (2014). *Global Gender Gap Report.* Retrieved from http:// reports.weforum.org/global-gender-gap-report-2014/.

World Health Organization. (2004). *Health statistics and information systems: Maternal mortality.* Retrieved from http://www.who.int/health info/statistics/indmaternal mortality/en/.

CHAPTER 21

Are Financial Incentives for Breastfeeding Feasible? A Mixed-Methods Field Study in the UK of a Shopping Vouchers for Breastfeeding Scheme

Clare Relton, Barbara Whelan, Mark Strong, Kate Thomas, Heather Whitford, Elaine Scott, Patrice van Cleemput, and Mary Renfrew

T he UK has one of the lowest breastfeeding rates in the world with regards to duration and exclusivity. On average, just over half (55%) of all UK babies are receiving any breastmilk by the time they are 6 to 8 weeks old. UK breastfeeding rates vary widely by area, and are strongly socially patterned, with young women in areas of high-deprivation being less likely to breastfeed than women living in areas of low deprivation (McAndrew et al., 2010).

The causes of these low rates are complex, but include inadequate support for mothers, lack of motivation to breastfeed, and growth of the formula-milk industry, coupled with extensive advertising of infant formula. Despite many strategies being implemented to improve breastfeeding rates (e.g., UNICEF Baby-Friendly Initiative http://www. unicef.org.uk/BabyFriendly/), there has been no increase in the duration of breastfeeding in the UK in recent decades.

The potential of financial incentives to influence health behaviors has been studied in a number of areas (e.g., tax levies upon tobacco to discourage smoking, particularly in pregnant women, and monetary incentives to tackle obesity levels). Research has found that if the incentive is large enough and paid immediately, financial incentives are more effective at encouraging healthy behavior changes compared to usual or no care (Giles, 2014).

Though government funded breastfeeding financial incentive programms for women on unemployment benefit exist in Quebec and Saskatchewan in Canada, to date, there has been no primary research into using financial incentives to encourage women to breastfeed. This study tested the feasibility of offering a financial incentive intervention to increase breastfeeding in UK areas with 6 to 8 week breastfeeding rates of 40% or less. Prior to the feasibility stage, the intervention—the financial incentive scheme—had been developed by the researchers, in close consultation with women and health care providers in the local area (Whelan et al., 2014; Whitford et al., 2014).

Method

The intervention studied was a structured financial incentive scheme offered to women with babies aged up to 6 months old who were living in areas with low breastfeeding rates. The intervention was described as a "Vouchers for Breastfeeding Scheme," and given the short title, NOSH – NOurishing Start for Health (see Figure 1).

Women could apply to join the Vouchers for Breastfeeding Scheme, and claim the shopping vouchers, if they were breastfeeding their baby at any of five different time points—i.e., when their baby was 2 days, 10 days, 6 weeks, 3 months, and 6 months old. Women could check if they were eligible, using an online postcode checker http://www.nosh-vouchers.org/.

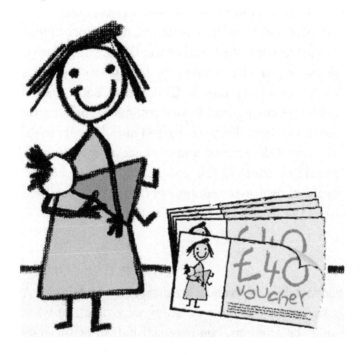

Signed statements from the mother and health care professional (after a discussion had been had about breastfeeding) were used to verify that the baby was being fed breastmilk (partial or exclusive). Mothers sent in claim forms, and those eligible were sent the shopping vouchers. Vouchers were for supermarkets, and high street shops, where women could buy a very wide range of goods (including food, clothes, household goods, and toys), to the value of £40 ($60) for each eligible claim, up to a maximum of £200 ($304).

Starting in November, 2013, the Vouchers for Breastfeeding scheme was offered to women with babies born during a 16-week period resident in three small geographically defined areas in Derbyshire and South Yorkshire in the north of England in the UK. The areas chosen all had historically persistent low 6 to 8 week breastfeeding rates (these ranged from 21% to 29%).

The feasibility (acceptability and deliverability) of the incentive scheme to key stakeholder groups (women, midwives, health visitors, and all others involved in infant feeding services) was assessed with both quantitative and qualitative methods, in advance of undertaking a full randomized controlled trial of the financial incentive. A total of 36 health care providers (midwives, health visitors, breastfeeding support workers, nursery nurses, Children's Centre managers, and Public Health specialists), and 19 women, gave semi-structured interviews to the researchers. They were asked questions about their views and experiences of the scheme and to suggest any changes that they thought should be made to the Vouchers for Breastfeeding scheme. The feasibility study also tested some of the proposed methods for the full-scale trial that was being planned at that time.

Findings

All the relevant UK National Health Service and Local Authority approvals and permissions for the study were obtained without problems, despite the apparent controversial nature of the intervention. The Vouchers for Breastfeeding scheme was launched in November 2013, and was met with an unexpectedly loud media coverage (print, radio, social media) at both the local and national level (with some international coverage as well), much of which expressed concern regarding the effectiveness of the scheme, and the ethics of what was often described as "bribing" mothers to breastfeed.

Of a total of 108 women who were eligible for the scheme, 58 (53.7%) joined the scheme, 48 (44.4%) claimed 2-day vouchers, 45 (41.7%) claimed 10-day vouchers, and 37 (34.3%) claimed 6 to 8 week vouchers. Though some women heard about the scheme from their midwife or the media, many heard about the scheme from their midwife. Some midwives seemed to be more enthusiastic and knowledgeable about the scheme than others. A total of 53 health care providers co-signed the claim forms for the vouchers. Satisfaction with the scheme (including the method used to verify whether the baby was receiving breastmilk) was high amongst both mothers and the health care staff participating in the scheme.

Women interviewed generally spoke about the scheme in terms of it being a "reward" or "a nice treat" or something that made them feel "valued."

> I felt rewarded, especially when you get the letter that says congratulations for breastfeeding at such and such days … you hold your head up and you think, yes, it's worth the sleepless nights because somebody, even in letter form, is saying congratulations (Woman on Scheme).

Women didn't think the vouchers influenced their decision to breastfed, but some mothers did report that it had helped them breastfeed for longer by using the claim points (2 days, 10 days, 6 weeks, 3 months, and 6 months) as goals to achieve.

> Midwives and health visitors tended to question whether the scheme was encouraging women to breastfeed or not, but some did think that it had influenced women's infant feeding decisions, particularly in continuing to breastfeed.

> I think the early days, because of the way it went, and because of the amount that was given quite early, definitely got her to that 6-week (point) … I reckon that's probably what got her through really (Health visitor).

> The fact that it involved payment felt a little bit uncomfortable I guess … dissipated quite a lot cause I think we've seen how pleased the women have been … how positive they've been about it (Midwife).

The Vouchers for Breastfeeding scheme provided a talking point for women about breastfeeding with family and friends and it provided the opportunity for some health care providers to "affirm" what women were doing. While some women did feel that the scheme gave women the incentive to try breastfeeding, it did not help when things went wrong, and there was not enough breastfeeding support. Some women suggested that breastfeeding support should be combined with the scheme.

Generally, women found that applying for and claiming Vouchers for Breastfeeding "straightforward" and "self-explanatory," and they liked getting a text from the NOSH office, which ran the Vouchers for Breastfeeding Scheme to say that their vouchers had been sent. They found getting the claim form signed convenient as it usually coincided with them having an appointment with their midwife or health visitor. Many appreciated that verification was based on trust, and that they did not have to show themselves breastfeeding. However, some women made a point of breastfeeding in front of their health care provider in order to "prove" that they were breastfeeding. Health care providers did not think that the scheme impacted on their workload and that it fitted in with their usual care of women and promotion of breastfeeding.

Interpretation

Despite considerable concern about the scheme expressed in the media, in the feasibility study, the financial incentive scheme was found to be both deliverable and acceptable to mothers and health care staff. No problems were identified that required any alteration of the scheme itself for the next stage of the research—the full-scale trial. All the key stakeholders in the feasibility areas were keen to continue the scheme in all three areas.

Financial incentives are a potentially powerful method to encourage people to adopt healthy behaviors, and have been used with varying success in a range of settings, such as stopping smoking in pregnancy, losing weight, and attending health screening. Building on the findings of the feasibility study (Relton et al, 2015), a large cluster (area-based) randomized controlled trial is currently testing the clinical/ public health and cost effectiveness of the scheme in 88 clusters with an estimated 10,500 babies born between February 2015 and February 2016 in five urban and rural areas in northern England.

Funding

Medical Research Council: National Prevention Research Initiative (MR/J000434/1).

Acknowledgments

We would like to thank all the women, babies, and health care providers who participated in this field study.

References

Giles E.L, Robaline S., McColl E., Sniehotta F.F., & Adams J. (2014). The effectiveness of financial incentives for health behaviour change: Systematic review and meta-analysis. *PLOS ONE*, *9*(3), 1-16.

McAndrew F., Thompson J., Fellows L., Large A., Speed M., & Renfrew M.J. (2012). *Infant Feeding Survey: 2010*. IFF Research, Health and Social Care Information Centre. Retrieved from http://www.hscic.gov.uk/catalogue/PUB08694/Infant-FeedingSurvey-2010-Consolidated-Report.pdf

Relton C., Whelan B., Strong M., Thomas K., Whitford H., Scott E., & Van Cleemput P. (2014). Are financial incentives for breastfeeding feasible in the UK? A mixed-methods field study. *The Lancet* 384, S5. Available at: http://www.thelancet.com/journals/lancet/article/PIIS0140-6736%2814%2962131-0/abstract.

Whelan B., Thomas K.J., Van Cleemput P., Whitford H., Strong M., Renfrew MJ., Scott E., & Relton C. (2014). Healthcare provider's views on the acceptability of financial incentives for breastfeeding: a qualitative study. *BMC Pregnancy and Childbirth, 14*, 355. Available at http://www.biomedcentral.com/content/pdf/1471-2393-14-355.pdf.

Whitford H., Whelan B., Van Cleemput P., Thomas K., Renfrew M., Strong M., Scott E., & Relton C. (2015). Encouraging breastfeeding: Financial incentives. *The Practising Midwife, 18*(2), 18-21.

Section 2

Advancing Public Support

Addressing Discomfort with Seeing Breastfeeding: Suggestions for a New Approach to Improving Future Breastfeeding Duration Rates

Erin L. Austen

Across Canada and the United States, progress is slow in changing breastfeeding duration rates; although rates have improved somewhat over the years, they remain well below targeted levels (Centers for Disease Control and Prevention, 2014; Gionet, 2013). This is the case, despite an increase in efforts to promote breastfeeding. Why is this? What barriers remain that are so pervasive that even large-scale efforts to promote breastfeeding are insufficient in making significant improvements in breastfeeding duration rates?

One likely possibility is that while these efforts are effective in communicating the benefits of breastfeeding, and in increasing the intention to breastfeed, they have been ineffective in addressing or changing the structural constraints around breastfeeding (e.g., efforts do not address a lack of public support for breastfeeding anytime and anywhere). Further, if you consider geographic regions where breastfeeding rates are low, and where, as a direct consequence of low breastfeeding rates, there are limited opportunities to see breastfeeding, existing breastfeeding promotion efforts may perpetuate the unintended message that while breastfeeding is something to be done, it is not something to be seen. In other words, people living within geographic locations where breastfeeding duration rates are low, likely grapple with conflicting messages; on the one hand, they may get the message that breastfeeding is a healthy infant feeding choice that has long-term benefits, but by not seeing positive examples of breastfeeding firsthand, they are also getting the message that breastfeeding is something that should be done privately.

This creates two problems. One, we know that if mothers feel restricted in when and where they can breastfeed, breastfeeding duration rates are likely to remain low (Li, Fein, Chen, & Grummer-Strawn, 2008). Two, we also know that when people get a chance to see breastfeeding, many report feeling uncomfortable because they think they are seeing something they are not meant to see (Spurles & Babineau, 2011). This problem is a circular one that requires a significant change in the way that we approach breastfeeding promotion.

What does that change entail? I believe that breastfeeding promotion efforts need to be focused, at least in part, on young adults, as they are the next generation of potential mothers and fathers. As a first step, exposure to breastfeeding is key to decreasing the discomfort associated with seeing breastfeeding, and to changing perceptions of social norms around breastfeeding. Secondly, by introducing innovative and age-appropriate efforts around breastfeeding promotion, we can challenge current thinking about breastfeeding, paving the way for more receptive responses to seeing breastfeeding. Research conducted in my lab focuses on perceptions of breastfeeding among young adults; this research was conducted in Northeastern Canada, where breastfeeding rates tend to be low, but where typical breastfeeding supports at both the hospital level (e.g., lactation consultants), and community-level (e.g., mother-to-mother support groups, La Leche League) are available.

Intentions versus Perceptions of Social Norms: An Argument for Increasing Exposure to Breastfeeding

Over the last number of years, we have assessed intentions to breast-feed in large educated samples of young adults. It is our view that if current breastfeeding promotion efforts are reaching young people, there should be some evidence of that within this particular group. From 2007 to 2011, we found that 87% of the respondents that we surveyed reported the intention to breastfeed (Austen, in prep). On its own, this data paints a positive picture of future breastfeeding rates. It is clear that the message that breastfeeding is a healthy choice is reaching young people. They are, at this early stage, making up their minds to breastfeed. However, the picture is less positive when we look at other predictors of breastfeeding behavior, such as comfort level to see breastfeeding, and one's perception of how members of the public will react to seeing breastfeeding or breastfeeding promotion images. Even among our samples of educated young adults, many reported that they would be uncomfortable to see a stranger breastfeeding her baby, and the majority indicated that other people would react negatively to seeing images of breastfeeding, such as those used in breastfeeding promotion campaigns (Austen, Dignam & Hauf, in prep). These types of reactions stem, in part, from the view that breastfeeding is a private act between a mother and baby that, if done in a public space, needs to be done discreetly. Further, participants report a strong sense that breastfeeding is not intended for other people to see, nor is it something that people want to see.

How can it be that the majority of young adults in the samples that we tested intend to breastfeed, but are uncomfortable to see breast-feeding, and perceive social norms around breastfeeding to be largely negative? Some would argue that this is because we live in a hypersex-ualized society where our exposure to breasts is limited to a sexualized view of the breast (Wolf, 2008). This may be true, but it does not explain why breastfeeding rates are still lower than expected in countries where breasts are less sexualized. An alternative explanation is that in locations where breastfeeding rates are low, people have limited opportunities to see positive images of breastfeeding. If breastfeeding is not seen, but is being widely promoted, the message that people may take away from this is that breastfeeding is something that one should do, but not publicly. If this is the case, then we should be able to improve breastfeeding rates by increasing exposure to breastfeeding. We have some promising data to suggest that this is the case. That is, when we repeatedly present images of breastfeeding to young adults who previously reported being uncomfortable to see breastfeeding, we see a small, but significant, improvement in reported comfort levels to see breastfeeding (Beadle & Austen, in prep). This data is consistent with research on the Mere Exposure Effect, which suggests that the more we see something the more we tend to like it (Bornstein, 1989).

Innovative and Age-Appropriate Approaches to Breastfeeding Promotion

There is no doubt that technology is a significant component of many young adults' lives, and that the Net Generation and iGeneration rely on social media outlets not only to connect with people but to inform them of what is going on in the world. Hence, promoting breastfeeding through social media sites, such as Facebook, and through public sites, such as YouTube, might be a particularly effective way to reach people in this age group. My colleagues and I have new data to support that this approach (Beadle, Aquino, Lukeman, Lukeman & Austen, in prep). We began by recruiting a group of young adults to brainstorm ideas on how to tackle discomfort associated with seeing breastfeeding. They suggested that a music video parody would be a good way to capture the attention of young adults and to make any breastfeeding promotion message more memorable. Following their ideas, we created a novel music video parody, *Breastfeeding My Baby*, using the music from the popular song *Call Me Maybe*. The video was filmed in the local area with a cast of identifiable young adults, and shows "mothers" (played by young adults) breastfeeding their "babies" (dolls, in this case) in a variety of public and private locations. The video relied on humor and song as a way to challenge viewers to consider breastfeeding as appropriate anytime and anywhere. The video was uploaded to YouTube for public viewing and shared on Facebook; based on statistics provided by both of these sites, it was clear that the video gained widespread attention.

To test the effectiveness of the novel music video parody in improving reactions to breastfeeding, we first assessed comfort levels with seeing breastfeeding among a large sample of young adults using a Picture Rating Scale; participants rated comfort levels seeing breastfeeding and bottle-feeding images. Two months later, we showed the music video to half of our original sample. After another two-month delay, we reassessed comfort levels among the entire sample. One of our key manipulations was that some of these participants were given the post-test Picture Rating Scale before we surveyed them about the music video, while others were surveyed about the music video first, and then completed the post-test.

In the former group, there was very little change in comfort level ratings. This was discouraging, but maybe not surprising with such a brief intervention. However, looking at the data from latter group, there was a clear improvement in comfort ratings when participants were first reminded about the video. This cannot be just a test-retest effect, because if it were, the improvement would have been present in the entire sample. Instead, it is likely that the video effectively got participants to think about, and reevaluate, their attitudes and comfort levels, and when reminded of the video, this is what they did. What was also encouraging was that the survey results indicated that for participants who saw the video, the video was memorable, and the intent of the video was understood. Further, almost all participants indicated that a video was an effective approach to talk about breastfeeding. This research is an important first test of using this type of approach to address discomfort with seeing breastfeeding.

References

Austen, E.L. An assessment of young adults' breastfeeding intentions and comfort levels over a five-year span: Are we making progress? *Manuscript in preparation.*

Austen, E.L., Dignam, J., & Hauf, P. Assessing the potential risks of using breastfeeding images to promote breastfeeding among young adults. *Manuscript in preparation.*

Beadle, J., Aquino, N., Lukeman, E., Lukeman, S., & Austen, E.L. Using a music video parody to promote breastfeeding and increase comfort levels. *Manuscript in preparation.*

Beadle, J., & Austen, E.L. Is discomfort viewing breastfeeding detectable? *Manuscript in preparation.*

Bornstein, R.F. (1989). Exposure and affect: Overview and meta-analysis of research, 1968-1987. *Psychological Bulletin, 106 (2),* 265-289.

Centers for Disease Control and Prevention. (2014). *Breastfeeding report card: United States, 2014.* Retrieved from: http://www.cdc.gov/breastfeeding/pdf/2014breastfeedingreportcard.pdf.

Gionet, L. (2013). Breastfeeding trends in Canada, *Health at a Glance.* November Statistics Canada Catalogue no. 82-624-X. Retrieved from: http://www.statcan.gc.ca/pub/82-624-x/2013001/article/11879-eng.pdf.

Li, R., Fein, S.B., Chen, J., & Grummer-Strawn, L.M. (2008). Why mothers stop breastfeeding: Mothers' self-reported reasons for stopping during the first year. *Pediatrics, 122,* S69-S76.

Spurles, P.K., & Babineau. J. (2011). A qualitative study of attitudes toward public breastfeeding among young Canadian men and women. *Journal of Human Lactation, 27(2),* 131-137.

Wolf, J.H. (2008). Got milk? Not in public! *International Breastfeeding Journal, 3 (11).*

CHAPTER 23

Breastfeeding in Public: Success, Failure, and the Way Forward

Jodine Chase

S exualization of breasts, and moralizing about sex, collide every day with mothers simply living their lives while feeding their children. Conflict hotspots include churches, airlines and airports, retail stores, restaurants, and beaches: every summer, for example, droves of women take off almost all of their clothing at swimming pools to beat the heat, provoking a culture clash between breastfeeding and bikini culture. And in the virtual world, social media networks heighten conflict over boobs-for-sex vs. boobs-for-baby.

Research shows early weaning is linked to lack of support for breastfeeding in public; in one study, women who felt comfortable breastfeeding in public, or in front of their friends, were about three times more likely to be breastfeeding at 6 months (Jessri et al., 2013; Makin, Timmings, & McKeown, 2010). Unfortunately, support from the community lags behind legal rights. As more women breastfeed, and breastfeed longer, conflicts have led to legislation in every U.S. state but one (Idaho) protecting this right. In Canada, protection came when gender rights were entrenched in its constitution in 1982 (Sterken, n.d.; U.S. Department of Health and Human Services, 2015).

Despite protective laws, breastfeeding women are still harassed (Best for Babes, 2012). Lifeguards, store managers, and security staff deal with these situations without policy, education, or training. Frequently these incidents play out a familiar, but unfortunate way: a woman is asked to cover or move, she shares her experience, and the resulting outrage prompts online criticism, and even on-site protests and nurse-ins. Attempts at resolution usually start with an apology. Sometimes this will come with a change in policy and procedures in an effort to keep it from happening again (*Huffington Post,* 2013). Occasionally, articulated policy, procedures, training, and public education will create safe and welcoming spaces for breastfeeding. Full resolution is rare, and so the cycle repeats itself with every incident (Friedman & Grossman, 2013).

There are real and perceived barriers to accommodating breastfeeding in public. In churches, barriers are everywhere. Even a progressive church may have elders who don't want breastfeeding in the sanctuary, and a culture of modesty is likely to amplify concerns. In the U.S., state laws protecting breastfeeding may not apply in the church, synagogue, or mosque (*USA Today,* 2014). Pope Francis's decision to speak out to encourage his faithful to breastfeed at the Sistine Chapel opened the sanctuary doors to breastfeeding for Catholic families everywhere. Women are forming grassroots breastfeeding policy groups within their faith communities (Fletcher Stack, 2013; Linshi, 2015).

There are bureaucratic barriers to policy changes in all arenas. Municipalities and state governments, federal health protection agencies and national non-profit recreation agencies and lifeguard certification organizations all have their own red tape. There may be very poor public and institutional awareness that women's legal right to breastfeed, without being asked to cover or move, extends to restaurants, retail stores, and the swimming pool deck (Strange,

2002). Myths about the lack of safety of breastmilk also abound that has resulted in breastmilk being categorized as blood, fecal matter, or vomit, when it should be equated to perspiration, or tears (Centers for Disease Control and Prevention, 2007; Strange, 2002; World Health Organization, 2006,).

When recreational facilities are closely aligned with public health departments, change is often swift and positive—a recent incident at a pool in West Vancouver resulted in retraining and a public poster campaign, "Of course, you can" (breastfeed here) within hours of the incident. Recreational facilities are beginning to post breastfeeding policies on their websites in the hope that public education will lead to fewer incidents (City of Edmonton, 2014; West Vancouver Aquatic Centre, 2014). Grassroots leadership has had a substantial impact when efforts are shared between communities. There are some strong policies and examples now in Canada, including YMCA Canada's release of national model breastfeeding policy (YMCA Canada, 2014).

There have been multiple high profile incidents at places like Walmart, Target, Applebee's, and airline companies like Delta (CBC, 2015; Friedman & Grossman, 2013; LKCTV-5 News, 2012/13; *Time,* 2011). Unfortunately, despite major pressure, including lawsuits and continent-wide nurse-ins, these organizations have not adopted a full set of policies, procedures, training, and signs and systems to welcome breastfeeding.

Starbucks has had a number of high-profile breastfeeding discrimination incidents, and while it may have changed its policies, and provided training to its staff, its efforts have been opaque to customers. Recently, an Ottawa customer asked a barista to force a woman to stop breastfeeding. However, instead, the barista upheld the right of the woman to feed her child in the store, and offered her a free coffee for her troubles. This positive outcome received widespread, global coverage. We do not know whether this was the result of Starbuck's new policy, or the actions of the individual barista. We do not know because, sadly, Starbucks is not talking about this issue. Follow-up news coverage indicates the barista took his initiative, and publicity came from the breastfeeding customer's post on social media, which went viral (Luscombe, 2014).

Social media is the new frontier. The millennial generation uses smartphones to share the details of their lives, and that includes breast-feeding (Mashable, 2015). Facebook has been the leading social media network for the last decade, and it has taken the brunt of criticism for its poor handling of user reactions to breastfeeding images (Breastfeeding Basics, 2014; Moms Pump Here, Aug. 2015). Facebook has over a billion active users and hundreds of thousands of images shared each hour (Facebook, 2015).

The barriers to supporting breastfeeding in the virtual public space are significant. The concentration of young, mostly male workers in the tech world amplifies the bias of approval of sexually charged images of women (Losse, 2014). In Facebook's early years, sharing a breastfeeding photo could result in the automatic disabling or dele-tion of accounts, and Facebook was accused of rejecting breastfeeding, while allowing sexually charged images, and even of promoting a rape culture (Chemaly, 2013; Salon, 2013). While the network has evolved and now allows breastfeeding images, including those that display a fully bare breast, there is still work to be done (Facebook, 2015). Facebook approves most breastfeeding images reported, and uses a system of escalating warnings and temporary bans when it doesn't approve. But the sheer volume of photos means mistakes are made, and accounts are blocked even when the image should be approved. There is no mechanism for review. and Facebook confirms a person-to-person solution is not scalable across its network. Facebook's changes represent one of the most significant shifts in the last decade around public breastfeeding policy. It consistently indicates its support for the sharing of breastfeeding images in public communication, and its policies are more transparent than most multinational entities.

Action in three key areas could result in fundamental change: lead-ership, research, volume tracking, and increased public awareness.

- Leadership works when respected leaders speak up in support of breastfeeding; it can cause a major shift in public attitudes, as we have seen since Pope Francis started speaking out.

- Research is important when women wean because of a lack of support for breastfeeding in public, it becomes not just a rights issue, but a public health one as well. More is needed in this area: when we ask women why they did not meet their breastfeeding goals, we must include an assessment of their comfort level with breastfeeding in public as a weaning factor. It is important to track the volume of incidents, especially since many are not reported, or they may be amplified by mainstream or social media coverage. We must explore the impact that high profile news stories have on attitudes and behavior: for example, it would be useful to survey Catholic churchgoers to determine the Pope's impact on their ability or comfort with breastfeeding at church.

- Public attention given to breastfeeding discrimination is controversial; some believe public action does more harm than good by radicalizing breastfeeding, and by amplifying discrimination, as well as provoking fear and anxiety in new mothers (Flam, 2013). However, it is often not until negative publicity surrounding an incident occurs that organizations take action. Public pressure, combined with behind-the-scenes negotiations, is an accepted and proven formula for success. Women who do go public must be warned to expect revictimization in the media, and advocates should know nurse-ins are just one tool in the toolbox, and it shouldn't be the first tool used. As U.S. community organizer Saul Alinsky noted, it's the threat of action that produces results.

Leading breastfeeding organizations must make it a priority to change policies, procedures, training, and public education around breastfeeding rights. Good practices include a written policy, publicly articulated, and backed by training and public education, and publicity; knowledge of the existing federal and state laws; training and education to shift attitudes to be welcoming; a desire to keep families safe from harassment; and efforts to keep breastfeeding visible, both in person and in imagery. Until all women and all children are supported to comfortably breastfeeding in public, the provision of alternative spaces for privacy and comfort may be needed. These self-sustaining practices will lead to more comfort for women, more babies being breastfed, healthier infants and children, and ultimately, less drag on our health care system.

References

Best for Babes Foundation. (2012). *NIP hotline news: 8 harassment incidents in first week.* Retrieved from http://www.bestforbabes.org/nip-hotline-news-8-harassment-incidences-in-first-week/

Breastfeeding Basics. (2014). *Breastfeeding professionals silenced by Facebook censorship.* Retrieved from https://www.breastfeedingbasics.com/unlatched/breastfeeding-professionals-silenced-facebook-censorship

Canadian Broadcast Corporation. (2015). *Breastfeeding mom says she was berated by Walmart employee.* Retrieved from *http://www.cbc.ca/news/canada/montreal/breastfeeding-mom-says-she-was-berated-by-montreal-walmart-employee-1.3177242*

Centers for Disease Control and Prevention. (2007). *Infectious diseases and specific conditions affecting human milk.* Diseases and Conditions. Retrieved from http://www.cdc.gov/breastfeeding/disease/index.htm.

City of Edmonton. (2014) *Recreation facility safety and use guidelines: General use guidelines.* Retrieved from http://www.edmonton.ca/activities_parks_recreation/rec-use-safety-guidelines.aspx.

Chemaly, S. (2013). *Facebook rejects rape culture. Can you?,* CNN. Retrieved from http://www.cnn.com/2013/05/30/opinion/chemaly-facebook/

Facebook. (2015). *Stats.* Retrieved from http://newsroom.fb.com/company-info/

Facebook. (2015). *Does Facebook allow photos of mothers breastfeeding?* Retrieved from https://www.facebook.com/help/340974655932193.

Flam, L. (2013). *Breast is best...for ap rotext? "Lactivists" debate whether nurse-ins help the cause. Today Parents.* Retrieved from http://www.today.com/parents/breast-best-protest-lactivists-debate-whether-nurse-ins-help-cause-1B8002725.

Fletcher Stack, P. (2013). *Battles break out over breastfeeding at Mormon meetings.* Salt Lake Tribune. Retrieved from http://www.sltrib.com/sltrib/lifestyle/55921668-80/breast-church-feeding-lds.html.csp.

Friedman, L.M., & Grossman, J.L. (2013). A private underworld: The naked body in law and society. *Buffalo Law Review, 61.* Retrieved from http://www.buffalolawreview.org/past_issues/61_1/Friedman.pdf

Huffington Post. (2013). *Walmart apologizes to Kayla Andre, Mom, After Refusing to Print Breastfeeding Photo.* Retrieved from http://www.huffingtonpost.com/2013/05/16/walmart-breastfeeding-photo-kayla-andre_n_3285988.html

Jessri, M., Farmer, A., Maximova, K., Willows, N., Bell, R., & APrON Study Team. (2013). Predictors of exclusive breastfeeding: observations from the Alberta pregnancy outcomes and nutrition (APrON) study. *BMC Pediatrics, 13,* 77. doi:10.1186/1471-2431-13-77.

Linshi, J. (2015). *Pope Francis reaffirms support for of public breastfeeding. Time* Magazine. Retrieved from http://time.com/3662983/pope-francis-breastfeeding//

LKCTV-5 News. (2012/13). *Many speak out after woman asked to leave Georgia Applebee's while breastfeeding,* Retrieved from http://www.kctv5.com/story/19649252/many-speak-out-after-woman-asked-to-leave-georgia-applebees-while-breastfeeding

Losse, K. (2012). *The boy kings: A journey into the heart of the social network.* New York: Simon and Schuster.

Luscombe, B. (2014). *What Starbucks tells employees about breastfeeding. Time* Magazinee. Retrieved from http://time.com/2954739/starbucks-breastfeeding-mom-barista-ottawa/.

Makin, S. Timmings, C., & McKeown, D. (2010). *Breastfeeding in Toronto: Promoting supportive environments, Toronto Public Health.* Retrieved from http://www.toronto.ca/legdocs/mmis/2010/hl/bgrd/backgroundfile-28171.pdf and http://www.toronto.ca/legdocs/mmis/2010/hl/bgrd/backgroundfile-28423.pdf.

Mashable. (2015). #Brelfie: *The breastfeeding selfie that's taken over social media.* Retrieved from http://mashable.com/2015/02/25/brelfie-breastfeeding-selfie/#R1SDpM3cvmqR

Moms Pump Here. (2015). *Facebook's negative stance on breastfeeding ads needs updating.* Retrieved from http://www.momspumphere.com/blog/entry/facebooks-negative-stance-on-breastfeeding-ads-needs-updating

Salon. (2013). *Facebook finally addresses its rape culture.* Retrieved from http://www.salon.com/2013/05/29/facebook_finally_addresses_its_rape_culture/

Sterken, E. (n.d.). *Breastfeeding, it's your right, INFACT Canada.* Retrieved from http://www.infactcanada.ca/breastfeeding_rights.htm.

Strange, B. (2002). *Breastfeeding at municipal pools in Canada. A report from the Breastfeeding Action Committee of Edmonton.* Retrieved from http://www.breastfeedingalberta.ca/images/pdf%20files/BREASTFEEDING%20AT%20MUNICIPAL%20POOLS%20IN%20CANADA.pdf and http://www.breastfeedingalberta.ca/images/pdf%20files/BREASTFEEDING%20AT%20MUNICIPAL%20POOLS%20IN%20CANADA-Appendices.pdf.

Time. (2011) *Moms breastfeed in 250 Target Store. Can a nurse-in change perceptions of public breastfeeding?* Retrieved from http://healthland.time.com/2011/12/29/target-nurse-in-did-it-change-perceptions-of-public-breast-feeding/

West Vancouver Aquatic Centre. (2014). *"Of Course, You Can!"* Retrieved from http://westvancouver.ca/parks-recreation/community-centres/aquatic-centre.

World Health Organization. (2006). *Guidelines for safe recreational waters.* Retrieved from http://www.who.int/water_sanitation_health/bathing/srwe2chap3.pdf.

YMCA Canada. (2014). *Guideline regarding breastfeeding in YMCA facilities.* YMCA Canada newsletter to member associations.

U.S. Department of Health and Human Services. (2015). *Breastfeeding state laws.* Retrieved from http://www.ncsl.org/research/health/breastfeeding-state-laws.aspx

USA Today. (2014). *Breastfeeding is on the rise, but in church it's still an issue.* Retrieved from http://www.usatoday.com/story/news/nation/2014/01/03/breast-feeding-church-pope-francis/4307037/

CHAPTER 24

Toronto Public Health Breastfeeding in Public Campaign

Jill Mather and Susan Gallagher

Toronto is Canada's largest city, the fourth largest in North America, and home to a diverse population of about 2.8 million people. There are approximately 30,500 births every year in Toronto (Toronto Public Health, 2013). In January 2013, Toronto Public Health (TPH) became the largest public health unit in Canada to receive the Baby-Friendly Initiative (BFI) designation. BFI is a globally recognized standard of best practices for infant feeding.

Breastfeeding has a number of well-documented health benefits for both the mother and baby. This evidence prompted prominent health organizations, including The World Health Organization, to recommend exclusive breastfeeding to 6 months of age, the introduction of complementary foods at 6 months, and continued breastfeeding for the first 2 years and beyond (TPH, 2013).

A few years ago, TPH conducted a Breastfeeding Study. The findings were released in a report entitled *Breastfeeding in Toronto: Promoting supportive environments* (Toronto Public Health, 2010). This study found that almost all first-time Toronto mothers initiated breastfeeding, and at 6 months postpartum, almost three quarters of these mothers were still breastfeeding. However, fewer than one in five mothers who initiated breastfeed continued to exclusively breastfeed their babies to 6 months. A number of factors were found to be associated with any and/or exclusive breastfeeding at various points in time. In particular, younger mothers (less than 25 years old), and recent immigrants (living in Canada 5 years of less), were identified as less likely to exclusively breastfeed to 6 months. In addition, the study found that mothers who felt comfortable breastfeeding in public locations, and/or in the presence of friends, were 2.9 times more likely to continue to breastfeed to 6 months than mothers who were not comfortable, or did not breastfeed in public (TPH, 2010).

The Ontario Human Rights Commission (OHRC) supports women's right to breastfeed undisturbed in public places (OHRC, 2014). In addition, the City of Toronto allows and supports breastfeeding mothers to breastfeed in all public places controlled by City Agencies, Boards, Commissions, and Divisions (City of Toronto, 2007). TPH also has the Baby-Friendly Initiative Compliance policy in place outlining staff responsibilities to support mothers to breastfeed their infants and young children in public (TPH, 2012).

The *Registered Nurse Journal* (November/December 2013) had an article about a "stigma-fighting initiative" conducted by Algoma Public Health. This health unit developed a campaign which placed life-sized cut-outs of breastfeeding women throughout the region to normalize breastfeeding in public (Punch, 2013). TPH recognized that this type of campaign would fit our mandate to protect, promote, and support breastfeeding. TPH began exploring the possibility of doing something similar in Toronto, and sought permission from Algoma Public Health to adapt their campaign.

Campaign Overview

This campaign was conducted during World Breastfeeding Week 2014, celebrated the first week of October in Canada. This campaign was intended to promote mothers' rights to breastfeed in public spaces and advocated for community support of breastfeeding women. The objectives of the campaign included:

- Educating the public on the right to breastfeed in public,
- Promoting the acceptance of breastfeeding in public, and
- Promoting breastfeeding as the cultural norm.

The audience for this campaign was all women of reproductive age and their social support networks, with a specific focus on young mothers, new immigrants, and women with older babies. The secondary audience included the general public, and businesses—in particular, retailers that are frequented by families and college/university students. The slogan, *"It's OK to brEAsTfeed in public. Support breastfeeding anywhere, anytime,"* was selected as the message to positively reflect the campaign goals and objectives.

Campaign Components

Signage and Outreach

Nine "breastfeeding models" were recruited to be photographed. These "breastfeeding models" were a combination of staff and TPH clients which represented Toronto's diverse population, including a younger mother, and a mother with an older baby. Photos of five "breastfeeding models" were selected to be made into life-size cut-outs. Thirty cut-outs were placed in 20+ high-traffic areas around Toronto, including City buildings, subway stations, malls, community centers, outdoor squares, and post-secondary institutions. Each cut-out held a sign with the campaign slogan and provided the campaign website (www.tph.to/breastfeeding) for more information.

TPH staff accompanied the cut-outs to several of the venue,s and met with members of the public to promote the campaign message, answer questions, and share information about TPH breastfeeding and infant feeding services. Each staff wore a T-shirt that promoted the campaign slogan and website. A question and answer (Q & A) document was created to support the staff when meeting with the public or responding to media inquiries.

Digital Media Advertising

A YouTube video was created by an in-house creative team and posted on the campaign website. This video raised the question, "What if eating a sandwich in public got the same reaction as breastfeeding in public?" It was played on the largest screen in downtown Toronto on a continuous loop throughout the week-long campaign. It was also screened in 62 waiting rooms at physicians' offices across the city for approximately 6 weeks.

Testimonials of Breastfeeding Women

All nine "breastfeeding models" were also interviewed about their breastfeeding experiences and why breastfeeding in public was important to them. A video collage of these testimonials was created and posted on the campaign website.

Social Media, Including Contest

TPH posted regular messages on Twitter and Facebook about the campaign. The public was encouraged to take selfies with the cut-outs, and tweet the photos using the hashtag #BFingInPublic for a chance to win an Apple iPad.

Public Campaign Web Breastfeeding in Site

A Breastfeeding in Public campaign website was developed (www.tph. to/breastfeeding). The new website was an online vehicle to promote the campaign's slogan, "It's OK to breastfeed in public. Support breast-feeding anywhere, anytime," and to house elements of the campaign, including YouTube videos, mothers testimonials, Twitter, and Facebook feeds, as well as contest rules.

Promotional Materials

Approximately 1,250 water bottles were ordered with the campaign slogan to raise awareness about the right to breastfeeding in public. These water bottles were distributed among TPH pre- and postnatal clients.

Promotion of the Campaign

In House

Prior to the launch of the campaign, TPH staff were emailed the details of the campaign,, and were encouraged to inform their clients and promote participation. In addition, prior to and following the campaign, articles were published in various TPH and city-wide staff newsletters.

External

Prior to the launch of the campaign, an email was sent to key community stakeholders such as Toronto birthing hospitals, local community health centers, and neighboring health units as well as those who we identified as "influencers," such as WHO and Health Canada, encouraging them to promote the campaign amongst their networks and to join the conversation on social media.

An owner of several local retail malls was also sent an e-mail with details about the campaign as they agreed to promote the campaign through their social media networks. In addition, at the request of University of Toronto and Ryerson University, articles to promote the campaign were provided for their internal newsletters/web.

Traditional Media

A "soft launch" of this campaign was planned, given a number of other high profile health stories that were occurring simultaneously and limited staff resources. A News Release was issued, and a photo shoot was conducted with the Medical Officer of Health at a prominent downtown square on the first day of the campaign. A national radio interview was subsequently conducted in support of the campaign.

Campaign Outcomes

Signage and Outreach

Staff met with approximately 600 members of the public at over 20 venues across the city.

Digital Media Advertising

In less than 5 days, the Breastfeeding in Public campaign video became TPH's most- watched video on YouTube. The video continues to be viewed with over 6,500 views to date. The video was played 2,199 times, and had 1,009,659 impressions during its run on the largest video screen in downtown Toronto. It also had 428,488 impressions while showing in waiting rooms at physicians' offices.

TPH Breastfeeding Website

The TPH Breastfeeding website almost doubled the number of views during the campaign, from 3,892 in September 2014 to 7,086 in October 2014.

Social Media

There was significant social media activity in support of the campaign, as well as sharing and retweeting. TPH gained nearly 500 new followers on Twitter and saw a spike in user engagement. Campaign tweets had over 11,000 engagements, which demonstrated an increase of 685% compared to average weekly engagements of 1,400. Since launching the campaign, TPH gained nearly 500 new Facebook fans. Facebook posts for this campaign generated nearly 300,000 impressions. Over 100 Twitters users entered our #BFingInPublic contest.

Summary Statement

TPH implemented a successful multi-faceted breastfeeding in public campaign during World Breastfeeding Week. This campaign was intended to help women feel more comfortable breastfeeding in public places and advocated for community support of breastfeeding women. The campaign consisted of life-size cut-out photographs of breastfeeding women appearing in high traffic areas around Toronto, a fun online YouTube video and testimonials of breastfeeding mothers posted on the TPH website (www.tph.to/breastfeeding). It was also promoted through social media and the distribution of water bottles with the campaign slogan. The campaign had significant reach in person, through digital media and online.

References

City of Toronto. (2007). *Breastfeeding in public policy.* Retrieved from http://www.toronto.ca/legdocs/mmis/2007/hl/bgrd/backgroundfile-4311.pdf.

Ontario Human Rights Commission. (2014). *Policy on preventing discrimination because of Pregnancy and breastfeeding.* Retrieved from http://www.ohrc.on.ca/sites/default/files/Policy%20on%20preventing%20discrimination%20because%20of%20pregnancy%20and%20breastfeeding_accessible_2014.pdf.

Punch, D. (2013). Bringing breastfeeding to life with cardboard cutouts. *Registered Nurse Journal, November/December,* 9-10. Available at http://rnao.ca/resources/rnj/issues/novemberdecember-2013.

Toronto Public Health. (2010). *Breastfeeding in Toronto: Promoting supportive environments.* Retrieved from http://www.toronto.ca/legdocs/mmis/2010/hl/bgrd/backgroundfile-28171.pdf.

Toronto Public Health. (2012). Baby-Friendly Initiative compliance policy. Retrieved from http://insideto.toronto.ca/health/policies/pdf/baby_pol.pdf.

Toronto Public Health. (2012). *Baby-Friendly Initiative compliance; Support of breastfeeding on city premises.* Retrieved from http://insideto.toronto.ca/health/policies/pdf/breastfeeding_pro.pdf.

Toronto Public Health. (2013). *Baby-Friendly Initiative Update 2013.* Retrieved from http://www.toronto.ca/legdocs/mmis/2013/hl/bgrd/backgroundfile-55580.pdf .

CHAPTER 25

Assessing Changes in Public Attitudes Toward Breastfeeding: 1999-2014

Barbara Hormenoo, Melanie Pringle, and
Paige Hall Smith

The public's attitudes about breastfeeding and breastfeeding women reflect important social and cultural norms. By extension, these norms have an effect on women's infant feeding decisions, as they shape women's perceptions of the level of support they may receive for breastfeeding and other forms of infant feeding (Hannan et al., 2005; Li et al., 2002; Matich et al., 1992). Such attitudes may also shape three concurrent levels of breastfeeding support in U.S. society: the willingness of individual women to breastfeed in public or at work; the willingness of employers to enact workplace lactation support (Hannan et al., 2005); and, most broadly, the willingness of legislators to support breastfeeding-friendly legislation (Li et al., 2004).

To increase our understanding of general attitudes toward, and knowledge about breastfeeding, the Centers for Disease Control and Prevention (CDC) collaborates with Porter Novelli on HealthStyles, an annual survey of a nationally representative sample of U.S. adults aged 18 and up to learn about their attitudes, or orientations, and practices around health. HealthStyles, conducted annually since 1999 (except for 2008), has included questions to assess public attitudes toward breastfeeding.

Findings from previous analyses of these data indicated large geographic, racial, and income variation in breastfeeding knowledge and opinions about breastfeeding duration and public breastfeeding; men and women were found to have similar attitudes (Hannan et al., 2005). Li and colleagues (2007) reported that while survey data indicated a generally positive view of women breastfeeding, even in public, the rate of positivity appeared to be declining over. Li also found that a greater percentage of the population in 2003 (25.7%) than in 1999 (14.3%) believed that formula is an appropriate substitute for, if not actually as healthy as, breastmilk. They also found that African Americans, and people with lower income viewed breastfeeding as something that is difficult to do successfully without additional support, particularly with barriers to breastfeeding at work and in public (Li et al., 2004).

No papers have been published that have analyzed public attitudes toward breastfeeding using HealthStyles data since 2007. Using data from the 1999-2014 HealthStyles Survey, the goals of this study were to identify: (1) changes and variations in the categories of attitudes assessed by CDC over this time period; and (1) changes in public attitudes over time.

Method

We created a dataset of results from the HealthStyles surveys from 1999-2014 using data publically available on the CDC website (CDC, 2015a). (As we went to publish this article, the 2015 HealthStyles data were posted on the CDC website.) Our dataset included the survey year, the question item, and the percent of individuals who agreed with each item. The questions assessing the public's attitudes toward breastfeeding were different each year; hence, we cannot examine changes in attitudes by comparing responses to the same questions over time. However, the surveys did include multiple items that assessed attitudes about similar ideas over time. To determine changes in attitudes over time, we categorized the items that represented similar ideas together and created unique categories. The study authors, along with other colleagues, individually categorized the items; we then reviewed the different approaches and collectively arrived at a final categorization.

Results

Over the period of study (1999-2014), the HealthStyles Survey included 50 different items assessing the public's attitudes toward breastfeeding. We classified these 50 items into 12 categories (see Table 1). Over this 15 year period, the number of items representing each category ranged from a high of 21 items (Attitudes about the relative value of breastmilk) to a low of two items (Personal infant feeding recommendations; Attitudes about the impact of breastfeeding on the family).

Centers for Disease Control and Prevention Priority Areas

To the extent that the number of items, and the time frame they were asked, were reflective of CDC's priority areas regarding public attitudes toward breastfeeding, four categories stand out as priorities: (1) Attitudes about the relative value of breastmilk (21 items); (2) Attitudes about accommodations in the workplace for breastfeeding mothers (19 items); (3) Attitudes about breastfeeding in public spaces (15 items); and (4) Attitudes about harm to infants for not breastfeeding (14 items).

Combining items across categories suggest that there three areas have been assessed significantly more than others: (1) attitudes the public holds about the relative value and health benefit of human milk compared to infant formula (35 items across categories 1 and 3); (2) attitudes about employer and the governmental support for policies and practices that accommodate the needs of working mothers who want to breastfeed (29 items across categories 2 and 4); most of these items focused on attitudes related to support for pumping at work rather than breastfeeding, at work; and (3) attitudes about breastfeeding in public (15 items in Category 3).

The time frame covered by the items in these areas suggests that CDC continues to be interested in issues related to the relative value of human milk and workplace support. Indeed, their interest in the public's attitudes about the importance of governmental polices supporting breastfeeding may be growing. While these data indicate that CDC continues to be generally interested in public attitude about the relative value of human milk, their more specific interest in attitudes about harm to infants *not* breastfeeding has waned. After 2010, the only questions included in *any* of the HealthStyles surveys were items assessing the relative value of human milk and workplace support (prior to 2015). Although CDC's interest in the public's attitudes toward women breastfeeding in public was strong in the early years, their interest in this waned over time; 2010 was the last year that any questions related to this category were included.

Categories of less interest to CDC over time include attitudes about: breastfeeding challenges (7 items); the impact that breastfeeding has on women's lives (4 items); the impact that breastfeeding has on the family (2 items). Only one category, consisting of 4 questions, concerned the role of the health care system in breastfeeding promotion and support (attitudes about the influence doctors have on infant feeding decisions). These data suggest that CDC's interest in all these categories has waned.

Changes over Time in Public Attitudes

Changes over time across the 12 categories are summarized in Table 2. We identify the following themes from our analysis:

1. **The public's attitudes about breastfeeding may be independent of their attitudes about infant formula.** While the vast majority agreed that breastfeeding is healthier, that it is specifically designed to meet a baby's needs, and few agreed that

infant formula is as good as breastmilk, only about ¼ believed formula will make the baby sick, and very few believed that *not* breastfeeding will cause harm. Hence, these data suggest that, although, the public believes breastfeeding "may be best," they also believe that using formula does not cause harm.

2. **There may be more public support for pumping/expressing milk in the workplace than for strategies that keep mothers and babies together to allow breastfeeding at work.** The public's support for workplace accommodations to help women pump at work has increased (private room; break time), yet support for employers providing maternity leave for women who want to breastfeed has decreased. In contrast, however, support for governmental support for a federal law providing paid maternity leave has increased. Evidence supporting this theme is compromised by the fact that most of the items address pumping, and none directly ask about women breastfeeding at work with the infant present.

3. **Breastfeeding in public is fine if "I don't have to see it."** Overall individuals believed that mothers have the right to breastfeed in public, but most were uncomfortable seeing it, and agreed that it is embarrassing for a mother to breastfeed in front of others. The public's support for private lactation places in public places (malls, public buildings) could indicate that they believe women need these places, or it could mean that they, the public, are more comfortable when breastfeeding women are hidden. Since no questions were asked about breastfeeding in public after 2010, it is not clear whether these attitudes changed in the last half decade.

4. **The public's view of the impact of breastfeeding on women and challenges they experience are inconsistent with women's experiences.** Six of the eight questions, across two categories (categories 7 and 8), addressing attitudes about breastfeeding challenges and the impact of breastfeeding on women's lives, were asked only in

2000, so we cannot say whether these attitudes have changed. The data from that one year indicated that public attitudes did not necessarily correspond to what we know about women's experiences. Specifically, few agreed that women experienced the breastfeeding challenges (pain, difficulties producing milk, infants crying), while a nearly 45% agreed that women would have to give up too many lifestyle habits, such as favorite foods, smoking, or alcohol). Yet, data from the Infant Feeding Practices Study II (IFPS11; 2005-7) (CDC (2015b) on why women did not initiate, or weaned, suggests the opposite: the proportion of women who did not initiate, or who weaned in order to reclaim these lifestyle behaviors (smoking, diet), was low, while the proportion weaning because of these other difficulties, such as insufficient milk, pain, or other bodily challenges, was much higher (CDC, 2015).

In addition, HealthStyles data indicated that very few believed that a mother "can't breastfeed her baby and go to work or school" (10.4%), yet around 43.5% of mothers in the IFPSII data indicated that "work or school" was an important reason why she did not initiate (the IFPSSII survey did not include work or school related reasons for weaning).

Conclusions and Recommendations

Most (76%) of the 50 items included in the annual HealthStyles survey since 1999 addressed one primary area: the public's attitudes about the relative value and health benefits of breastfeeding compared to human milk. The survey has included many items that identified public attitudes in two categories important to helping women succeed with breastfeeding, specifically employer and governmental support for working mothers, and breastfeeding in public. The HealthStyles survey include few questions that will help us learn about the public's attitudes toward other categories relevant to women's breastfeeding experiences, specifically, impact of breastfeeding on the family and on women's lives, and the challenges women face while breastfeeding. While a few items (N=4) addressed public attitudes about the influence doctors have on infant feeding decisions, no other items addressed attitudes toward health care responses.

These data suggest that the public remains squeamish about women breastfeeding in public spaces, and that they may have a poor understanding of the challenges women face while breastfeeding, particularly trying to combine breastfeeding with work or school. Nevertheless, around half agree that employers should support policies and spaces that make it easier for women to pump at work.

Going forward, we recommend that HealthStyles surveys:

1. Decrease the number of items assessing attitudes about the relative value of breastmilk/breastfeeding compared to formula;

2. Reinstate items that assess the public's attitudes toward women breastfeeding in public;

3. Continue to ask questions about workplace accommodations for pumping, maternity leave (both employer and government supported);

4. Create new questions that address breastfeeding, as well as pumping, at the workplace;

5. Reinstate items that address the challenges that women experience while breastfeeding, and the impact that breastfeeding has on women's lives;

6. Create new items that assess public attitudes toward emerging public health breastfeeding support strategies, including breastfeeding-friendly maternity care practices, baby- friendly hospitals, childcare centers, and breastfeeding education in public schools, and posting of "breastfeeding welcome here" signs in public spaces.

As we went to publish this article, the 2015 HealthStyles data were posted on the CDC website.

References

Centers for Disease Control and Prevention. (2015a). *Breastfeeding.* Centers for Disease Control and Prevention. Retrieved from: http://www. cdc.gov/breastfeeding/data/healthstyles_survey.

Centers for Disease Control and Prevention. (2015b) *Infant Feeding Practices Study II and its Year Six Follow Up.* Retrieved from: http://www.cdc. gov/breastfeeding/data/ifps/results.htm#ch3.

Hannan, A., Li, R., Benton-Davis, S., & Grummer-Strawn, L. (2005). Regional variation in public opinion about breastfeeding in the United States. *Journal of Human Lactation, 21*(3), 284-288. http://jhl. sagepub.com/content/21/3/284.full.pdf+html.

Li, R., Fridinger, F., & Grummer-Strawn, L. (2002). Public perceptions on breastfeeding constraints. *Journal of Human Lactation, 18*(3), 227-235. http://jhl.sagepub.com/content/18/3/227.full.pdf+html.

Li, R., Hsia, J., Fridinger, F., Hussain, A., Benton-Davis, S., & Grummer-Strawn, L. (2004).

Public beliefs about breastfeeding policies in various settings. *Journal of the American Dietetic Association, 104,* 1162-1168. http://www.ncbi.nlm. nih.gov/pubmed/15215778.

Li, R., Rock, V.J., & Grummer-Strawn, L. (2007). Changes in public attitudes toward breastfeeding in the United States, 1999-2003. *The Journal of the American Dietetic Association, 107,* 122-127. http:// www.ncbi.nlm.nih.gov/pubmed/17197280.

Matich, J.R., & Sims, L.S. (1992). A comparison of social support variables between women who intended to breast or bottle-feed. *Social Science & Medicine, 34,* 919-927.

Table 1

Public Attitudes Toward Breastfeeding 1999-2014: Categories, Items, and Change over Time

Category	Items in Category	Total no. of times items appeared[1]	Most recent year[2]	Conclusion
1. Attitudes about the relative value of breastmilk	Infant formula is as good as breastmilk. Feeding baby formula instead of breastmilk increases the chances the baby will get sick. Breastfeeding is healthier for babies than formula feeding. Breastmilk is specifically designed to meet a baby's nutritional needs.	21	2014	• CDC continues to have strong interest in this category • The belief that formula is as good as breastmilk increased between 1999 (14%) and 2005 (28%) then decreased to a similar starting percentage in 2014 (16%) • Between 1999 and 2010, there was an increase in belief that breastfeeding was healthier than formula (68% to 73%).
2. Attitudes about accommodations in the workplace for breastfeeding mothers	I believe employers should provide extended maternity leave to make it easier for mothers to breastfeed. I believe employers should provide a private room for breastfeeding mothers to pump their milk at work. I believe employers should provide flexible work schedules, such as additional break time, for breastfeeding mothers. Breastfeeding or pumping milk at work is a personal choice, not something a manager should have to deal with. It is inconvenient for others at work when women take time to breastfeed or pump milk during work hours.	19	2014	• CDC continues to have strong interest in this category • Questions primarily on workplace accommodations for milk expression/pumping but not for breastfeeding (with infant present). • Overall (2001-2014) there has been an increase in beliefs that employers should provide the opportunity for women to pump work. • There has been an increase in belief that employers should provide flexibility in work schedules, and time for breastfeeding mothers. • There has been a decrease in support for maternity leave (from 47% in 2001 to 36% in 2010).

217

3. Attitudes about breastfeeding in public spaces	I am comfortable when mothers breastfeed their babies near me in a public space, such as a shopping center, bus station, etc. Mothers who breastfeed should do so in private spaces only. It is embarrassing for a mother to breastfeed in front of others. It is appropriate to show a woman breast-feeding her baby on TV programs. Shopping malls should provide private places to help women breastfeed. I believe women should have the right to breastfeed in public places. Public buildings need to have room where women could breastfeed and pump milk for their babies.	15	2010	• CDC has had minimal interest in this issue and interest has waned. • There was an increase (2001, 2010) in the belief that public buildings need to have a room where women could breast-feed/pump and that women have the right to breastfeed in public (41% in 2001 to 55% in 2010 and 43% in 2001 to 59% in 2010, respectively). • There was increase (2000, 2010) in percent who find it embarrassing for a mother to breastfeed in public (27% in 2000 to 32% in 2010).
4. Attitudes about harm to infants not breastfeeding	If a child is not breastfed, she/he will be more likely to get diarrhea. If a child is not breastfed, she/he will be more likely to get diabetes. If a child is not breastfed, she/he will be more likely to become overweight. If a child is not breastfed, she/he will more likely to get ear infections. If a child is not breastfed, she/he will be more likely to get respiratory infections, such as bronchitis, or pneumonia.	14	2013	• CDC had strong interest in this category between 2003-5; interest has waned. • Respondents did not support "harm" statements, meaning that a low percentage believed that children who are *not* breastfed are more likely than those breastfed to develop problems.

Category	Statements	#	Year	Notes
5. Attitudes about importance of governmental policy supporting breastfeeding	I believe breastfeeding education should be available as a part of a high school health education curriculum. I would support tax incentives for employers who make special accommodations to make it easier for mothers to breastfeed. There should be laws that protect a mother's right to pump breastmilk while at work. There should be a federal law providing paid maternity leave to workers.	10	2013	• CDC continues to have moderate interest in this category and interest may be growing. • Between 2006 and 2009 there was a decrease in support for tax incentives for employers who make special accommodations for breastfeeding mothers (30% to 25%). • Between 2010 and 2012, there was an increase in support for a federal law providing paid maternity leave to workers (46% to 54%).
6. Attitudes about breastfeeding duration	Babies ought to be fed cereal or baby food by the time they are three months old. Babies should be breastfed at least for the first 6 months. Babies should be exclusively breastfed (fed only breastmilk) for the first 6 months. One-year-old children should not be breastfed by their mother.	8	2010	• CDC has had moderate interest in this category and interest has waned. • From 2004 to 2005, about twice as many individuals believed that babies should be breastfed at least for the first 6 months as believed infants should be *exclusively* breastfed for the first 6 months. • The percent (30%) who believed infants over 12 months should *not* be breastfed remained stable (2000, 2010).
7. Attitudes about breastfeeding challenges	Breastfeeding is painful to the mother. Breastfeeding doesn't come naturally—it needs to be learned. Women commonly have problems making enough milk for their babies. Breastfed babies cry a lot more than bottle fed babies. Breastfeeding a baby correctly is hard to learn. Breastfeeding will spoil a baby. A mother needs lots of support to breastfeed her baby.	7	2002	• CDC has had minimal interest in this category and interest has waned. • Through 2002, few believed that women experienced any breastfeeding challenges (pain, difficulties producing enough milk, babies crying). • Yet, in 2002 a high percentage (41%) believed that breastfeeding mothers need lots of support • Changes overtime cannot be assessed.

Category	Items	[1]	[2]	Findings
8. Attitudes about impact of breastfeeding on women's lives	A mother can't breastfeed her baby and work or go to school. Breastfeeding will tie the mother down and interfere too much with her. A mother who breastfeeds has to give up too many lifestyle habits like favorite foods, cigarette smoking, and drinking alcohol.	4	2010	• CDC has had minimal interested in this category and interest has waned. • Overtime (2000, 2010) there was a small increase in the percent who believed that breastfeeding mothers have to give up too many lifestyle habits (food/smoking/drink); about half agree. • In 2000, few believed that women would have difficulty combining breastfeeding with work/school (10%). • Changes overtime cannot be assessed.
9. Attitudes about non-medical influences on women's infant feeding decisions	A mother's mother has a lot of influence on whether or not she breastfeeds her baby. A mother's friends have a lot of influence on whether or not she breastfeeds. A father has a lot of influence, whether or not his baby is breastfed. A mother's decision to breastfeed is influenced by what she sees.	4	2002	• CDC has had minimal interest in this category; interest has waned. • In 2002, more believed that a mother's friends (31%) and her mother (39%) have more influence on her decision to breastfeed than the father (26%); less than half agreed that any sources would have an influence (25%). • Changes overtime cannot be assessed.
10. Attitudes about influence doctors have on women's infant feeding decisions	Doctors have a lot of influence on whether a mother breastfeeds her baby. Doctors don't always support a mother's decision to breastfeed her baby. Doctors look down on a mother if she bottle-feeds her baby.	3	2002	• CDC has had minimal interest in this category; interest has waned. • In 2002, most seemed to believe that doctors would support women's infant feeding decisions: both breastfeeding and formula feeding. • Changes overtime cannot be assessed.
11. Personal infant feeding recommendations	Women should be encouraged to breastfeed. If a close friend or relative was having a baby, I would recommend she breastfeed.	2	1999	• CDC had minimal interest in this category and interest had waned. • In 1999 about half agreed that women should be encouraged to breastfeed (55%) and would recommend it (52%). • Changes overtime cannot be assessed.
12. Attitudes about the impact breastfeeding has on family	A father can feel left out if the mother breastfeeds the baby. Breastfed babies do not feel as close to their fathers and grandparents as bottle fed babies.	2	2002	• CDC has had minimal interest in this issue and interest has waned. • From 2001 to 2002, few believed that the father would feel left out if the mother breastfeeds (19%) and that while breastfeeding, the baby will not feel as close to their fathers or grandparents as bottle-fed babies (7%).

[1] This number refers to the total number of times any of the items in the category appeared across all items

[2] This represents the most recent year in which the HealthStyles survey included a question relating to an attitude in this category.

Religious and Cultural Context of Breastfeeding Among Immigrant Muslim Women

Wafa Khasawneh

B reastfeeding disparities have been documented in vulnerable populations, particularly among immigrant and minority cultural groups, and may contribute to social, economic, cultural, and political challenges impeding successful breastfeeding. Religious minority groups with health disparities often have religious values that may influence their health behaviors. Immigrant Muslims women are a fast-growing, and underserved minority group in the United States. The Islamic practices of American immigrant Muslims women play a significant role in how breastfeeding promotion needs to be approached in this population. Muslim immigrant women often lack social support and have difficulties accessing health care services that support breastfeeding. Overcoming these cultural, social challenges, and disparities requires health care providers to develop a better understanding of how religious values influence breastfeeding behaviors. The purpose of this paper is to describe Muslim religious and cultural context of breastfeeding beliefs and practices, identify key barriers affecting immigrant

Muslim women breastfeeding, and suggest culturally specific interventions to support and promote breastfeeding within this population.

Islamic Contexts of Breastfeeding

Religious teachings are strong principles influencing Muslim's health perceptions and actions (Zaidi, 2014). Although these are taught across many different Muslim countries, the ways that the Islamic religion shapes many aspects of people's health across national boundaries are not a homogenous, due to differences in ethnicity and local customs (Ott, Al-Khadhuri, & Al-Junaibi, 2003). Despite these cultural and ethnic differences, more similarities in health behavior exist among Muslim people than differences. These views have their origins in the *Quran*, which is believed by Muslims to be a direct revelation from God through the angel Gabriel to the Prophet Muhammad (Peace be Upon Him) for all human kind.

Breastfeeding is mentioned in seven verses in the *Quran*. Five of the *Quranic* verses contain instruction and rules that are considered mandated aspects of breastfeeding in Islam. In *Surah Al-Baqarah,* the *Quran* mandates women to breastfeed their babies for up to 2 years, if possible, and states that every newborn infant has the right to be breastfed. The translation (Khan & Al-Hilali, 1999) of the verse states:

> The mothers shall give suck to their children for 2 whole years, (that is) for those (parents) who desire to complete the term of suckling, but the father of the child shall bear the cost of the mother's food and clothing on a reasonable basis. No person shall have a burden laid on him greater than he can bear. No mother shall be treated unfairly on account of her child, nor father on account of his child. And on the (father's) heir is incumbent the like of that (which was incumbent on the father). If they both decide on weaning, by mutual consent, and after due consultation, there is no sin on them. And if you decide on a foster

suckling-mother for your children, there is no sin on you, provided you pay (the mother) what you agreed (to give her) on reasonable basis. And fear Allah and know that Allah is All-Seer of what you do (*Quran* 2:233).

In the second verse the duration of breastfeeding is addressed: "And We have enjoined on man (to be dutiful and good) to his parents. His mother bore him in weakness and hardship upon weakness and hardship, and his weaning is in 2 years, give thanks to Me and to your parents, unto Me is the final destination" (*Quran* 31:14). The duration of breastfeeding in months is clearly stated in the third verse: "And We have enjoined on man to be dutiful and kind to his parents. His mother bears him with hardship and she brings him forth with hardship, and the bearing of him, and the weaning of him is thirty (30) months" (*Quran* 46:15).

As outlined in the above verses, the recommended time in Islam for breastfeeding is approximately 2 years. This is congruent with current research and World Health Organization (WHO) recommendations (World Health Organization, 2015). From the above verses, *Quran* teachings identified that breastfeeding is a shared responsibility of the child's parents. If it is decided that the biological mother cannot nurse the baby, the mother and the father can mutually agree to let a wet nurse feed the child (Mohamad, Ahmad, Rahim, & Pawanteh, 2013).

In *Surah At-Talaaq* (The Divorce), Islam outlines the breastfeeding regulations in case of divorce as:

Lodge them (the divorced women) where you dwell, according to your means, and do not treat them in such a harmful way that they be obliged to leave. And if they are pregnant, then spend on them till they deliver. Then if they give suck to the children for you, give them their due payment, and let each of you accept the advice of the other in a just way. But if you make difficulties for one another, then some other woman may give suck for him (the father of the child) (*Quran* 65:6).

The verse explained that breastfeeding should be continued, even if a couple is divorced. *Quran* teachings emphasized that breastfeeding is a mother's responsibility, and the infant's father has an obligation to provide shelter and financial support so that his ex-wife can continue nursing the child, including paying for a wet nurse if it is necessary (Khattak & Ullah, 2007). This demonstrates the strong and long-standing preference in Islamic teachings regarding feeding children human milk instead of animal milk (Shaikh & Ahmed, 2006).

The other three *Quranic* verses focus on wet nursing practices and challenges in Islam. According to Islamic law, the wet nurse becomes the child's "mother in lactation." Children who have been regularly breastfed by the same woman are considered siblings, and hence, are prohibited from marrying each other (*Quran* 4:23). This may be a significant issue when offering a donor human milk to Muslim families.

The story of Moses (Peace be Upon Him), and God's suggestion to his mother to suckle him to calm her emotions, is presented in *Surah Al-Qasas* (The Narration). *Surah Al-Hajj* (Pilgrimage) refers to breastfeeding as maternal instinct. Both of these teachings are congruent with our current understandings of the hormonal effects of nursing (Groër & Kendall-Tackett, 2011).

Cultural Contexts of Breastfeeding

The religious beliefs of Muslim women serve as a contributing factor to their breastfeeding success. Nevertheless, Muslim women hold breastfeeding cultural practices or myths that hinder successful breastfeeding. For example, some Middle Eastern mothers believed that colostrum is harmful to the baby, as it can cause stomach ache or jaundice (Ergenekon-Ozelci, Elmaci, Ertem, & Saka, 2006; Hizel, 2006). Therefore, water sweetened with sugar is given for the first 3 days after delivery to cleanse the bowels of a newborn until the production of white milk. Prelacteal feeding (e.g., water, sugar water, salt solution, crushed dates, artificial milk, animal milk, yogurt, grippe water, herbal tea, and black tea) is a common traditional practice, and interferes with exclusive breastfeeding (Al-Hreashy et al., 2008; Al Ghwass, 2011; Radwan, 2013).

Muslim women use the concept of "bad milk" to refer to the mother's ability to harm her baby through breastfeeding. For example, several mothers believed that mother's illness, such as respiratory infection, cracked nipple, or maternal abdominal cramp can harm the baby through breastfeeding (Osman, El Zein, & Wick, 2009). Another cultural myth is that the mothers' negative emotions and stress can impact the quality of the milk, and can cause abdominal pain for the baby (Hizel, 2006). These beliefs reflect women's views of breastfeeding as a method for feeding and transmission of feeling and emotions between the mother and baby. Turkish mothers believe that if a breastfeeding mother works under the direct sun, and becomes tired, her milk will be harmful to the baby (Ergenekon-Ozelci et al., 2006).

Several mothers believed that the infant can harm the mother through breastfeeding. For instance, if the baby burped while breastfeeding, the mother can develop a breast infection (Osman et al., 2009). Breastfeeding during pregnancy can harm the fetus and infant (Ergenekon-Ozelci et al., 2006; Hizel, 2006; Oweis, Tayem, & Froelicher, 2009; Saka, Ertem, Musayeva, Ceylan, & Kocturk, 2005). Many women believed that "evil eye" can affect the quality of breastmilk if the mother nurses near other mothers (Hizel, 2006; Osman et al., 2009; Saka et al., 2005). These cultural beliefs influence mothers' breastfeeding ability in front of other women, and may encourage the mother to supplement with formula.

A common belief is that mother's inadequate intake of food contributes to lack of production of enough milk for the baby (Abdul Ameer, Al-Hadi, & Abdulla, 2008; Amin, Hablas, & Al Qader, 2011; Nabulsi, 2011; Yesildal, 2008). Therefore, mothers need to eat more to produce more milk and thus, breastfeeding causes maternal obesity. Some mothers were concerned that their inability to breastfeeding was inherited from their mothers (Osman et al., 2009). These women are discouraged from breastfeeding because they were told by their mothers and sisters that this issue runs in the family, and their milk is not nutritious (Osman et al., 2009; Saka et al., 2005). These folk's beliefs highlight the importance of discussing a Muslim woman's understanding of what affects her milk and its production.

Muslim Immigrant Women Breastfeeding Challenges

Muslim women face breastfeeding challenges when they immigrate to the U.S. These challenges are related to religious, cultural, linguistic, and health care barriers. The religious values and cultural challenges already explained. The religious values may not be respected for new mothers who are Muslim and immigrants, or she may not know how to access breastfeeding services if she has difficulties creating not only the risk of breastfeeding failure, but also feelings of religious guilt and failure to meet religious expectations. These challenges highlight the importance of assessing women's reasons for breastfeeding and their family's expectations.

Muslim women's lack of knowledge about the effects cultural practices may have on breastfeeding may pose additional obstacles, which non-Muslim health care providers need to address. Linguistic barriers also contribute to the increased difficulties experiences by new immigrant Muslim mothers. Health care agencies frequently do not have interpreters skilled in working with this population, and this population is not linguistically homogeneous. Immigrant Muslim women are less likely to have prenatal and childbirth classes available within their native language, further disadvantaging their breastfeeding course. Available community resources are even more limited, which further emphasizes the need to work with these religious communities that have a strong pro-breastfeeding value structure to create resources for this population that too often are unable to realize their breastfeeding goals, and have unmet needs.

Interventions to Promote Breastfeeding Among Muslim Immigrant Mothers

An ecological perspective on interventions is needed. Interventions are needed to raise women's awareness of the importance of exclusive breastfeeding. Educational interventions should be targeted to support religious beliefs. Culturally tailored intervention to the specific breastfeeding concerns and needs of Muslim immigrant women could promote breastfeeding initiation, duration, and exclusivity for this vulnerable population.

References

Abdul Ameer, A. J., Al-Hadi, A. H., & Abdulla, M. M. (2008). Knowledge, attitudes and practices of Iraqi mothers and family child-caring women regarding breastfeeding. *Eastern Mediterraean Health Journal, 14*(5), 1003-1014.

Al-Hreashy, F. A., Tamim, H. M., Al-Baz, N., Al-Kharji, N. H., Al-Amer, A., Al-Ajmi, H., & Eldemerdash, A. A. (2008). Patterns of breastfeeding practice during the first 6 months of life in Saudi Arabia. *Saudi Medical Journal, 29*(3), 427-431.

Al Ghwass, M. M. E. (2011). Prevalence and predictors of 6-month exclusive breastfeeding in a rural area in Egypt. *Breastfeeding Medicine, 6*(4), 191-196. doi: 10.1089/bfm.2011.0035.

Amin, T., Hablas, H., & Al Qader, A. A. (2011). Determinants of initiation and exclusivity of breastfeeding in Al Hassa, Saudi Arabia. *Breastfeeding Medicine, 6*(2), 59-68.

Ergenekon-Ozelci, P., Elmaci, N., Ertem, M., & Saka, G. (2006). Breastfeeding beliefs and practices among migrant mothers in slums of Diyarbakir, Turkey, 2001. *Eurpean Journal Public Health, 16*(2), 143-148.

Groër, M. W., & Kendall-Tackett, K. A. (2011). *Clinics in Human Lactation: How Breastfeeding Protects Women's Health Throughout the Lifespan: The psychoneuroimmunology of human lactation.* Amarillo, TX: Praeclarus Press.

Hizel, S. (2006). Traditional beliefs as forgotten influencing factors on breast-feeding performance in Turkey. *Saudi Medical Journal, 27*(4), 511-518.

Khan, M. M., & Al-Hilali, M. T.-u.-D. (1999). *Interpretation of the Meaning of the Noble Qur'an.* Retrieved from http://noblequran.com/translation/index.html.

Khattak, I., & Ullah, N. (2007). Fundamental rights of infants are guaranteed in Islam—breastfeeding is mandatory. *Saudi Medical Journal, 28*(2), 297-299.

Mohamad, E., Ahmad, A. L., Rahim, S. A., & Pawanteh, L. (2013). Understanding religion and social expectations in contemporary Muslim society when promoting breastfeeding. *Asian Social Science, 9*(10), 264-273.

Nabulsi, M. (2011). Why are breastfeeding rates low in Lebanon? A qualitative study. *BMC Pediatrics, 11*(1), 75. doi: 10.1186/1471-2431-11-75.

Osman, H., El Zein, L., & Wick, L. (2009). Cultural beliefs that may discourage breastfeeding among Lebanese women: A qualitative analysis. *International Breastfeeding Journal, 4*(1), 12.

Ott, B. B., Al-Khadhuri, J., & Al-Junaibi, S. (2003). Pediatric ethics, issues, & commentary. Preventing ethical dilemmas: Understanding Islamic health care practices. *Pediatric Nursing, 29*(3), 227-230.

Oweis, A., Tayem, A., & Froelicher, E. S. (2009). Breastfeeding practices among Jordanian women. *International Journal of Nursing Practice, 15*(1), 32-40. doi: 10.1111/j.1440-172X.2008.01720.x.

Radwan, H. (2013). Patterns and determinants of breastfeeding and complementary feeding practices of Emirati Mothers in the United Arab Emirates. *BMC Public Health, 13*, 171. doi: 10.1186/1471-2458-13-171.

Saka, G., Ertem, M., Musayeva, A., Ceylan, A., & Kocturk, T. (2005). Breastfeeding patterns, beliefs and attitudes among Kurdish mothers in Diyarbakir, Turkey. *Acta Pædiatrica, 94*(9), 1303-1309. doi: 10.1111/j.1651-2227.2005.tb02092.x.

Shaikh, U., & Ahmed, O. (2006). Islam and infant feeding. *Breastfeeding Medicine, 1*(3), 164-167.

World Health Organization. (2015). *Health topics: Breastfeeding.* Retrieved from http://www.who.int/topics/breastfeeding/en/.

Yesildal, N. (2008). Breastfeeding practices in Duzce, Turkey. *Journal of Human Lactation, 24*(4), 393-400. doi: 10.1177/0890334408322265.

Zaidi, F. (2014). Challenges and practices in infant feeding in Islam. *British Journal of Midwifery, 22*(3), 167-172.

CHAPTER 27

The Inequities of Nighttime Breastfeeding

Cecilia Tomori

The majority of breastfeeding advocacy and policy initiatives to date have focused on enabling and protecting women's rights to breastfeed in public spaces, and to express breastmilk at work. Significantly less attention has been devoted to facilitating breastfeeding at night since it is a practice that takes place at the home, out of public view, at a time when most mothers and babies are together. Yet nighttime breastfeeding, which plays a crucial role in the physiology of breastfeeding, and is intimately tied to the physiology of mother-infant sleep, has been mired in controversy in the U.S. Cultural norms of autonomy and independence, reinforced by strict public health recommendations for solitary sleep, clash with many parents' experience, who have found bedsharing, and continued proximity and night-feedings helpful in facilitating and sustaining breastfeeding (Ball, 2009; Ball & Volpe, 2013; McKenna, Ball, & Gettler, 2007; McKenna & McDade, 2005).

After many years of debate, the American Academy of Pediatrics (AAP) task force now includes breastfeeding as a protective factor against Sudden Infant Death Syndrome (SIDS), but the blanket recommendation against bedsharing remains (Task Force on Sudden Infant

Death Syndrome, 2011; Tomori, 2014). Moreover, pediatric advice often emphasizes reducing or eliminating nighttime breastfeeding in order to facilitate "sleeping through the night" (Ferber, 2006; Henderson, France, Owens, & Blampied, 2010; McKenna & Ball, 2010). Biological anthropologists and breastfeeding researchers have questioned these recommendations, which rely on cultural ideologies of solitary sleep and infant feeding with artificial breastmilk substitutes, and undercut breastfeeding (Ball & Volpe, 2013; McKenna et al., 2007).

Nevertheless, parents continue to receive conflicting advice about breastfeeding and solitary infant sleep, and have little practical support for navigating nighttime infant care. Just as breastfeeding during the daytime is facilitated or hindered by unequal social positions, sustaining nighttime breastfeeding in the face of these challenges requires social privileges. This chapter examines the inequities of nighttime breastfeeding through the lens of an anthropological study of nighttime breastfeeding (Tomori, 2014).

Method

The methods for this study have been discussed in detail elsewhere (Tomori, 2014). In brief, this study comprised two years of ethnographic research with 18 middle-class, White, first-time mothers and their families in the Midwestern U.S., who planned to breastfeed their children. In addition to participant observation and interviews with families, I engaged in a series of other research activities, including interviews and observations with childbirth education and lactation professionals, participant observation of community events related to childbirth and breastfeeding, and training as a postpartum doula, among others. I examined my ethnographic findings in comparative cross-cultural, historical, and evolutionary perspectives using anthropological and feminist analysis.

Results

Participants in my study encountered numerous challenges in their attempt to sustain breastfeeding at night while also conforming to infant sleep recommendations. They found that their babies had a difficult time falling asleep without being held and breastfed, and often woke up as soon as put down, only to need to be breastfed again. Some parents also had trouble falling asleep without their baby being nearby. While they were all concerned about the safety of bedsharing and SIDS, they were also exhausted and, ultimately, nearly all of them brought their babies into bed for at least part of the night.

Although these initial bedsharing practices were often unplanned, falling asleep while breastfeeding in their beds prompted parents to rethink their nighttime practices. These early decisions led some parents to habitually share their beds with their babies, while many others engaged in part-night bed-sharing and room-sharing. Nearly all parents kept their babies in the same room with them to facilitate nighttime breastfeeding for far longer than they had planned.

To address the dilemmas brought about by the challenges of night-time breastfeeding, the participating couples in my study drew on a constellation of social privileges they possessed. Socioeconomic resources were pivotal in the participants' childbirth and breastfeeding journeys, including quality health insurance plans that covered child-birth and lactation education, and a choice of pediatricians who were supportive of breastfeeding. Moreover, couples possessed educational resources that enabled them to learn more about sleep recommendations and their relationship to breastfeeding.

The ability to seek out and identify relevant material in the literature also enabled couples to question current infant sleep recommendations, and to develop their own plans for sleeping that were more compatible with breastfeeding. For instance, when one couple encountered a physician during their hospital stay who stated that "babies die when they sleep in beds" (Tomori, 2014, p. 133), they quickly reviewed the pediatric literature, and identified the tension between the pediatric guidance on breastfeeding and SIDS, and located literature that questioned the blanket recommendations to never bedshare. Although the early postpartum weeks remained fraught partly because of the fears instilled by this physician, this knowledge ultimately helped this couple make decisions about their sleep arrangements that consisted of part-night bedsharing to facilitate breastfeeding and sleep.

The knowledge parents acquired also facilitated locating, and even switching to pediatricians who were supportive of breastfeeding, and continuing to breastfeed babies at night when pediatricians encouraged nighttime separation and night-weaning. The selection of pediatricians was crucial, since they were the primary form of medical authority participants encountered who asked about sleep practices. Although pediatricians could not be openly supportive of bedsharing because of the AAP guidelines, some were far more tolerant than others. For instance, one couple had switched to a second pediatrician with the explicit purpose of finding better breastfeeding support. When the mother was explicitly asked about whether her child spent much time in the crib at night, her response was met with understanding, and no authoritative effort to intervene.

Race was a silent privilege in interactions with pediatricians and other medical professionals. African American mothers, who tend to bedshare more often and breastfeed less than White women, have been particularly targeted by sleep interventions (Hackett, 2007). Participants' ability to avoid further scrutiny by simply remaining silent about their nighttime practices, or by selectively sharing information to supportive physicians they were able to access, was partly due to their race, which enabled them to escape assumptions of "problematic" parenting.

Despite the relative privileges that my research participants possessed, they nevertheless struggled with the misalignment of expectations and embodied realities of nighttime breastfeeding and infant sleep, and with the cultural stigmatization of bedsharing, continued nighttime proximity, and nighttime breastfeeding by friends, relatives, and medical professionals. There was also heterogeneity among couples' financial, educational, social, and emotional resources, which had an impact on their ability to navigate the challenges they encountered. For instance, one mother was extensively questioned about her baby's sleep and nighttime feeding practices at the baby's 6-month pediatric visit. Upon discovering that the baby slept in a portable play yard next to the parents' bed to facilitate nighttime breastfeeding, the mother was told that she needed to move her baby to a separate room and eliminate night-feedings. Since the mother was working outside the home during the day, and had limited opportunities to express her milk using a breast pump, cutting out nighttime breastfeeding had a significant impact on her breastfeeding frequency. The mother did not link the marked reduction in her milk supply, or her perception that the baby was not interested in breastfeeding, to this advice, and did not question the physician's authority. The physician's advice played a critical role in ending this dyad's breastfeeding around 9 months.

Discussion

My anthropological study of nighttime breastfeeding in the U.S. confirms that when parents attempt to breastfeed, they find pediatric recommendations for breastfeeding and solitary sleep at odds with one another. White, middle-class parents, such as participants in my study, have significantly greater social, economic, and educational resources to seek out and evaluate advice about infant feeding and sleep, and make decisions that facilitate and sustain breastfeeding, often by creating a safe space in or near their bed for their babies, keeping their sleep practices secret, and finding breastfeeding-friendly pediatricians. Defying pediatric sleep advice is less risky for these parents, since they fit class- and race-based cultural norms for parenting. These practices enable them to continue to breastfeed during the night, and thereby support the continuation of the breastfeeding relationships, despite cultural norms and medical recommendations promoting solitary sleep.

Those with fewer resources, however, may not be able to access information about how to bedshare safely, which may result in more dangerous sleeping situations (such as sleeping on the couch in order to avoid bedsharing). Alternately, they may be less able to resist pressure to conform to norms of nighttime separation, which can lead to difficulties maintaining breastfeeding over time, especially when mothers and babies are separated during the daytime. Finally, parents of color may face greater pediatric scrutiny, and have less access to supportive pediatricians. To provide equal opportunities for breastfeeding success across social groups in the U.S., breastfeeding advocacy needs to consider the sociocultural context of nighttime breastfeeding and infant sleep, and the quality of advice and support given to families about navigating nighttime challenges.

References

Ball, H. L. (2009). Bed-sharing and co-sleeping: Research overview. *NCT New Digest, 48*, 22-27.

Ball, H. L., & Volpe, L. E. (2013). SIDS risk reduction and infant sleep location: Moving the discussion forward. *Social Science & Medicine, 79*, 84-91.

Ferber, R. (2006). *Solve your child's sleep problems* (Vol. Revised and Expanded Edition). New York: Fireside.

Hackett, M. (2007). *Unsettled sleep: The construction and consequences of a public health media campaign.* New York: The City University of New York.

Henderson, J. M. T., France, K. G., Owens, J. L., & Blampied, N. M. (2010). Sleeping through the night: The consolidation of self-regulated sleep across the first year of life. *Pediatrics, 126*(5), e1081.

McKenna, J. J., & Ball, H. L. (2010). Early infant sleep consolidation is unnecessary barrier to breastfeeding: E-letter in response to Henderson et al 2010. *Pediatrics, 126*(5), e1081.

McKenna, J. J., Ball, H. L., & Gettler, L. T. (2007). Mother-infant cosleeping, breastfeeding and Sudden Infant Death Syndrome: What biological anthropology has discovered about normal infant sleep and pediatric sleep medicine. *American Journal of Physical Anthropology Supplement, 134*(S45), 133-161.

McKenna, J. J., & McDade, T. (2005). Why babies should never sleep alone: A review of the co-sleeping controversy in relation to SIDS, bedsharing and breast feeding. *Paediatric Respiratory Reviews, 6*(2), 134-152.

Task Force on Sudden Infant Death Syndrome. (2011). SIDS and other sleep-related infant deaths: expansion of recommendations for a safe infant sleeping environment. *Pediatrics, 128*(5), e1341-e1367.

Tomori, C. (2014). *Nighttime breastfeeding: An American cultural dilemma*. New York, London: Berghahn Books.

"Mixed Feeding, Mixed Messages": Using Qualitative Methods to Understand Low Exclusive Breastfeeding Rates in Newfoundland and Labrador, Canada

Julia Temple Newhook, Leigh Anne Newhook,
William K. Midodzi, Janet Murphy Goodridge,
Lorraine Burrage, Nicole Gill, Beth Halfyard,
and Laurie Twells

Many regions of the world report high levels of intention to breast-feed, but very low exclusive breastfeeding (EBF) duration rates. Data in the Canadian province of Newfoundland and Labrador (NL) indicate that although 65% of pregnant individuals report an intention to EBF their infants for 6 months, the rate of EBF to 6 months is just 5.8% (Statistics Canada, 2014). Initiation rates are also consistently the lowest in the country, at 69.6% (Provincial Perinatal Program, 2013), compared to 90.4% nationally (Statistics Canada, 2012).

Experiences of breastfeeding are shaped by cultural context and knowledge (Stuart-Macadam & Dettwyler, 1995). In NL, as in many parts of the world, breastfeeding knowledge that had previously been passed on through generations of lived experience has been rapidly lost in the past half-century. Breastfeeding became equated with poverty, yet formula was often not available or affordable, and canned evaporated milk became the preferred infant food from the 1950s to 1970s (CWA Annual Reports, 1939-1962). Breastfeeding rates of close to 100% in the 19th century dropped to less than 5% by the 1960s (Severs, Williams, & Davies, 1964).

Purpose of this Study

This study used a feminist, intersectional, mixed-methods approach to examine perceptions of reasons for cessation of EBF and early weaning among breastfeeding parents who had intended to EBF for 6 months. Our study combined data from multiple sources including: (1) statistical analysis from a population-based survey, (2) qualitative analysis of survey participants' accounts of their experiences of infant feeding, and (3) a reflexive auto-ethnographical account of my own experiences as a breastfeeding peer support volunteer. This paper focuses on analysis of the qualitative data.

Methodology

The qualitative data were derived from the Feeding Infants in NL (FiNaL) Study, a province-wide, population-based, prospective cohort survey, administered to individuals in the third trimester (N=1,204), at 1 to 3 months postpartum, and at 6 to 12 months postpartum (Twells et al., in press). This analysis focuses on the population who intended to EBF for 6 months, and who had given birth to a healthy, full-term singleton infant, and completed all three phases of the study (n=284). Data was analyzed manually and organized by theme.

Results and Discussion

Five themes were identified relating to participants' perceptions of the reasons for cessation of EBF and early weaning: (1) cultural expectations of infant behavior, (2) the myth of insufficient milk, (3) artificial nipples, (4) public shame, and (5) medical mixed messages and misinformation.

Cultural Expectations of Infant Behavior

The cultural pressure to produce an independent, scheduled infant, who makes minimal demands on caregivers, was a dominant theme. This pressure often contrasts with infants' normal physiological development: for example, devaluing infant needs for comfort and attachment.

> My [4-month-old] baby was very attached to me, to the point that she would not even stay in her father's arms when I was near. I weaned her in an attempt that she would be more content with her father and other family members. I felt that if they could bottle- feed, they would be able to spend more time with her, rather than just me ... I very much enjoyed breastfeeding, and this was a very difficult decision.

The pressure to "schedule" a baby's feedings was also frequently mentioned: "It's frustrating when people tell me to get the baby on a schedule." Often, scheduling concerns were connected to sleep:

> I absolutely love breastfeeding! She is sleeping well, wakes one to two times per night. However, I do believe that if she was fed formula, or maybe even supplemented with some formula at night, that she would sleep better. All of my friends that formula-feed, their babies are sleeping through the night and are the same age as my daughter.

This finding is echoed in a recent American study, noting that parental beliefs concerning "spoiling" infants were linked to early breastfeeding cessation (Burnham et al., 2014).

Participants also revealed that the pressure to reduce infant demands was combined with strongly gendered childcare and domestic workloads.

> Baby (was) not gaining enough weight, I would have
> had to feed [him] every 2 hours, or less, and wasn't able
> to do that with another little one at home.

This divide may be exacerbated in NL by high rates of father absence due to employment-related migration and rotational work in male-dominated occupations (e.g., offshore oil fields, resource-based work in other provinces).

The Myth of Insufficient Milk

The myth of insufficient milk as a frequent physiological occurrence is widespread in bottle-feeding cultures (Gatti, 2008). The perception of low milk supply was a second theme in this study.

> I wasn't producing enough milk for my son, and he was
> hungry all the time. I tried to supplement with formula,
> and then he didn't want any breastmilk at all. I tried to
> get him to feed and he wouldn't.

This belief coincides with a lack of knowledge about growth spurts, with increased feeding frequency and fussy behavior, as physiologically normal breastfed-infant development.

> My little guy is an excellent feeder. We have had some
> problems … a period of constant crying, where I thought
> my milk supply was low, but we made it through.

Artificial Nipples and Bottles

Frustration with artificial nipples, or preference of the infant for an artificial nipple, was a third theme. Participants described turning to nipple shields when they were unable to find support to help their infant latch to the breast: "My child has difficulty latching and will not feed without a shield."

Pumping was also mentioned as an alternative to latching an infant to the breast, but it was almost invariably described as time-consuming and tiring:

> Pumping was an absolute nightmare. I wish I had never started it. I have so much guilt about not spending the first 6 weeks holding my baby instead of pumping around the clock. My worst decision since his birth was to pump. I would never recommend it on a permanent basis.

Public Shame

In Canada, a breastfeeding parent has the right to breastfeed anywhere they are legally allowed to be present. However, some participants described feeling unwelcome in certain public spaces. First-time parents, in particular, mentioned public embarrassment as a challenge to EBF.

> The only thing I dislike about breastfeeding is feeling as though I am not welcome to breastfeed at other people's houses or in public in certain places.

> I find [breastfeeding] hard on the mom, mostly because of the inconvenience when in public. I am glad I chose this but I am finding it hard to remain exclusive for 6 months.

243

Medical Mixed Messages and Misinformation

A recent study from Malta revealed that incorrect advice from health care providers was the most significant negative determinant of breastfeeding (Montalto et al., 2010). It is of great concern in our data that incorrect and inconsistent breastfeeding advice from health care providers was a dominant theme in the reasons given for cessation of EBF and early weaning.

> I really enjoy breastfeeding. I wish I had less interference from health care. I feel that I would not be giving formula if it was not for the doctor at the hospital.

Incorrect advice related to the safety of breastfeeding while taking medications was evidenced. One participant reported being instructed to cease breastfeeding because she was taking antibiotics for a dental infection. Participants also reported being told to introduce formula for a myriad of non-evidence-based reasons. For example, to improve mild reflux symptoms, "the doctor suggested trying formula because it is thicker."

Additionally, participants reported "mixed messages" and "conflicting information" from health care providers that made learning to breastfeed as "a very confusing and overwhelming process."

> I wish the nurses in the hospital gave me more information and support with breastfeeding. I did not understand the process of milk "coming in," and how little the baby needed to be satisfied … As a first-time mom, I read a lot of books and information on breastfeeding, but this did not completely prepare me for the real thing. I did not realize how difficult it was going to be.

Emotional Health

Finally, participants expressed considerable distress regarding the cessation of EBF and early weaning. Although a detailed discussion is beyond the scope of this paper, the data indicated that for those who intended to EBF, the decision to cease EBF, or to wean, may have substantial negative impact on one's own emotional health:

> I feel that if I had better help in the beginning at the hospital, I would not have experienced the problems I've faced since. She never latched properly in the beginning. She didn't get any milk. I had sore cracked nipples by the time I was discharged, and she wasn't gaining weight. I started pumping. But she still wouldn't latch. After infections, and two terrible bouts of mastitis, sore painful nipples, and many tears, I just had to throw in the towel. It broke my heart because I really wanted to breastfeed.

Conclusions and Recommendations

Our research indicated that intention to EBF can be undermined by cultural and social context, including the loss of generations of breast-feeding knowledge, and the current lack of knowledge and support for normal breastfeeding, and the behavior of normal breastfed infants.

Health care also takes place within a particular cultural and social context, and health care providers are not immune to the bottle-feeding culture in which they live and practice. Particularly disturbing, in our results, was the perception of health care providers as a source of "mixed messages" and "misinformation" regarding breastfeeding.

Our recommendations for public health practice include:

- Implementation of Baby-Friendly policies and 10 Steps (Breastfeeding Committee of Canada, 2012).

- Creation of a comfortable, relaxed atmosphere for learning to breastfeed.

- Education of health care providers and the public about normal physiological breastfeeding, and newborn nursing behavior, and the safety of medications while lactating.

- Increase in peer breastfeeding and doula support in hospital (Spiby et al., 2015).

- Education of the public on normal breastfeeding, importance of "mothering the mother," and challenging gendered childcare roles.

- Increase in availability of childcare support in the postpartum period.

Funded by the Canadian Institutes of Health Research and the Research Development Corporation of Newfoundland and Labrador.

We intentionally use language that is inclusive of all gender identities, and recognize the existence of birthing and breastfeeding individuals who identify as fathers, or as parents, but not as mothers. We cannot confirm the gender identities of participants, as we unfortunately did not include this question in our questionnaires.

References

Abdul Ameer, A. J., Al-Hadi, A. H., & Abdulla, M. M. (2008). Knowledge, attitudes and practices of Iraqi mothers and family child-caring women regarding breastfeeding. *East Mediterraen Health Journal, 14*(5), 1003-1014.

Breastfeeding Committee of Canada. (2012). *Integrated 10 steps and WHO code practice outcome indicators for hospitals and community health services: Summary.* Retrieved from http://breastfeedingcanada. ca/documents/2012-05-14_BCC_BFI_Ten_Steps_Integrated_ Indicators_Summary.pdf.

Burnham, L., Buczek, M., Braun, N., Feldman-Winter, L., Chen, N., & Merewood, A. (2014). Determining length of breastfeeding exclusivity: Validity of maternal report 2 years after birth. *Journal of Human Lactation, 30*(2), 190-194.

CWA Annual Reports. (1939-1962). Child Welfare Association Collection. *Centre for Newfoundland Studies. Memorial University.* COLL-002.

Gatti L. (2008). Maternal perceptions of insufficient milk supply in breastfeeding. *Journal of Nursing Scholarship, 40*(4), 355-363.

Montalto, S., Borg, H., Buttigieg-Said, M., & Clemmer, E.J. (2010). Incorrect advice: The most significant negative determinant of breastfeeding in Malta. *Midwifery, 26,* e6-e13.

Nickel, N.C., Martens, P.J., Chateau, D., Brownell, M.D., Sarkar, J., Chun, Y.G., Burland, E., Taylor, C., Katz, A., & The Paths Equity Team. (2014). Have we left some behind? Trends in socioeconomic inequalities in breastfeeding initiation: A population-based epidemiological surveillance study. *Canadian Journal of Public Health, 105*(5), e362-e368.

Pérez-Escamilla, R., & Sellen, D. (2015). Equity in breastfeeding: Where do we go from here? *Journal of Human Lactation, 31*(1), 12-14.

Provincial Neonatal Screening Program, Perinatal Program, Newfoundland Labrador. Newfoundland and Labrador. (2013). *Breastfeeding Rates, 2006-2013*. Retrieved from http://www.easternhealth.ca/Professionals.aspx?d=2&id=1981&p=1972.

Severs, D., Williams, M., & Davies, J. (1964). Infantile scurvy: A public health problem. *Canadian Journal of Public Health, 52,* 214-220.

Spiby, H., Green, J.M., Darwin, Z., Willmot, H., Knox, D., McLeigh, J., & Smith, M. (2015). Multisite implementation of trained volunteer doula support for disadvantaged childbearing women: A mixed-methods evaluation. *Health Services and Delivery Research, 3,* 8.

Statistics Canada. (2012). *Health trends*. Statistics Canada Catalogue No. 82-213-XWE. Ottawa. Retrieved from http://www12.statcan.gc.ca/health-sante/82-213/index.cfm?Lang=ENG.

Stuart-Macadam, P., & Dettwyler, K.A. (Eds.) (1995). *Breastfeeding: Biocultural perspectives*. New York: Aldine de Gruyter Press.

Twells, L., Ludlow, V., Midodzi, W.K., Murphy-Goodridge, J., Burrage, L., Gill, N., Halfyard, B., Temple Newhook, J., Morgan, B., & Newhook, L.A. [Accepted with revisions]. The feeding infants in Newfoundland and Labrador (FiNaL) study: Design and Methodology. *International Journal of Breastfeeding*.

CHAPTER 29

Practicing the Multiplicity of Donor Milk in Neonatal Intensive Care

Katherine Carroll

Imagine that you work with donor milk as a neonatal nurse. How would you classify donor milk? Is it a food that you need to provide on a regular basis to tiny infants? Do you handle it as a bodily fluid that has to be shared between two people? Or perhaps you tell worried parents that donor milk is like a medicine for their preterm infants. Now imagine you are a manager of the neonatal intensive care unit (NICU), and you are in charge of administering the budget. How would you classify donor milk? Is it a food that the NICU must provide for its smallest infants when a mother cannot feed her own child? Or is donor milk a precious commodity that also must be monitored for its cost to the unit? Now imagine that you are a new mother who has just given birth to a very premature infant weighing 1,200 grams, and you are struggling to produce enough milk to feed your baby. What is donor milk to you? Is it simply a food, or does donor milk bring about strong associations with motherhood?

As a medical sociologist and hospital ethnographer, I adopt a social constructivist perspective regarding "what" donor milk is. Therefore, all these perspectives may be true. At the foundation of social constructionism is the belief that "all knowledge, and therefore all meaningful reality as such, is contingent upon human practices, being constructed in and out of interaction between human beings ... and developed and transmitted within an essentially social context" (Crotty, 1998, p. 42). Thus, how we work with donor milk, the activities that we draw on, the conversations we have about it, and the social roles that we are expected to fill when we use it all contribute to what donor milk becomes. Put simply, the different classifications of donor milk are brought into existence by what we do with donor milk and by the context in which we live, communicate, and work. The outcome of a social constructivist approach is that we cannot claim there to be one, singular or universal classification of what donor milk actually is. Instead, a social constructivist approach enables us to see that donor milk can shift classifications depending on context, social interactions, and practices. In this way, donor milk can be considered "multiple." By drawing on research observations of everyday NICU practices, in this chapter, I show that it is precisely this multiplicity that enables us to advocate for the use of donor milk in a way that appeals to different people, in different contexts, at different times. Thus, a social constructionist approach reveals the utility of donor milk's multiplicity for championing its worth, while alerting us to the unintended or preconscious effects of our own routinized perspective as to what donor milk "is."

Method

This chapter draws on research from 6 months of observations of the use of donor milk in two level-III NICUs in the USA, details of which have been described elsewhere (Carroll, 2014). During these periods of observation, I recorded health professionals' practices, conversations, and meetings, in addition to interactions with parents, and medical artifacts as handwritten field notes. I subsequently analyzed these field notes using a matrix coding system. The matrix was structured so that I could detail the day-to-day practices of parents, nurses, doctors, and lactation consultants in the NICU, along the following classifications of donor milk: a food, a therapeutic agent, a shareable resource, a commodity, and a fluid rich in sociocultural connotations of motherhood and kinship. This matrix coding assisted in revealing how the different classifications of donor milk in NICUs shift during the everyday, routine practices enacted by health professionals, and by the communications with parents within the broader medicalized culture of neonatal intensive care.

Findings

Table 1 offers a summary of the everyday practices that occur in NICU that give rise to the multiple perspectives or classifications of donor milk. It shows how donor milk is shaped into a food, a shareable human tissue, a medicine, a commodity and a fluid that is rich in social and cultural connotations by the very way that it is talked about, handled, experienced, and managed by nurses, doctors, lactation consultants, and parents in the NICU. Table 1 also provides an example of how these shifts in classifications occurred over time by providing a brief case study of an NICU mother and her premature infant who needed donor milk.

Table 1 displays the different perceptions of donor milk, and the routines that support the use of donor milk. It reveals that donor milk is more than merely a food or a therapeutic resource for preemie babies. The many people involved in the care of a NICU baby, and his or her parents, bring this diversity of donor milk into existence. The case of Melanie and her infant, in Figure 1, makes this clear. On the day of birth, donor milk is cast as a food when Melanie is asked by the doctor to make an infant feeding choice. On the same day, donor milk is cast as a human tissue when Melanie is asked to sign the consent form. Donor milk is also cast as a therapeutic when it is presented as something that can help prevent a severe medical condition. Melanie's initial disgust at the idea of donor milk also points to the sociocultural connotations that surround donor milk. On the day after Melanie gave birth, donor milk as a body tissue became evident because a milk donor's lifestyle behaviors, donor screening, and milk pasteurization were discussed with the mother.

On Day 2, donor milk was cast as a medicine through the doctor's writing of a prescription. While earlier that day, donor milk can be classified as a human tissue because of the consent process, and through the nurses' recording the batch number of the donor milk in the patient file to ensure milk could be traced from donor to recipient. Donor milk as a commodity was also highlighted through the nurse's careful practice in trying not to spill a drop of this expensive item as she goes about measuring the exact amount of milk from the bottle.

Table 1
Coding Matrix Summary

Classification	Daily NICU practices involving donor milk	Example NICU case study: Melanie and her baby
Food	Donor milk is referred to as "feedings" in ward rounds and in medical discussions questions, such as "how is s/he eating?" and "what do we feed him/her" are raised.	Melanie gave birth to her son who was born at 28 weeks gestation, weighing 1,200 grams. A neonatologist attended, and the baby was immediately admitted into the NICU. Melanie is 22 years old and a single mother. As part of routine, neonatologists, neonatal nurses, and lactation consultants started gentle discussions with Melanie about Ray's health and prognosis, including what to feed Ray. The neonatologist asked Melanie if she had plans for how she planned to feed Ray. Melanie had bottle-fed formula to both of her other children, and was not intending to breastfeed her third child. She had not considered expressing her milk for Ray, and explicitly stated that she did not want to.
Medicine	Doctors and nurses advocate donor milk to parents of very low birthweight infants as donor milk being "like a medicine," and the bioactive factors in donor milk are promoted as helping with gastrointestinal development. The way donor milk is measured, counted, recorded, and prescribed by nurses and doctors is like a medicine.	On the day Melanie gave birth to her baby, the neonatologist explained that human milk is the best option for premature babies like hers. The doctor explained the feeding donor milk helped to prevent complications with the gastrointestinal system. Melanie reiterated that she did not want to pump her milk. The neonatologist then explained that an exclusive human milk diet is the best choice for such premature infants, and as a next step asked her to consider the use of donor milk to feed Ray for the first month of his life.
Human Tissue	There is a consent process for donor milk because it is a human tissue. The consent and parent education component highlights pasteurization and freezing to inactivate viruses and diseases, because it is a human tissue. Some nurses used gloves when handling donor milk. North American human milk banks pooling donor milk to reduce the variability of breastmilk between women.	The day after Melanie gave birth to her son, she was adamant that she did not want to pump as she had never planned to breastfeed. Although she knew donor milk was the next best option for her baby, she was also worried because she didn't know the donor, and whether the donor was a drinker or a smoker. Melanie found the acts of donor screening and milk pasteurization by the human milk bank "settling," but she still did not want to use donor milk. The neonatologist explained that if donor milk was chosen by Melanie, the nurse would bring a consent form for Melanie to read and sign, in order to allow doctors to prescribe donor milk.

253

Sociocultural	Some parents and staff react with the "yuck factor" when presented with donor milk, and will exhibit a preference for mother's own milk or formula. Some mothers view the option of donor milk as one way to achieve breast-milk feedings for their babies. The use of donor milk casts reflections on "normal" motherhood by some NICU mothers.	The day after Melanie gave birth to her son, Melanie explained that although she was considering the option of donor milk, but that she really didn't want him to have somebody else's milk. She felt that her own breastmilk would provide a connection between herself and her baby, and that he would come to learn that the milk was hers. She stated that she simply didn't feel comfortable with another woman pumping her milk and giving it to her baby. She was worried the baby would connect with somebody else instead of her.
Commodity	Donor milk attracts a processing fee and postal costs, which must be absorbed by hospital budget, or reimbursed in insurance. Some NICUs ask parents to pay for donor milk. Due to expense, some NICUs may limit donor milk to those most in need. NICUs that are human milk bank depots may also have financial arrangements with regard to postage and dry ice reimbursements.	On the third day after Melanie's son was born, it was time for the nurse to feed him donor milk. The nurse needed to go to the milk room and measure the 3 mLs of donor milk into a syringe. The nurse did this carefully: a spill of donor milk is costly as the hospital paid US$4 per ounce to the milk bank for the milk. In the past year, the hospital had spent US$18,000 on donor milk as a non-billable expense.

Concluding Thoughts for Policy and Practice

The social constructivist approach, and the matrix coding of research observations in NICUs reveals the multiplicity of donor milk. Rather than reducing the multiple classifications of donor milk to one single type, the multiplicity of donor milk can be celebrated and respected as a complex female bodily fluid. This multiplicity can be used to appeal to different people, in different contexts, and in different times to offer parents, health professionals, policy makers, and activists a toolkit of new and different ways to analyze and use donor milk. A key example of this is when health professionals advocate for donor milk as medicinal, and at the same time downplaying donor milk as a body-tissue to enhance acceptability among new mothers (Carroll, 2014).

In this chapter, I have presented donor milk as a slippery, fluid substance that can be difficult to pin down. Yet, in advocating for the recognition of this multiplicity, there is an important caveat. We must also ask ourselves, what are the hierarchies implicit in each context and classifications? Does the uneven power of one classification silence the importance of others? Are there any frictions between them, and how does this affect a mother and her infant?

To conclude, I ask you to reflect once more. Take a moment to envisage how you currently work with donor milk. How do you classify it? Can the notion of donor milk having multiple classifications change the way you think, talk about, or handle donor milk in your working day? I invite you to recall and to use the concept of multiplicity as you go about your daily work to enhance the acceptability of donor milk in the hospital, the community, and in health policy.

References

Carroll, K. (2014). Body dirt or liquid gold? How the 'safety' of donated breastmilk is constructed for use in neonatal intensive care. *Social Studies of Science, 44*(3), 466-485.

Crotty, M. (1998). *The foundations of social research: Meaning and perspective in the research process.* Sydney: Allen & Unwin.

"An Empty Sack Does Not Stand": Community Perspectives on Exclusive Breastfeeding in Léogâne Commune, Haiti

Lauren Zalla

Sak vid pa kanpe is a proverb in Haitian Creole that means "an empty sack does not stand," or equivalently, "you can't do much on an empty stomach." Hunger was a theme that frequently arose in a study of exclusive breastfeeding practices in rural Léogâne Commune, Haiti. Conversations with mothers and community health workers revealed how, in this context, the ability to practice exclusive breastfeeding is determined, in part, by maternal nutritional status, which is in turn inextricably tied to socioeconomic position.

In this paper, I hope to highlight how the choices women make regarding infant feeding in rural Haiti may be shaped by their surrounding physical and social environments, and particularly by the effects of poverty and food insecurity.

Method and Context

From May to July 2014, a mixed methods study of exclusive breast-feeding practices and infant growth outcomes was conducted in rural Léogâne Commune, Haiti. The study included an assessment of the prevalence and determinants of exclusive breastfeeding, and its effect on infant growth through a cross-sectional survey of mothers with infants younger than 8 months. In addition, community health workers completed written questionnaires and participated in focus groups to explore the barriers to exclusive breastfeeding in their communities.

The 10 rural communal sections within Léogâne Commune have a combined population of about 97,000 (Institut Haïtien de Statistique et D'Informatique, 2009). The area is mountainous and very physically isolated. The primary economic activity is small-scale agriculture. However, most households do not produce enough to satisfy their food needs (Desamours et al., 2009). As a result of policies that have destabilized the agricultural economy, and caused persistent environmental degradation, food insecurity is widespread in rural Haiti. Consequently, rural communities suffer an elevated prevalence of malnutrition, particularly chronic malnutrition. Among children under five, 24.7% are estimated to suffer from chronic malnutrition in rural Haiti, compared to 15.8% in urban Haiti (Cayemittes et al., 2013).

In rural Haiti, breastfeeding is nearly universal, and the median duration of breastfeeding is nearly 18 months (Cayemittes et al., 2013). Breastfeeding is viewed as part of being a good mother and necessary to achieve developmental milestones, such as walking (Alvarez & Murray, 1981; Dornemann & Kelly, 2012). However, mixed feeding from birth is the norm in Haiti. In the study sample of 119 infants in Léogâne Commune, 98% of infants were breastfed, but only 11% were exclusively breastfed to 6 months (Zalla, 2015).

Results

Thirty-two community health workers participated in the study. In general, community health workers reported that mothers in their communities believe that breastmilk is the best food for an infant. However, most women perceive *exclusive* breastfeeding as a modern phenomenon, and associate it with the biomedical system. Traditionally, infants are administered a castor oil purgative, called *lòk,* immediately after birth, and within a few weeks, they are given porridges, or *labouyi,* made from locally ground plantains, manioc, corn, rice and other starches. Community health workers reported greater exposure to public health messages about the importance of exclusive breastfeeding in recent decades, and consequently, a decrease in the use of *lòk,* and an increase in the proportion of mothers practicing exclusive breastfeeding. While few mothers make it to 6 months, more than half of infants in the study sample were exclusively breastfed for at least 2 months.

The community health workers described several barriers that prevent the widespread adoption of exclusive breastfeeding to 6 months in Léogâne Commune. One key barrier they identified was skepticism of exclusive breastfeeding among older women in the community. In rural Haiti, many mothers live in extended family households, or *lakou,* and their mothers and grandmothers may discourage them from practicing exclusive breastfeeding. As one community health worker put it,

> There are so many who still have a myth in their minds that says, when their mothers were raising them, they didn't breastfeed, they gave them food, and nothing bad happened, they didn't die, nothing happened to them.

This reported barrier to exclusive breastfeeding is related to cultural tradition. However, most of the other barriers that the community health workers described were not cultural, but institutional, having to do with social position and access to resources. For example, mothers who did not have enough money to eat well often doubted the quality of their breastmilk, and felt obligated to supplement. One community health worker explained,

> People are always saying that they have no food, so they
> can't breastfeed...there are people who say "Oh, I am
> already anemic. I can't breastfeed my baby. I myself
> don't have any food, so I can't give my baby the breast."
> We often encounter these problems.

In addition, mothers who work to support their families are often
forced to leave their babies at home in the care of older siblings or
grandmothers because of the long distances they travel on foot. In the
words of one community health worker,

> There are mothers who have such a great burden on
> their backs, sometimes they have children, and they
> would really like to spend time admiring them, truly
> breastfeeding them for 6 months, but there is a problem.
> They have other children they are responsible for, older
> ones, and they have to go sell at the market, if they have
> a garden they have to tend to it, so they have to leave the
> child in the care of another older one in order to make a
> life for them. Sometimes they aren't even together with
> the father, and that promises a lot of difficulties.

The need to work prevents many women, especially single mothers and
women whose families rely on them for financial support, from staying
home for 6 months to practice exclusive breastfeeding.

Unfortunately, the alternatives to breastfeeding are also inaccessible to many women because of their socioeconomic position. For
example, infant formula is very costly in Haiti. Of mothers in the
study sample who supplemented, half reported supplementing with
unmodified powdered milk. The community health workers noted this
double bind, reporting that mothers who lack the means to breastfeed
successfully also lack the means to purchase formula.

> Often, the mothers know what type of milk they ought
> to give a baby. But the economic problem, it counts
> more. Meaning, when they buy a little can of infant for-

mula, it won't even last them four days. When they buy a big can of powdered milk, that gives them more time. That's one of the reasons why the economic problem crushes them, because the milk for them to give their babies, whatever lasts longer, whatever gives them a few more days, that's what they use.

Discussion and Conclusion

In summary, this study yields new insights for policy and practice through qualitative exploration of the barriers to exclusive breastfeeding in rural Léogâne Commune. Despite a growing proportion of women wishing to practice exclusive breastfeeding to 6 months, there are several barriers preventing its widespread adoption in Haiti. While previous studies, and public health efforts, have largely focused on cultural barriers to exclusive breastfeeding, citing the need to educate women about the importance of exclusive breastfeeding, and address their "misunderstandings," this study suggests that education is not a complete solution. Behavior change may be impossible in the face of the institutionalized processes that systematically marginalize poor women in rural Haiti. The inability to eat well and the need to work are two key barriers that limit the ability of these mothers to practice exclusive breastfeeding, even if they wish to do so. Indeed, these institutionalized processes may explain the seemingly paradoxical attitude toward breastfeeding in rural Haiti. On the one hand, the belief that breast is best, and on the other, the supposed unwillingness of mothers to practice exclusive breastfeeding.

In conclusion, this study prompts questions about the sensitivity of efforts to promote exclusive breastfeeding to the lived experiences of women in Haiti. To be successful, these efforts will need not only to educate women about the importance of exclusive breastfeeding, but also to acknowledge and work to remove structural constraints on individual autonomy.

References

Alvarez, M. D., & Murray, G. F. (1981). *Socialization for scarcity: Child feeding beliefs and practices in a Haitian village*. Report Submitted to USAID. Retrieved from http://users.clas.ufl.edu/murray/research/haiti/Haiti.index.html.

Cayemittes, M., Busangu, M. F., Bizimana, J. de D., Barrère, B., Sévère, B., Cayemittes, V., & Charles, E. (2013). *Enquête Mortalité, Morbidité et Utilisation des Services, Haïti, 2012*. Calverton, Maryland. Retrieved from http://dhsprogram.com/publications/publication-FR273-DHS-Final-Reports.cfm.

Desamours, A., Delbaere, J., Horjus, P., Papavero, C., Norciede, J. C., Sirois, R., & Coordonnateur, L. (2009). *Analyse Compréhensive de la Sécurité Alimentaire et de la Vulnérabilite en Milieu Rural Haïtien*. Port au Prince, Haiti. Retrieved from http://www.wfp.org/content/haiti-analyse-comprehensive-securite-alimentaire-vulnerabilite-en-milieu-rural-haitien-2009.

Dornemann, J., & Kelly, A. H. (2012). "It is me who eats, to nourish him": A mixed-method study of breastfeeding in post-earthquake Haiti. *Maternal & Child Nutrition, 9*, 74–89.

Institut Haïtien de Statistique et D'Informatique. (2009). *Population Totale, Population de 18 Ans et Plus Menages et Densites Estimes en 2009*. Port-au-Prince, Haiti. Retrieved from http://www.ihsi.ht/produit_demo_soc.htm.

Zalla, L. (2015). *The prevalence and social determinants of exclusive breastfeeding and implications for infant growth in rural Haiti: A mixed-methods study*. (Thesis). Durham, NC: Duke University.

CHAPTER 31

Fighting Social Norms
for Better Health Outcomes
in Bihar, India

Rajshree Das

Project Concern International (PCI) is implementing a community mobilization and accountability project, Ananya initiative, funded by the Bill and Melinda Gate's Foundation (BMGF) in Bihar, India. ("Ananya" is the name of the umbrella project.) The overall objective of this initiative is to increase adoption of key Maternal, New born and Child Health and Sanitation (MNCHS) behaviors among women of reproductive age (WRA) in the most marginalized (MM) communities of Scheduled Castes (SC), Scheduled Tribes (ST), and Backward Muslims (BM) in Bihar, India. (Scheduled Castes is the official name given in India to the lowest caste, considered "untouchable" in orthodox Hindu scriptures and practice, officially regarded as socially disadvantaged. The term "Scheduled Tribe" first appeared in the Constitution of India. Article 366 (25) defined scheduled tribes as such tribes or tribal communities or parts of or groups within such tribes or tribal communities as are deemed under Article 342 to be Scheduled Tribes for the purposes of this constitution.)

The Ananya Initiative is based on the *Parivartan* theory of change; this theory seeks to effectively combine economic and social empowerment with community- and individual-level attitudes and behaviors by promoting participatory learning and collective action in women's groups. (*Parivartan* is a Hindi word that means Change or Transform.) This approach aims to provide a real sense of possibility for change, ultimately liberating the power of marginalized women and communities to be effective agents of transformation that will result in improved and sustained MNCHS behaviours.

About the Area

With nearly 103 million people (The Registrar General & Census of India, 2011), Bihar is the third most populous state in India with per capita income of $398, which is the second lowest among the states. The female literacy rate of Bihar is 53%. Bihar faces a major equity related challenge because of extreme poverty and deep rooted caste division. For example, nearly 40% of its population is living below poverty line, and 16% belonging to schedule caste and schedule tribes (SC/ST). Among them, there are around 5 million extremely backward castes or *Mahadalits.* There are 21 low Dalit castes, which have been included in the list of *Mahadalits.* This gives an opportunity to these listed castes special provisions and facilities provided by the state government. Refer to Table 1 for key demographic indicators of Bihar, in comparison to India.

Table 1. Key Demographic Indicators of Bihar and India

Indicator	India	Bihar
Infant Mortality Rate	57	62
Neonatal Mortality Rate	39	40
Under 5 Mortality Rate	74	85
Total Fertility Rate	2.4	3.6

We encountered the deep-rooted social norms linked with infant- and young-child feeding practices (IYCF), many of which run counter to recommended breastfeeding practices. These include:

- Colostrum should be discarded and not fed to newborn infants.
- It is acceptable to feed newborn infants milk from some other nursing and/or lactating mother than feeding "colostrum milk."
- A mother will start producing milk 2 to 2.5 days after giving birth.
- There are some religious rituals to be followed after that only the child should be given breastmilk, like *ajan* among the Muslim communities.
- Since the child has not developed teeth, there is no need to feed them semi-solid foods after 6 months of age.
- Infants have small stomachs, so they should only be given milk, and this is sufficient for the child.
- Infants should only be given boiled food.
- Young children should not be given any vegetables.

Project Parivartan Theory of Change

Figure 1 depicts the theory of change that guided the three-year implementation of Parivartan project. Project Parivartan had developed this theory of change to bring as part of the implementation design for desired results. This theory incorporates the following:

- Shifting the power to the women who participate in the self-help groups through a blend of social and economic empowerment.
- Women self-help groups become the Change Agent for health, nutrition, and sanitation issues.
- Capacitated women self-help groups bring in change in behavior at individual, family, and community level.
- Leaders of these capacitated women self-help groups negotiate and demand for their entitlements.

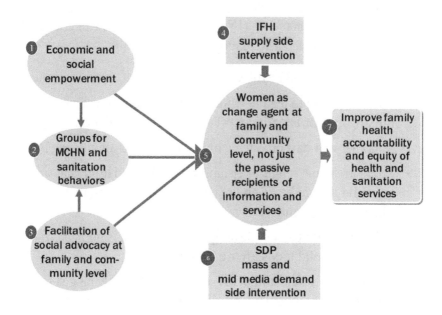

During this time, women from the most marginalized communities, who are in the reproductive age group, were mobilized to form self-help groups. Intensive efforts were made so to conduct weekly meetings to allow members to develop the habit of sitting once in a week as a "group" or "collective." These meetings gave them opportunity to talk about different issues at the household and community level. The community health workers, called *Saheli*, facilitated meetings. *Saheli* is a local word, which means friend. Under the project the health volunteers are called as *Sahelis*. One *Saheli* is responsible to support around 8 to 10 groups.

With this process, the social cohesion at the group level increased. Gradually, the community health workers (*Sahelis*) provided group members with modular training on health, nutrition, and sanitation behaviors linked with maternal and child health outcomes. These trainings had engaging, interactive, and pictorial tools like songs, stories, puzzles, which helped the illiterate and semi-literate women understand the messages on maternal and child health. In the self-help groups, there were elderly women (mothers-in-law and sisters-in- law), who play vital roles in addressing the social norms. There was an explicit emphasis on helping the *Saheli* build their facilitation skills. This included classroom sessions followed by the handholding support of *Saheli* facilitators by the PCI trainers on regular basis for around 2 years. During the handholding session, the trainers observed the *Saheli's* facilitation and delivery of content to the women self-help group members. Based on the observation, the trainers gave feedback to the *Saheli's*, and were capacitated on the specific areas of improvement.

Parivartan Project has collaborated with the Government supported Livelihoods program so that the women self-help groups get linked with the economic empowerment activities. Ministry of Rural Development, Government of India, and State Government in Bihar is committed to improving rural livelihoods and driving social and economic empowerment of poor on a sustainable basis through creation of SHGs through project Jeevika implemented by Bihar Rural Livelihoods Promotion Society (BRLPS).

Evaluation

In 2014, a midterm evaluation was conducted for the project and the results are encouraging (Figure 2 and 3).

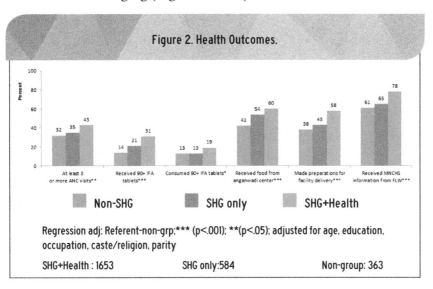

Figure 2. Health Outcomes.

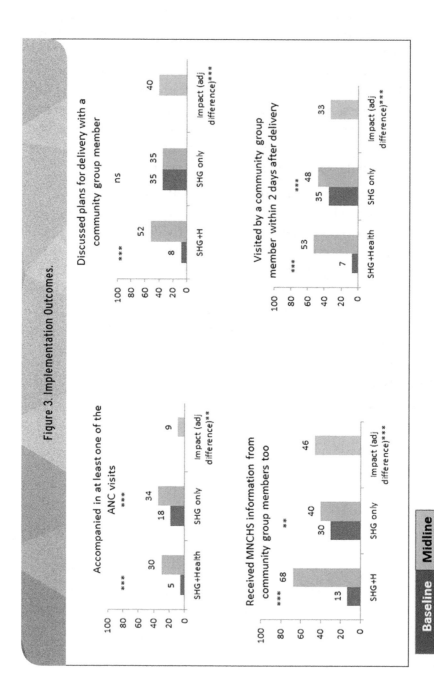

Figure 3. Implementation Outcomes.

Source: Parivartan Midline. Notes: Impact (DID method) - */**/*** =adjusted difference significant at the 10/5/1 percent level. ns – not significant Chi-sq test for association between outcome indicators and time within each group. */**/*** =significant at the 10/5/1 percent level

Apart from the health outcome, there has been changes in the self-efficacy of the women self-help group members. Many women self-help group members helped other group members seek services, and also gave information linked with mother and child health (Figure 4).

Parivartan Pathway

The Parivartan Pathway believes that community mobilization, with a strong focus on collective action and social accountability, plays a vital role in shifting social norms. The journey of community mobilization starts with building self-esteem and confidence among the members of the groups, which enables them to speak in group meetings and talking to other group members. The confidence of the member then helps to improve the individual agency followed by social cohesion among the group members. With change at the member level, the changes could be seen at the collective level that starts from collective efficacy, and moves toward the collective action. The final step is social accountability, wherein the group, or group members, works as agents of change in the larger community and diffusion in an organized manner (see Figure 5).

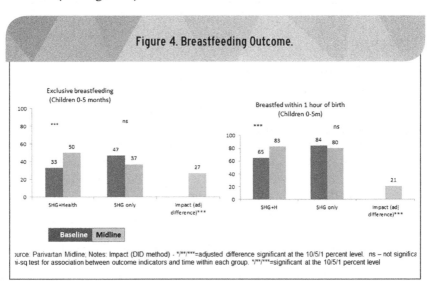

Figure 4. Breastfeeding Outcome.

Source: Parivartan Midline; Notes: Impact (DID method) - */**/***=adjusted difference significant at the 10/5/1 percent level. ns – not significa
i-sq test for association between outcome indicators and time within each group. */**/***=significant at the 10/5/1 percent level

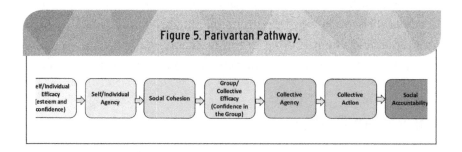

Figure 5. Parivartan Pathway.

There is still much to learn about this approach to community change, including:

- What's a realistic time span between the different steps in the pathway?
- What are the inputs (behavior change communication/facilitation/other) required to get the best result in different steps?
- How could we improve the negotiating power of the women at the household level (especially with the husband), and community level, for changing the social norms?
- What is the retention level of this "change" or "transformation?"

References

Government of Bihar Finance Department (2011). *Economic survey 2010–11.* Retrieved from http://gov.bih.nic.in/documents/economic-survey-2011-english.pdf.

The Registrar General & Census Commissioner, India, New Delhi, Ministry of Home Affairs, Government of India; Census of India (2011). *Population of Bihar.* Retrieved from http://censusindia. gov.in/2011-prov-results/data_files/bihar/Provisional%20 Population%20Totals%202011-Bihar.pdf.

CHAPTER 32

Innovative Projects to Support Breastfeeding Beyond the Hospital

Kathleen L. Anderson

O ptimal breastfeeding—that is, exclusive breastfeeding for the first 6 months, with the introduction of complementary solid foods at 6 months, and continued breastfeeding for 1-to-2 years and beyond (American Academy of Pediatrics [AAP], 2012; World Health Organization, 2011)—significantly impacts the health of children and their mothers (Ip et al., 2007). Breastfeeding initiation rates have risen, yet the number of children who are exclusively breastfed for the first 6 months, and who continue to be breastfed at 1 year of age continues to be lower (Centers for Disease Control and Prevention, 2014). This paper describes two projects that are providing interventions to support mothers in the continuum of breastfeeding beyond the hospital stay: during the vulnerable periods of the first 6-to-12 weeks postpartum, and after the mother returns to work.

Reaching Beyond the Hospital: Supporting Breastfeeding in Wake County

This stakeholder-driven project explores breastfeeding support and care as experienced by vulnerable groups of women, in particular, minority women and those with low-resources, during the early days and weeks postpartum. The project is designed to further coordination of breastfeeding services among health care providers, agencies, and organizations that offer breastfeeding services and messages in a large, urban county in North Carolina during these critical time periods, and to identify specific messaging and program adaptation to provide consistent and pertinent breastfeeding education to support cultural and social needs of African American and Hispanic women, and those from low-resource families.

The prenatal and early postpartum period encompasses a broad range of health care and community services. The stakeholders in this project reflect that range of services, and include state and county agencies (i.e., Wake County Human Services, and NC Department of Human Services Women's Health Branch and Nutrition Services Branch), as well as breastfeeding support organizations in the county. We also enlisted the support of the North Carolina physicians' societies, in particular, the Pediatric Society, Obstetrical and Gynecological Society, and Academy of Family Physicians, as well as local hospitals.

Through community-based participatory planning among stakeholders, a two-prong approach was developed to learn about the services and messages that are offered by health care providers and support organizations. Key informant interviews are being conducted among stakeholders and others who serve, or are in contact with, pregnant and postpartum women and their families. In addition, mothers, fathers, and other family supporters are being recruited to participate in focus groups about their breastfeeding experiences.

Data collection from the key-informant interviews and focus groups continues. Preliminary data indicate differences among health care providers around the accessibility of their services and messages, as well as their expectations related to mothers' breastfeeding needs in the early weeks. Preliminary information from mothers suggests that messages regarding breastfeeding in the early weeks postpartum may not be consistent or clear, such as those related to maintaining an adequate milk supply in the early weeks.

The overall strategy of the project is to foster increased coordination of services, and the consistency and pertinence of breastfeeding messages through community-based participatory methods and formative exploration with mothers/families and health care providers/community organizations. Implementation of new elements into ongoing services and messages may emerge to meet the goal of helping women make the informed decision to initiate breastfeeding, exclusively breastfeed, and achieve longer durations of breastfeeding.

Ten Steps to Breastfeeding-Friendly Child Care (BFCC)

The statewide scale-up project is designed to provide interventions designed to increase breastfeeding support in the Early Care and Education setting. More than half of mothers with infants under a year of age are entering the workforce (U.S. Department of Labor, 2015), and going back to work is a barrier to breastfeeding (U.S. Department of Health and Human Services, 2011). In addition, research shows that infants who are routinely cared for by someone other than their mothers are significantly less likely to be breastfed (Kim & Peterson, 2008).

National Early Care and Education (ECE) standards recognize the importance of providing breastfeeding support in the ECE setting (AAP, 2011). In addition, many states have developed breastfeeding-friendly childcare designation programs to encourage ECE facilities to support breastfeeding. However, many ECE professionals find it challenging to provide adequate support for breastfeeding families in their facilities. The Ten Steps to BFCC was developed to support ECE professionals to better meet the needs of their breastfeeding families.

BFCC is built upon the positive results from a pilot study in one North Carolina County, and the collaboration of North Carolina State and local agencies that provide training in the ECE setting. The collaborators encompass the many statewide agencies and organizations that are involved in supporting breastfeeding in childcare, including the NC Child Care Health and Safety Resource Center, the NC Infant Toddler Enhancement Project, Shape NC, Health Starts for Young Children, and the NC Department of Health and Human Services, as well as county agencies and organizations within North Carolina.

As part of the scale-up, a Training of Trainers (TOT) curriculum model has been developed to meet the ECE training needs within the many counties in the state. The TOT curriculum includes two hours of online pre-training to provide background information about breastfeeding, and the Ten Steps to BFCC intervention for ECE providers, as well as a three-hour/in-person Training of Trainers. Materials have been updated for statewide applicability, and vetted to align with NC childcare licensing standards. The additional breastfeeding pre-training was incorporated into the TOT training, because breastfeeding was not part of many trainers' professional trainings, backgrounds, or experiences. Pretest and post-test data have been collected to measure the efficacy of the TOT.

Trainers include Child Care Health Consultants, Infant-Toddler Specialists, WIC Regional Breastfeeding Coordinators, Shape NC Hub Specialists, and others who provide training for Early Care and Education providers. One of the challenges, as described earlier, was that breastfeeding was not part of many Trainers' professional backgrounds or personal experiences. Even with training, some knowledge and attitude gaps persisted and required additional discussion, such as whether gloves are required when handling human milk in the ECE setting. In addition, there was continued Trainer turn-over, and maintaining a Trainer pool was another challenge.

Interest in the Ten Steps to BFCC training has increased with the launch of the NC Breastfeeding-Friendly Child Care designation.

A growing number of Early Care and Education professionals, both teaching staff and directors, in ECE programs across the state have completed the Ten Steps to BFCC provider training, which includes a two-hour/in-person training, and materials to support optimal infant feeding practices for all families, and for breastfeeding families. During the two-hour training, participants reflect on their own beliefs and feelings about breastfeeding, gain knowledge and information about breastfeeding and human milk, and become familiar with the BFCC materials for families and providers. Preliminary results indicate an increase in knowledge and attitude regarding breastfeeding and support for breastfeeding in the ECE setting.

The purpose of this scale-up project was to increase statewide support for breastfeeding in childcare through expanded access to breastfeeding-friendly childcare training and materials for ECE providers. An important next step will be to integrate best practices in breastfeeding-friendly childcare into state licensing and rating systems to better meet the needs of breastfeeding mothers to be able to continue to breastfeed after returning to work or school.

The Surgeon General's Call to Action to Support Breastfeeding (U.S. Department of Health and Human Services, 2011) includes a call to communities beyond the hospital to support mothers to be able to continue to breastfeed their children. Two important and critical times for mothers are the early days and weeks postpartum, and the return to work. Breastfeeding support during these critical times will help a mother exclusively breastfeed, and continue to breastfeed her child for as long as the mother and child desire.

References

American Academy of Pediatrics. (2012). Policy statement: Breastfeeding and the use of human milk. *Pediatrics, 129*(3). Retrieved from http://pediatrics.aappublications.org/content/129/3/e827.full.pdf+html.

American Academy of Pediatrics, American Public Health Association, National Resource Center for Health and Safety in Child Care and Early Education. (2011). *Caring for our children: national health and safety performance standards; Guidelines for early care and education programs.* (3rd Ed.). Elk Grove Village, IL: American Academy of Pediatrics; Washington, DC: American Public Health Association. Retrieved from http://cfoc.nrckids.org/WebFiles/CFOC3_Book_6-10-14Update_.pdf.

Centers for Disease Control and Prevention. (2014). *Breastfeeding report card.* Retrieved from http://www.cdc.gov/breastfeeding/pdf/2014breastfeedingreportcard.pdf.

Ip, S., Chung, M., Raman, G., Chew, P., Magula, N., DeVine, D. et al. (2007). Breastfeeding and maternal and infant health outcomes in developed countries. *Evidence report/technology assessment No. 153. AHRQ Publication No. 07-E007.* Rockville, MD: Agency for Healthcare Research and Quality. Available at http://citeseerx.ist.psu.edu.libproxy.lib.unc.edu/viewdoc/download?doi=10.1.1.182.8429&rep=rep1&type=pdf.

Kim, J., & Peterson, K.E. (2008). Association of infant child care with infant feeding practices and weight gain among U.S. infants. *Archives of Pediatric and Adolescent Medicine (JAMA Pediatrics),* 162(7). Available at http://archpedi.jamanetwork.com.libproxy.lib.unc.edu/article.aspx?articleid=379824.

U.S. Department of Health and Human Services. (2011). *The Surgeon General's Call to Action to Support Breastfeeding.* Washington, DC: U.S. Department of Health and Human Services, Office of the Surgeon General. Retrieved from http://www.surgeongeneral.gov/library/calls/breastfeeding/calltoactiontosupportbreastfeeding.pdf.

U.S. Department of Labor. Bureau of Labor Statistics. (2015). *Employment characteristics of families summary – 2014.* Retrieved from http://www.bls.gov/news.release/famee.nr0.htm.

World Health Organization (WHO). (2011). *Exclusive breastfeeding.* Retrieved from http://www.who.int/mediacentre/news/statements/2011/breastfeeding_20110115/en/.

Section 4

***Advancing Health
Care Responses***

CHAPTER 33

Racializing Postpartum Mothers in Breastfeeding Promotional Contexts: An Ethnographic Account from Western Canada

Alysha McFadden

Narratives of "race" pervade everyday practices of biomedicine. (The term "race" is in quotation marks to remind the reader of its socially constructed nature.) The professionalization and expanded authority of medical practitioners has enhanced the legitimacy to ascribe race in particular ways (Porter, 1997). Social analysts have shown that clinical praxis is a rich field for the re-inscription of social stereotypes (Berry, 2010; Gilman, 1985), with bodies frequently becoming raced sites (Fassin, 2011). Recent ethnographic work within hospitals show how raced ideologies often operate unchallenged in clinical domains (Sargent & Erikson, 2014). Studying connections between race and infant feeding within this context is particularly revealing because reproduction and childrearing are intimate places where societal norms and expectations are enforced, as well as targeted sites of reformation for racialized groups (Berry, 2010; Jolly, 1998).

In everyday health care encounters in urban, Western Canada, I have observed how particular mothers are singled out for special concern among public health nurses based on judgments of perceived social and biological differences related to their infant feeding practices. My study examined how professional nursing practices "work on" and "create narratives about" specific bodies, particularly lactating and non-lactating mothers. I undertook an ethnographic study to understand if, and how, nursing praxis reinforces and reproduces "facts" of otherness, which has the potential to limit opportunities for particular mothers and infants. My findings indicated that, indeed, mothers are racialized, as seen through the conflation of race, ethnicity, and culture.

Theoretical Framework

Race is a fraught and controversial topic. Hence, it is imperative that I clarify what race and racialization meant in the context of this study. Scientific evidence indicates that that race is not biologically and genetically determined, but it is, in fact, a social construct (Marks, 2011). Yet, race—as experienced through racism and discrimination—can have biological consequences (Gravlee, 2009; Krieger, 2000). For example, processes that engender differential care and treatment can lead to poor health outcomes (Chapman & Berggren, 2005). Since breastfeeding disparities and inequities are often understood through categories of race and ethnicity, understanding how deployments of the race concept are used in health care contexts can provide insights into these inequities (Dodgson, 2012). Therefore, I focus on racialization as a way to understand how raced categories operate in breastfeeding promotion programs.

Racialization is contingent on context, social structures, history, place, space, and time (Fassin, 2011). By racialization, I am referring to identity attribution based on perceived racial characteristics in relation to the prevailing social hierarchy (Fanon, 1952). However, racialization is not a stand-in term for "racist" (Ahmad, 1993). As Didier Fassin explains,

> Ascribing someone racially is therefore not only impos-
> ing an identity upon [her]: it is also depriving [her] of
> possible alternative identifications, including the mere
> possibility of multiple belongings (2011, p. 423).

Thus, racialization is a way of exerting power over another, insisting superiority of one's own racial knowing over the lived experiences of the racialized person (Fanon, 1952). Racialization can be employed for many reasons: to label, appraise, or validate oppressive practices (Fassin, 2011). Thus, racialization is an important aspect to study when looking at social interactions, especially when the terms of contact are related to bodily processes and professional obligations.

Ethnographic Context

Over a seven-month period, I conducted ethnographic research in Western Canada. This research included 20 semi-structured interviews, and 30 participant-observation experiences in diverse settings, such as home visits, immunization clinics, committee meetings, and breastfeeding clinics. My study participants were public health nurses who provide home visitation services for postpartum mothers and their infants.

In Western Canada, the government provides universal community-based, public health services for postpartum mothers and their newborns. This means all mothers are eligible to have a telephone assessment and/or home visit within 24 to 48 after hospital discharge. This program is voluntary, and mothers can refuse home visitation services or telephone assessments. The hospital sends a liaison form to the public health unit—with information about the client, such as name, contact information, health and birth history, and feeding plan—letting the nurses know of discharged clients. The program aims to provide continuity of care and assess whether the mother and newborn are physiologically stable, aware of community supports and resources, and if they are in need of breastfeeding support services.

Method

I focused on nurses and their professional practices because biomedical research on breastfeeding primarily assumes that mothers' practices need analysis, not health care practitioners' beliefs and practices regarding particular mothers. This discursive reallocation moves us away from paying exclusive attention to racialized mothers' practices. By shifting the gaze to the culture of public health nurses in Western Canada, I was able to provide contextual accounts of how practitioners racialize mothers.

Throughout all stages of my research, I used Public Health Critical Race (PHCR) praxis in order to pay explicit attention to my own positionality as a clinically trained public health nurse, as well as to the institutional, disciplinary, and biomedical discourses in which I was first trained (Ford & Airhihenbuwa, 2010). PHCR praxis encouraged me to continually critique my research questions and findings in relation to my own positionality and social location as a female, middle-class, heterosexual, able-bodied, "White," public health nurse. The term White is also in quotations to signify its socially constructed nature. People who are considered White are constructed as such based on specific local histories, which can change over time (Fassin, 2011).

Findings

Most of my participants understood the complicated and multifaceted reasons why mothers may experience difficulties with breastfeeding, and, as a consequence, some of these difficulties were perceived to cause breastfeeding disparities. Yet, when asked who is in need of breastfeeding support, the majority of my participants provided stereotypical, racialized descriptions.

"Boxification" of Culture

During participant-observation and interviews, I observed and asked my participants about their public health nursing practices in relation to breastfeeding disparities and inequities. The issue of culture was a common refrain in relation to breastfeeding disparities. Yet the issue of breastfeeding inequities was typically not broached. The nurses cited that mixed feeding styles were indicative and unchangeable for particular racialized mothers. These behaviors were also equated to people who had particularly "ethnic" last names. As such, many public health nurses were racializing mothers by their last names and infant feeding styles by over-determining those attributes to the mothers' culture.

This essentializing practice is not unheard of. In fact, Van Esterik (2012, p. 56), a Canadian cultural anthropologist and breastfeeding advocate, argues that the main breastfeeding textbook for health professionals encourages the "boxification of culture" in an attempt to educate practitioners to be culturally competent. Instead of promoting quality care, the focus on cultural knowing creates essentialized, static groups by not recognizing the diversity amongst people. These cultural stereotypes concomitantly racially box particular mothers' infant feeding practices, because culture is commonly conflated with categories of race and ethnicity in health care contexts. In fact, culture has come to be known as a proxy for race (Hannah, 2011).

My aim is not to throw out the culture concept altogether, but I do want to highlight when it is used, and for whom. The problem of culture was suggested as a reason for breastfeeding disparities during all of my interviews, except for one. In fact, culture was typically brought up as a way to juxtapose non-White groups' infant feeding practices to normative—read White—Canadian mothering practices. Therefore, most discussions surrounding culture had to do with racialized mothers.

Conclusion

These examples show how infant feeding styles can be presumed fixed and unchangeable based on an assessment of a mother's culture-cum-race. Thus, racialized mothers' may experience victim-blaming because their real life, everyday breastfeeding challenges may not be acknowledged. Furthermore, the lack of acknowledgment may perpetuate the status quo based on the belief of culture-cum-race as pathology, not other more salient reasons, such as differential treatment and care based on static, essentialized, and racialized depictions.

Acknowledgements

My fieldwork and program of study were supported by the Government of Canada (SSHRC CGM, #GXSO118), the Canadian Nurses Foundation (Military Nurses of Canada Scholarship), and The Dr. Djavad Mowafaghian Foundation Endowment Fund (the Faculty of Health Sciences Child Health Practice and Research Award).

The content of this paper is solely the responsibility of the author, and does not necessarily represent the official views of the above funding agencies.

References

Ahmad, W.I.U. (1993). *'Race' and health in contemporary Britain*. Buckingham, UK: Open University Press.

Berry, N. (2010). *Unsafe motherhood: Mayan maternal mortality and subjectivity in post-war Guatemala*. New York: Berghahn Books.

Chapman, R., & Berggren, J. (2005). Radical contextualization: Contributions to an anthropology of racial/ethnic health disparities. *Health: An Interdisciplinary Journal for the Study of Health, Illness, and Medicine, 9*(2), 145-167.

Dodgson, J. (2012). Racism, race, and disparities in breastfeeding. In P. H. Smith, B. L. Hausman, & M. H. Labbok (Eds.), *Beyond health, beyond choice: Breastfeeding constraints and realities* (pp. 74-83). New Brunswick, NJ: Rutgers University.

Fanon, F. (1952). *Black skin, white masks*. New York: Grove Press.

Fassin, D. (2011). Racialization: How to do races with bodies. In F. E. Mascia-Lees (Ed.), *A companion to the anthropology of the body and embodiment* (pp. 419-434). Malden, MA: Wiley-Blackwell.

Ford C., & Airhihenbuwa C. (2010). The public health critical race methodology: Praxis for antiracism research. *Social Science & Medicine, 71*(8), 1390-1398.

Gilman S.L. (1985). Black bodies, white bodies: Toward an iconography of female sexuality in late nineteenth-century art, medicine, and literature. *Critical Inquiry, 12*(1), 204-242.

Gravlee, C. (2009). How race becomes biology: Embodiment of social inequality. *American Journal of Physical Anthropology, 139*, 47-57.

Hannah, S. (2011). Clinical care in environments of hyperdiversity. In M.D. Good, S.S. Willen, S.D. Hannah, K. Vickery, & L.T. Park (Eds.), *Shattering culture: American medicine responds to cultural diversity* (pp. 35-69). New York: Russell Sage Foundation.

Jolly, M. (1998). Introduction: Colonial and postcolonial plots in histories of maternities and modernities. In K. Ram & M. Jolly (Eds.), *Maternities and modernities: Colonial and postcolonial experiences in Asia and the Pacific* (pp. 1-25). Cambridge, UK: Cambridge University.

Krieger, N. (2000). Refiguring "race": Epidemiology, racialized biology, and biological expressions of race relations. *International Journal of Health Services: Planning, Administration, Evaluation, 30*(1), 211-216.

Marks J. (2011). *The alternative introduction to biological anthropology.* New York: Oxford University.

Porter, R. (1997). *The greatest benefit to mankind: A medical history of humanity.* New York: W.W Norton & Company.

Sargent C., & Erikson C. (2014). Hospitals as sites of cultural confrontation and integration. In J. R. Bowen, C. Bertossi, J. W. Duyvendak, & M. L. Krook (Eds.), *European states and their Muslim citizens: The impact of institutions on perceptions and boundaries* (pp. 29-53). Cambridge, UK: Cambridge University.

Van Esterik, P. (2012). Breastfeeding across cultures: Dealing with difference. In P. H. Smith, B. L. Hausman, & M. H. Labbok (Eds.), *Beyond health, beyond choice: Breastfeeding constraints and realities* (pp. 53-63). New Brunswick, NJ: Rutgers University.

CHAPTER 34

Why are Pediatricians Non-Compliant with the WHO Code?

Amanda L. Watkins and Joan E. Dodgson

Breastfeeding has long been a public health priority, both nation-ally and internationally. Leading health organizations agree that breastfeeding provides optimal nutrition for infants during the first year of life and beyond (Academy of Breastfeeding Medicine Board of Directors, 2008; Eidelman et al., 2012). Yet breastfeeding rates in the United States lag modest national goals set forth by *The Surgeon General's Call to Action to Support Breastfeeding* (U.S. Department of Health and Human Services [U.S. DHHS], 2011). The lack of primary provider support for breastfeeding has been a frequently cited barrier to successful breastfeeding (Eidelman et al., 2012). *The Surgeon General's Call* (U.S. DHHS, 2011) emphasizes the importance of ensuring appropriate lactation management education for all pediatric health care providers in changing the societal norms in the U.S. This prompted the Academy of Breastfeeding Medicine to develop a protocol for creating a breastfeeding-friendly pediatrician's office (Grawey, Marinelli, Holmes, & the Academy of Breastfeeding Medicine, 2013), based on the World Health Organization's *International Code for the Marketing of Breast-Milk Substitutes* (WHO Code, 1981), which is the gold standard for ethical presentation of infant feeding information.

It is well-established that the actions, or non-actions, that health care providers take toward promoting and supporting breastfeeding families make a difference in the success and duration of breastfeeding (Sinai, 2011). Despite more than 30 years of discussion in the professional literature, the lack of visible breastfeeding supportive materials, and the lack of compliance with the WHO Code (1981) continue to be the norm in pediatric waiting rooms (Dodgson et al., 2014). Why? Researchers seeking to better understand this question have used self-report surveys to collect data from health care providers and their patients. However, many of these surveys have methodological flaws related to reporter bias. We used a more objective methodology, direct observation by trained observers using a standardized tool. Study aims were used to describe the (1) WHO Code compliance, (2) demographic factors affecting WHO Code compliance, and (3) the breastfeeding supportive materials available to families within pedestrians' waiting rooms. The analysis has uncovered broader sociocultural contexts that may have driven the observed practice-related patterns and the subsequent undermining of breastfeeding success (Dodgson et al., 2014). Framed by a feminist approach, the purpose of this paper is to critically analyze the socioeconomic and historical factors that have affected, and continue to affect, physicians' non-compliance with the WHO Code (1981).

We found that non-compliance with the WHO Code (1981) was the norm for the vast majority of pediatric waiting rooms. One might think that this was due to a lack of knowledge on the part of the physicians. However, the American Academy of Pediatrics (AAP), and the Academy of Breastfeeding Medicine, have numerous statements and policies aimed at informing and recommending that pediatricians support breastfeeding families through complying with the WHO Code (Grawey et al., 2013; Sinai, 2011). Clearly, the situation is more complex than a simple knowledge deficit.

Significant differences occurred in the amount and types of formula promotion, and breastfeeding-supportive materials, available in the offices. Affluent communities had more formula giveaways, and low-income communities had fewer breastfeeding-supportive materials available, continuing the widening gap in available resources based on geographic and economic contexts prevalent throughout the U.S.

In unpacking the contextual factors that may have affected our findings, we discuss the tangled historical roots surrounding the relationship between pediatricians and formula manufacturers, and the implications of patriarchal socioeconomic models that underline the inadequacy of breastfeeding promotion practices, especially in low-income and minority communities. The ways new parents' attitudes and practices may be shaped by both overt and covert messages within pediatricians' offices are also discussed.

Historical Influences

Infant feeding practices throughout history have been affected by cultural, socio-political, and geographical influences (Smith, Hausman, & Labbok, 2012). Although infants have been fed with human milk (either mother's own or the milk of another mother) since our existence began, deviations from this optimal feeding practice have plagued the modern era, and have persisted despite indisputable evidence that exclusive and prolonged breastfeeding remains the superior method of infant feeding. For example, American women during Colonial times would typically breastfeed through two summers. However, it was common by the end of the 19th century for women to feed cow's milk shortly after giving birth, and to wean completely by 3 months of age (Wolf, 2003). Although physicians quickly took note of the dangers of artificial feeding, the deleterious effects of artificial feeding, and its impact on the most vulnerable within our societies persist today (Allen, 1889; Ip et al., 2007). One need only look more closely at the historical influences to understand the complexity of the situation.

Traditionally, women who were unable to produce enough milk, or who did not nurse for various reasons, used wet nurses (i.e., another woman nursing a baby who is not her own). It was common for wealthy or royal women to choose wet nursing or hand feeding to maintain their status in society, physical beauty, and reproductive capabilities. The conscious decision by women not to breastfeed their babies is not new, but the capability to mass-produce safer human milk alternatives is a 20th Century phenomenon.

The confluence of medicine, science, and technology during the 18th and 19th centuries produced significant changes in infant feeding (Hausman, 2003). Artificial milks were "safely" produced with the advent of pasteurization in the late 1800s, and the widespread household use of refrigerators in the 1920s. The Industrial Revolution allowed excess dairy products (and newly manufactured artificial baby milks) to be transported and distributed widely. The medicalization of birth practices also occurred, resulting in childbirth moving into hospitals. Previously, births were attended by female doulas (rather than male medical staff), and took place in the home with the support of female relatives. As childbirth practices underwent medicalization based on a patriarchal paradigm, physicians (predominantly male) embraced the role of infant feeding expert, usurping a domain that had always been women's knowledge. Along with this change, much of women's knowledge that had been passed through the generations was lost.

Social changes also influenced the use of artificial feeding. World War II brought large numbers of women into the workforce, leaving their infants in the hands of caregivers (Apple, 1987). Choosing formula became the norm, and was marketed as the "scientific" or "modern" way of feeding. Pediatricians, a new medical subspecialty, guided mothers on how to feed their babies by providing prescriptions for making infant formula (Brosco, 1999). Within a decade, mothers relied on pediatricians' advice; the formula industry arose facilitated by the pediatric profession (Nestle, 2013). The strong influence of the billion-dollar formula manufacturing companies within the pediatric profession continues today (Hausman, 2003; Smith et al., 2012). The largest purchaser of infant formula in the U.S. is the U.S. government, which supplies the WIC program (Greenway, 2011).

As the alliance between pediatricians and formula manufacturing companies continued to grow during the 1960s and 1970s, members of the public health community questioned the health outcomes related to this societal change. Unethical marketing practices by formula manufacturing companies, and subsequent high infant mortality deaths due to formula misuse (e.g., over dilution of formula to "stretch" the volume and use of unsafe water sources) led to the World Health Assembly (WHA) approving the WHO Code in 1981 (Dodgson et al., 2014; World Health Organization, 1981). The goal of the WHO Code is to safeguard breastfeeding while ensuring the appropriate marketing, distribution, and use of infant formula (World Health Organization, 1981). Despite significant efforts to promote, protect, and support breastfeeding over the past 30 years, violations of the WHO Code are frequently reported (Barennes, Slesak, Goyet, Aaron, & Srour, 2016). Particularly egregious, WHO Code violations (e.g., unethical formula marketing practices) are widespread in low- and middle-income countries where little or no enforcement of the Code exists (Barennes et al., 2016).

Code Compliance Today

Our observational study of pediatric waiting rooms was an initial attempt to understand how widespread Code noncompliance was within pediatricians' waiting rooms in a large metropolitan area. None of the 100 offices observed were Code compliant. Eighty-one percent of offices openly displayed formula promotional materials in their waiting rooms, and only a few offices made breastfeeding support information and materials available (in their waiting rooms). Clearly, Code non-compliance was the norm in the offices sampled in this study.

The ways new parents' attitudes and practices may be shaped by both overt and covert messages within pediatricians' offices are particularly concerning. The effects of the tangled relationship between pediatricians and formula manufacturers, and the implications of patriarchal health care models, are still evident, despite current public policy efforts, professional organization advocacy, and increasing breastfeeding knowledge among health professionals. The inadequacy of breastfeeding promotion practices, especially in low-income and minority communities, further widens the gap between available resources. Changes must occur to improve breastfeeding promotion efforts in physician offices. New strategies are needed to advance breastfeeding advocacy that promotes change in the face of sociocultural norms in a medicalized health care system that clearly run counter to stated national breastfeeding goal.

References

Allen, N. (1889). The decline of suckling power among American women. *Babyhood, 5*(March), 111-115.

Apple, A. D. (1987). *Mothers and medicine: A social history of infant feeding 1890-1950*. Madison, WI: University of Wisconsin Press.

Barennes, H., Slesak, G., Goyet, S., Aaron, P., & Srour, L. M. (2016). Enforcing the International Code of Marketing of Breastmilk Substitutes for better promotion of exclusive breastfeeding: Can lessons be learned? *Journal of Human Lactation, 32*(1), 20-27. doi: 10.1177/0890334415607816.

Brosco J. (1999). The early history of the infant mortality rate in America: A reflection upon the past and a prophecy of the future. *Pediatrics, 103,* 78-485.

Dodgson, J. E., Watkins, A. L., Bond, A.B., Kinatro-Tagaloa, C., Arellano, A., & Allred, P.A. (2014). Compliance with the International Code of Marketing of Breastmilk Substitutes: An observational study of pediatricians' waiting rooms. *Breastfeeding Medicine, 9,* 1-7. doi: 10.1089/bfm.2013.0096.

Eidelman, A.I., Schanler, R.J., Johnston, M., Landers, S., Noble, L., Szucs, K., . . . American Academy of Pediatrics Section on

Breastfeeding. (2012). Breastfeeding and the use of human milk. *American Academy of Pediatrics, 129*(3), e827-e841. doi: 10.1542/peds.2011-3552.

Grawey, A.E., Marinelli, K.A., Holmes, A.V., & the Academy of Breastfeeding Medicine. (2013). ABM Clinical Protocol #14: Breastfeeding-friendly physician's office: Optimizing care for infants and children, revised 2013. *Breastfeeding Medicine, 8*(2), 237-242. doi: 10.1089/bfm.2013.9994.

Greenway, D.A. (2011). WIC breastfeeding support at risk. *Breastfeeding Medicine, 6*(5), 247-248.

Hausman, B. L. (2003). *Mother's milk: Breastfeeding controversies in American culture.* New York and London: Routledge.

Ip, S., Chung, M., Raman, G., Chew, P., Magula, N., DeVine, D., . . . Lau, J. (2007). Breastfeeding and maternal and infant health outcomes in developed countries. *Evidence report/technology assessment, 153,* 1-186.

Nestle, M. (2013). *Food politics: How the food industry influences nutrition and health.* Berkeley, CA: University of California Press.

Sinai, L. (2011). Divesting from formula marketing in pediatric care. *2012 Annual Leadership Forum Rsolution #67SC.*

Smith, P.H., Hausman, B.L., & Labbok, M. (Eds.) (2012). *Beyond health, beyond choice: Breastfeeding constraints and realities.* New Brunswick, NJ: Rutgers University Press.

The Academy of Breastfeeding Medicine Board of Directors. (2008). Position on Breastfeeding. *Breastfeeding Medicine, 3*(4), 267-270.

U.S. Department of Health and Human Services. (2011). *The Surgeon General's Call to Action to Support Breastfeeding.* Washington, DC: U.S. Department of Health and Human Services, Office of the Surgeon General.

Wolf, J. H. (2003). Low breastfeeding rates and public health in the United States. *American Journal of Public Health, 93*(12), 2000-2010.

World Health Organization. (1981). *International Code of Marketing of Breastmilk Substitutes.* Geneva, Switzerland: World Health Organization Retrieved from http://www.who.int/nutrition/publications/code_english.pdf.

Developing Effective Strategies to Create Favorable Environments for Breastfeeding in Québec, Canada: Addressing the Challenges of Health Professionals' Initial Training on Breastfeeding

Isabelle Michaud-Létourneau, Julie Lauzière,
Laura Rosa Pascual, Sylvie Chiasson, Juliette Le Roy,
Micheline Beaudry, and Isabelle Gaboury

In the last decades, many strategies have been deployed in Québec, Canada, to create favorable environments to optimize breastfeeding practices and experiences. However, several challenges remain, especially to improve the health care response with respect to breastfeeding. The challenge of improving the basic training of health professionals must be tackled as it has an important influence on professional practices including the support offered to mothers and families. This paper describes ways by which a group of actors are working to develop effective strategies to that effect in a complex system.

Breastfeeding in Québec, Canada

In Québec, after having reached a dramatic prevalence of around 11% of mothers who were initiating breastfeeding in the late 1960s (Myers, 1979), this trend has been gradually reversed to reach a current initiation rate of 89% (Gionet, 2013). Facilitators to reverse the trend include: 1) increases in public awareness of the importance of breast-feeding (women's groups, researchers, health professionals); 2) a better understanding of the factors that influence breastfeeding success; and 3) the availability of different tools and strategies to protect and pro-mote breastfeeding, and to support breastfeeding mothers (Beaudry, Chiasson, & Lauzière, 2006). The Baby-Friendly Initiative (BFI) is one of the strategies that has made an important contribution. However, despite the fact that Québec has been a leader regarding the implemen-tation of the BFI in Canada, and has a high breastfeeding initiation rate, only 52% of mothers breastfeed exclusively at the time they leave the maternity: around 2 days after giving birth (Neill, Beauvais, Plante, & Haiek, 2006). A lack of, or ineffective, support for breastfeeding likely contributes to this situation (Renfrew, McCormick, Wade, Quinn, & Dowswell, 2012). Professional practices favorable to breastfeeding are critical to improve the experience of mothers who wish to breastfeed, and hence, the rates of breastfeeding. The literature clearly shows the benefits of improved training of health professionals and many recommendations exist to that end (Academy of Breastfeeding Med-icine, 2011; Renfrew et al., 2006; UNICEF UK, 2014; World Health Organization, 2009).

A group of strategic actors, members of the *Mouvement Allaitement du Québec* (Québec Breastfeeding Movement, 2012-2015), primarily through its committee on training, have taken on the task of improving this situation. They are carrying out a multidimensional action research initiative to assess current challenges, influence different stakeholders, and stimulate and strengthen the motivation of specific actors to improve the competency of health professionals on breast-feeding through their initial training. The following section presents several actions and outcomes resulting from this overall initiative. A framework for strategic system thinking, which has previously been shown to help develop effective strategies in complex environments (Michaud-Létourneau, 2014), is used to organize the actions carried out so far. Although this paper does not detail the framework, the questions and elements of the framework are used to illustrate several actions developed by this strategic group.

How to Develop Effective Strategies to Improve Health Professionals' Initial Training on Breastfeeding

The training committee of the Québec Breastfeeding Movement comprises a group of participants who represent different disciplines (medicine, nutrition, osteopathy, IBCLC), who work in diverse fields (academia, health system, community), and who come from different regions of the province. They are complementary and represent various perspectives on the issue at stake. They use informal and formal channels to achieve their goals and develop their actions. Such a group benefits from going through a systematic and iterative process, as detailed below.

Step 1: Assessment and Identification

Who needs to do what, where, and when? What are the missing or weak parts of the system?

The first step was to assess the situation and what needed to be improved, as well as to put the pieces of the larger puzzle together. Following an online survey of educational institutions across Québec in which 28 programs representing six health professions took part, the group has highlighted weaknesses in the health professionals' training regarding breastfeeding (Lauzière et al., 2014). This finding was similar to the results of another Canadian study focusing on physicians' training regarding breastfeeding (Pound, Williams, Grenon,

Aglipay, & Plint, 2014). The heterogeneity of curricula across health professions and the absence of many essential topics, such as the physiology of the mammary gland and the factors influencing milk production, also emerged from the survey.

Step 2: Strategic Dimensions

What are the complementary objectives we want to achieve?

Effective strategies can be created through incremental complementary tactics that address various strategic dimensions. For example, to act on the results of the survey, the group identified and started to work on the following objectives and activities, summarized here for each strategic dimension.

> **Systemic:** Using a participatory approach, the group plans to organize an interdisciplinary workshop that targets those responsible for the courses on breastfeeding in various programs in the province.

> **Motivational:** Through a periodic newsletter, the group maintains regular contact with 115 key actors engaged in training on breastfeeding in different programs so as to sustain their interest, and provide them with relevant resources. The group is also in the process of meeting with several key stakeholders to assess their needs regarding training for breastfeeding, and to gather their ideas for the development of the workshop. Such a consultation can help to foster a collective change process and to mobilize many actors.

> **Political:** To assist with the development of the initiative, the group has secured the support of a local former dean of a medical school, who is a national champion in medical education.

Technical: Two members of the group carried out a pilot project with a department of nutrition to upgrade its course on breastfeeding, and better understand the challenges at stake for such an endeavor.

Social: One objective of the workshop is to create social relationships between several key actors from programs that train different health professionals so they can work together to strengthen and harmonize the training on breastfeeding.

Step 3: Hierarchy of Processes

What kind of processes do we want to influence (to improve, advance, create, or develop)?

In the complex system, we seek to influence, it is important to recognize that there are a variety of processes taking place. Giving attention to diverse processes can increase the likelihood of obtaining valid, reliable, and more importantly, sustainable results (high-quality results). During the planning of the workshop, an inclusive consultation process will aim to develop a strong feeling of working towards a collective goal. During the workshop itself, we will pay a lot of attention to group processes so as to create a safe space where actors can develop relationships.

Step 4: Catalysts for Change

What are the catalysts we can take advantage of (create, incentivize)?

Catalysts allow for producing energy and stimulating activities or changes in a system. In our context, they include:

Engagement: Engaging diverse actors using a participatory approach throughout the project will help to awaken their interest and motivation to improve the health professionals' initial training on breastfeeding.

Connectors and Superhubs: The group will make sure to identify, reach out, and engage actors with many connections to other people (connectors), as well as actors who not only know many people, but are also skilled in connecting those people with one another (superhubs).

Windows of opportunity: Those are moments in which opportunities appear that we can take advantage of. For example, one member of the group has been solicited by several students for different projects. This has been an opportunity for sharing ideas and examining potential partnerships. As a result we are currently developing a project in which a Master's student is likely to engage professors from different programs and professions into this broad project.

Step 5: High-Quality Outcomes

What type of high-quality outcomes do we want to foster (develop, create)?

Such an approach endorses a constructivist paradigm in which intangible products (ideas, relationships, trust) are as valued as tangible products. Ultimately, the workshop would be a starting point for the development and implementation of an interdisciplinary curriculum for the initial health professionals' training on breastfeeding in the province. To get there, an intermediate outcome of the workshop could be the creation of a core group of actors in each school, as well as a network or community of practice for these actors to support each other. Therefore, keeping this in mind can help us go through those five steps again, and consider additional tactics that could be created.

Conclusion

This paper described ways by which a group of actors seek to influence a complex system, in this case, to create favorable environments for breastfeeding in Québec. To be able to provide adequate support to breastfeeding mothers and families, health professionals need to develop core breastfeeding-related competencies during their initial training. Using a framework based on strategic capacity can help to develop effective strategies to improve and harmonize such training, which in turn will have a positive impact on the health care system for the benefit of children, women, and families.

References

Academy of Breastfeeding Medicine. (2011). Educational objectives and skills for the physician with respect to breastfeeding. [Guideline]. *Breastfeeding Medicine, 6*(2), 99-105. doi: 10.1089/bfm.2011.9994.

Beaudry, M., Chiasson, S., & Lauzière, J. (2006). Introduction. *Un peu d'histoire*. In *Biologie de l'allaitement - le sein, le lait, le geste* (pp. 1-14). Québec: Presses de l'Université du Québec.

Gionet, L. (2013). *Breastfeeding trends in Canada*. Retrieved from http://www.statcan.gc.ca/pub/82-624-x/2013001/article/11879-eng.htm.

Lauzière, J., Beaudry, M., Chiasson, S., Pascual, L., Le Roy, J., Michaud-Létourneau, I., & Gaboury, I. (2014). *Portrait de la formation en matière d'allaitement dans les programmes de formation qualifiante en santé au Québec*. Poster presented at the Journées annuelles de santé publique (JASP), Montréal, Qc, Canada. http://jasp.inspq.qc.ca/portrait-formation-allaitement.aspx.

MAQ. (2015). *Québec breastfeeding movement*. Retrieved from www.AllaiterAuQuebec.org.

Michaud-Létourneau, I. (2014). *Operationalizing Multisectoral Nutrition In Mozambique: The Role Of Strategic System Thinking "Strategies And Insights From A Complexity Perspective"*. Doctoral dissertation, Cornell University, Ithaca, NY.

Myers, A. (1979). Retrospective look at infant-feeding practices in Canada: 1965-1978. *Journal of the Canadian Dietetic Association, 40*(3), 200-210.

Neill, G., Beauvais, B., Plante, N., & Haiek, L. N. (2006). *Recueil statistique sur l'allaitement maternel au Québec, 2005-2006* (pp. 92). Québec: Institut de la statistique du Québec.

Pound, C. M., Williams, K., Grenon, R., Aglipay, M., & Plint, A. C. (2014). Breastfeeding knowledge, confidence, beliefs, and attitudes of Canadian physicians. *Journal of Human Lactation, 30*(3), 298-309. doi: 10.1177/0890334414535507.

Renfrew, M. J., McCormick, F. M., Wade, A., Quinn, B., & Dowswell, T. (2012). Support for healthy breastfeeding mothers with healthy term babies. *Cochrane Database Syst Rev, 5*, CD001141. doi: 10.1002/14651858.CD001141.pub4.

Renfrew, M. J., McFadden, A., Dykes, F., Wallace, L. M., Abbott, S., Burt, S., & Anderson, J. K. (2006). Addressing the learning deficit in breastfeeding: Strategies for change. *Maternal & Child Nutrition, 2*(4), 239-244.

UNICEF UK. (2014). *Guidance notes for implementing the UNICEF UK Baby-Friendly Initiative standards in universities* (pp. 49). Retrieved from http://www.unicef.org.uk/.

World Health Organization. (2009). *Infant and young child feeding: Model Chapter for textbooks for medical students and allied health professionals* (pp. 99). Geneva: WHO.

http://whqlibdoc.who.int/publications/2009/9789241597494_eng.pdf .

Night-time Breastfeeding Challenges on a Postnatal Ward

Kristin P. Tully, Catherine E. Taylor, and Helen L. Ball

This paper provides an overview of three original, interrelated research projects to assess the nighttime breastfeeding challenges of mothers, newborns, and their hospital staff on a UK postnatal ward. Our methodology incorporated overnight, infrared filming of naturalistic behaviors and semi-structured interviews with mothers; methodological details and findings are described in full elsewhere (Ball et al., 2006, 2011; Taylor, Tully, & Ball, 2015; Tully & Ball, 2012).

Method

Maternal-infant dyads were prenatally randomized to different bassinet conditions or bedsharing during continuous rooming-in on the same UK tertiary-hospital postnatal ward between 2002 and 2010. The stand-alone bassinet, in a wheeled cart located adjacent to the maternal bed, is standard for rooming-in (see Figure 1). The sidecar bassinet is 3-sided and locks onto the maternal bed frame (see Figure 2). Ethical and institutional approvals were obtained from Durham University, and the local NHS Research Ethics Committees. Participants were enrolled after completing a written consent form prior to childbirth. Exclusion criteria across the studies included premature delivery (< 37 gestational weeks) and neonatal intensive care.

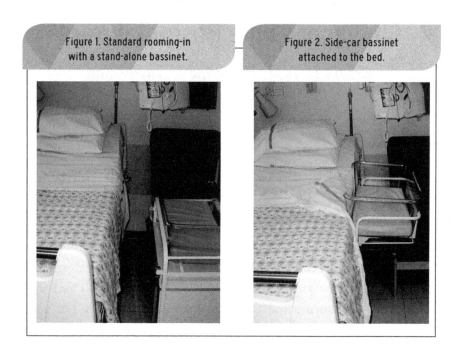

Figure 1. Standard rooming-in with a stand-alone bassinet.

Figure 2. Side-car bassinet attached to the bed.

The day after childbirth, each participant completed a semi-structured, face-to-face interview, and then a small camcorder and long-play videocassette recorder were set up. The camcorder's "night-shot" capability permitted filming in complete darkness and was mounted on a monopod clamped to the foot of the maternal bed. The videocassette recorder was housed in case positioned under the bed. Participants used the remote control to start recording once they were ready to sleep, and were requested to let the equipment record continuously for the duration of the tape. Mothers and their midwives could stop the recording at any point. Participants were encouraged to care for their infants as usual and disregard the camera. For the staff interviews, a purposive sampling strategy was employed to ensure that participants represented a range of professions. A small gratuity was offered to participants in the form of gift cards.

Analysis

A behavioral taxonomy was used with Noldus: The Observer to categorize behavioral states of mothers and infants, and the presence of midwives. Videotapes were coded from maternal sleep onset to last waking (or to the tape end, if still sleeping). The frequency and duration of behaviors were analyzed as proportions of the observation period, which ranged from 4 to 8 hours. Intra-observer reliability was assessed by recoding video segments. Interview responses were transcribed and thematically analysed through an iterative process of grouping and regrouping the data as themes became apparent.

Results

Five themes emerged: (1) maternal need for support, (2) response to infant cues, (3) negative experiences, (4) bedsharing as a way of coping, and (5) insufficient hospital staffing.

(1) Maternal Need for Support

Mothers with the stand-alone bassinet were hindered in accessing their infants while rooming-in at night. These women struggled to cope with fulfilling their infants' needs, and requesting midwifery assistance for non-medical issues made the mothers feel like a "nuisance." The majority of women who used the sidecar bassinets on the postnatal ward suggested these be the standard provision on postnatal wards. Both mothers who were assigned the sidecar bassinet, and those who allocated the stand-alone bassinet said that the sidecar makes a considerable, positive difference to mothers' postnatal ward experiences. Participant strongly emphasized the advantages of the close physical contact enabled by the sidecar bassinets.

(2) Response to Infant Cues

Postnatal ward rooming-infant arrangements had bidirectional impacts on mothers and their infants. Both mothers' responses to their infants' cues and the ability of the infants to bring their needs to their mothers' attention were impaired with the stand-alone bassinet arrangement. Mothers with the sidecar bassinets or bedsharing said that close physical contact with their infants enabled them to quickly respond to their infants and frequently offer time at the breast. The visual and physical connection also served to reassure mothers that their infants were safe and well. When women's movements were constrained after their deliveries, the mothers viewed the stand-alone bassinet as a direct impediment to their infant caretaking. Mothers allocated the stand-alone bassinet said that they were distressed about their infants suffering from impaired maternal access, which created breastfeeding challenges. The women sometimes worried whether infants could breathe when they coughed or displayed other concerning behavior. Some mothers were also anxious that their infants would disturb other dyads on the ward if they cried, and so they were tasked not only with the responsibility of newborn care, but also about keeping the peace during the night.

(3) Negative Experiences

A small proportion of women participating in the studies had infants taken out of their rooms for a period during the night. The explicit purpose of most of these separations was to enable the mother to get more sleep, without the burden of breastfeeding what one midwife described for "greedy" infants, or the perceived interruption of other caretaking behaviors. Well-meaning staff introduced the idea of non-continuous rooming-in for the mothers' wellbeing on multiple occasions. Although some women described welcoming the opportunity for the time apart from their infants, and one mother (allocated a stand-alone bassinet) said that she requested the midwives take her infant for part of the night, another mother attributed the actions by the midwifery staff as contributing to her early cessation of breastfeeding.

(4) Bedsharing as a Way of Coping

The inconvenience of the stand-alone bassinets led to many women unintentionally bedshare with their infants for sleep. One participant commented that she found it was getting "a bit silly," frequently getting in and out of bed, which was required when using the stand-alone bassinet. Women stated that when they removed their infant from the stand-alone bassinet to join them in the bed their intention was to stay awake. However, we observed several mothers who fell asleep with their infants in their arms, often on top of pillows, instead of returning them to the bassinet.

(5) Insufficient Staffing

Many women commented that care on the postnatal ward was compromised by the staff being too busy to offer them sufficient support, particularly with breastfeeding. The insufficient staffing level was not only a problem discussed by the mothers; all of the staff interviewed identified this constraint to the care they delivered. Several of the staff mentioned that the sidecar bassinet alleviated some of the demands on their time in addition to providing mothers with greater satisfaction of being able to independently meet their infants' needs. When discussing postnatal breastfeeding support, the staff lamented that although breastfeeding was high on their agenda, the reality of the postnatal ward demands meant that the time that staff devoted to infant feeding issues, and the quality the support they were able to offer, were inadequate.

Discussion

In deconstructing night-time postnatal ward interactions, we identify previously unknown or unacknowledged obstacles for new mothers and their infants, as well as the constraints on the staff involved in their care. Future steps to minimize these breastfeeding challenges on postnatal wards is important for health outcomes, the satisfaction of mothers and staff, and to better support the perinatal period for all those who are involved.

The research approach introduced in this summary enabled us to have unique insight into ways to make postnatal wards more family-friendly. The use of sidecar bassinets, having lactation support available and expected through the night, and facilitating partners to stay overnight are a few of the many protocol changes that are consistent with the 10 Steps to Successful Breastfeeding. These practices can be further examined to expand and implement evidence-based care. Our research findings suggested that projects utilizing the combination of extended, naturalistic filming and participant questioning to understand the observed behaviors are helpful for better understanding the difficulties that many new mothers experience while rooming-in on the postnatal ward. A key priority of women in our studies was their ability to respond to their infants' needs. Mothers who bedshared, or had the sidecar bassinets, were less reliant on hospital staff and reported that their overall postnatal ward experiences were greatly enhanced by access to their newborns. The stand-alone bassinet was found to be both a physical and emotional barrier between mothers and their infants.

References

Ball, H.L., Ward-Platt, M.P., Heslop, E., Leech, S.J., & Brown, K.A. 2006. Randomised trial of infant sleep location on the postnatal ward. *Archives of Disease in Childhood, 91,* 1005-1010.

Ball, H.L., Ward-Platt, M.P., Howel, D., & Russell, C. 2011. Randomised trial of sidecar crib use on breastfeeding duration (NECOT). *Archives of Disease in Childhood, 96,* 360-364.

Taylor, C.E., Tully, K.P., & Ball, H.L. (2015). Night-time on a postnatal ward: Experiences of mothers, infants, and staff. In F. Dykes &

R. Flacking (Eds.), *Ethnographic research in maternal and child health.* Abington, UK: Routledge Press.

Tully, K.P., & Ball, H.L. 2012. Postnatal unit bassinet types when rooming-in after cesarean birth: Implications for breastfeeding and infant safety. *Journal of Human Lactation, 28,* 495-505.

CHAPTER 37

Building a Better Breastfeeding Network (BBBN): Identifying IBCLC Training Needs in Florida

Erica H. Anstey, Aimee Eden, Deidre Orriola,
and Aynmarie Carter

Sub-optimal breastfeeding rates overall, and racial disparities in breastfeeding rates, in particular, are significant public health problems in the U.S. Black infants continue to have the lowest rates of breastfeeding initiation and duration when compared to White and Hispanic infants. The gap in breastfeeding initiation between Black and White infants is 19.5% (Centers for Disease Control and Prevention [CDC], 2015). However, despite these substantial disparities in breastfeeding initiation, duration, and exclusivity along racial and income-level lines, public health interventions and messaging have not succeeded in reducing these disparities (CDC, 2013, 2014a). The Maternity Practices in Infant Nutrition and Care (mPINC) survey is distributed biennially to maternity facilities to assess 10 evidence-based maternity care indicators that support breastfeeding (derived from the *Ten Steps to Successful Breastfeeding*). Studies have shown that maternity care practices have a significant effect on breastfeeding outcomes, yet hospitals located in areas with greater percentages of Black residents are significantly less likely to meet five of the 10 mPINC indicators for recommended practices that support breastfeeding (CDC, 2014a; DiGirolamo, Grummer-Strawn, & Fein, 2008; Grummer-Strawn et al., 2013).

One strategy identified in the 2011 *Surgeon General's Call to Action to Support Breastfeeding* identifies is that of creating opportunities to prepare and train more International Board Certified Lactation Consultants (IBCLCs) from racial and ethnic minority groups that are currently under-represented in the profession (U.S. Department of Health and Human Services, 2011). IBCLCs are the only health care professionals who are board-certified in lactation care, and their training includes didactic and clinical experiences that culminate in a board examination (International Board of Lactation Consultant Examiners, 2012). Studies have demonstrated that support from an IBCLC increases breastfeeding success among women in general (Bonuck, Trombley, Freeman, & McKee, 2005; Castrucci, Hoover, Lim, & Maus, 2006; Rishel & Sweeney, 2005), and those enrolled in WIC (Yun et al., 2010) and receiving Medicaid, in particular (Castrucci et al., 2006). Access to IBCLCs, however, is not equally distributed geographically or socio-demographically, which may exacerbate breast-feeding disparities.

Florida has fewer IBCLCs (2.45) per 1,000 live births than the national average (3.48), and the percent of live births at hospitals designated as "Baby-Friendly" (an international recognition of best practices in maternity care) in Florida was only 2.57, significantly below the national average of 7.79 (CDC, 2014b). These numbers mask disparities in professional lactation services between rural and urban areas, as well as IBCLC accessibility to other underserved populations, such as the un/underinsured and certain minority groups. These statistics also demonstrate a need for more IBCLCs in Florida, particularly in medically underserved areas.

Purpose

An important strategy to support breastfeeding entails creating opportunities to prepare and train IBCLCs from racial and ethnic minority groups. However, it can be difficult for individuals to access lactation education and gain clinical experience necessary to become an IBCLC. The Building a Better Breastfeeding Network (BBBN) project was a needs assessment designed, in part, to assess the demand for an academic IBCLC training program in Florida, and to get a sense of what would make such a program accessible.

Method

An online survey was administered via Qualtrics survey software. Participants were recruited through email lists and snowball sampling methods, and included undergraduate and graduate students, mother-baby nurses, members of professional and community-based mother-baby organizations, and WIC nutritionists and peer counselors. A total of 1,939 individuals from Florida met eligibility requirements (not already IBCLC and live, work, and/or attend school in Florida), and 1,668 completed the survey, though not all answered each question. Prior to beginning the survey, participants were asked to read and check a box consenting to participate. No names or other identifying information were collected. As an incentive, participants were invited to submit an email address (not linked to the survey) to enter into a raffle for a $25 gift card. The project was deemed a "community needs assessment" rather than research by our university's IRB, and, as such, did not require IRB oversight.

Survey data were exported into Microsoft Excel for analysis. Frequency distributions and descriptive statistics were completed on the entire data set. A qualitative thematic content analysis was applied to the open-ended comments. Team members read the comments and categorized them into appropriate themes.

Results

Most respondents identified as female (85% female and 5% male, though we had missing data for 10%), and the average age was 32. Most were White (70%), and others identified as Black (15%), Asian (5%), Alaska Native/American Indian (2%), and Native Hawaiian/ Pacific Islander (1%), (participants could check multiple boxes). Additionally, 17% identified as Hispanic. Many (60%) were students.

Of the 1,939 individuals who responded to the question, "If an IBCLC training program were offered through the University of South Florida, College of Public Health, would you be interested?" 61% (n=1,182) answered that they would be very interested or interested, and 25% (n=486) selected possibly interested. Another 25% were possibly interested/unsure. The 14% (n=271) who selected "not interested" did not complete the rest of the survey. Importantly, Black, Hispanic, and American Indian respondents more frequently expressed interest (over 50% of respondents in each of those groups) in an IBCLC training program than other groups (see Figure 1).

Respondents expressed interest in working in a variety of low-resource settings, such as WIC (58%) and a state or county health department (46%), as well as with underserved populations: teen moms (69%), low-income families (63%), working mothers (55%), and minority populations (53%), among others. For the didactic component of IBCLC training, participants clearly favored program formats with built-in flexibility, such as online or part-time options. Online learning was the most popular choice (74%), followed by part-time (52%), evening (39%), weekend extension (35%), and full-time (15%). Potential barriers to enrollment included cost (83%), time (55%), and travel/location (51%). Factors to facilitate enrollment included flexible class scheduling (85%), availability of scholarships (75%), and availability of financial aid (67%).

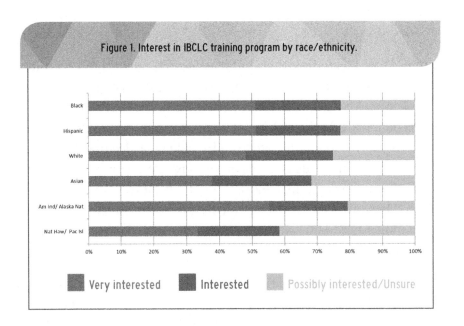

Figure 1. Interest in IBCLC training program by race/ethnicity.

Comments provided by respondents were overwhelmingly positive. A few examples of comments include:

- "I work on the postpartum unit at [X Hospital], and we are in desperate need of a program like this!"

- "This certification is an EXCELLENT opportunity for students to serve our community!"

- "These programs are needed. Not everyone that wants to study lactation wants to be a nurse. Unfortunately, until I found my current program, it seemed like that was the only way to do the things that I wanted to do. I wanted a degree in lactation, and my choices were very limited. I commend your school for pursuing this, and I am glad to help out in any way that I can."

- "Very interested in this program!! Looking forward to seeing your results implemented in a training/preparation program."

Conclusions

Eliminating racial disparities in breastfeeding rates requires a multi-dimensional approach. Providing access for more people, especially people of color and people who work with underserved populations, to become IBCLCs through an academic training program in human lactation may be one approach to addressing breastfeeding disparities. The results of this needs assessment demonstrate a strong interest in an IBCLC training program in Florida. The higher level of interest among Black, Hispanic, and American Indian respondents suggests that there is an unmet need of training opportunities available to individuals of color to become IBCLCs.

The profession of lactation consulting has been historically dominated by White women, but to address the unique cultural barriers and breastfeeding support needs of minority populations, IBCLC workforce diversification is essential. The results of this needs assessment suggest that affordability and flexibility would make an IBCLC training program more appealing and feasible for many individuals interested in becoming an IBCLC, and would potentially attract more individuals from underrepresented groups.

The need for more IBCLCs will continue to grow as public health and medical attention to breastfeeding and Baby-Friendly hospitals increases. A well-designed IBCLC training program that is responsive to the needs of future IBCLCs will address Florida's dearth of IBCLCs, including among underserved populations. A training program in Florida has the potential to draw students from across the state, thus increasing the number of IBCLCs in, and diversifying the IBCLC workforce throughout, Florida, and ultimately improving the state's breastfeeding rates and reducing breastfeeding disparities.

References

Bonuck, K. A., Trombley, M., Freeman, K., & McKee, D. (2005). Randomized, controlled trial of a prenatal and postnatal lactation consultant intervention on duration and intensity of breastfeeding up to 12 months. *Pediatrics, 116*(6), 1413-1426.

Castrucci, B. C., Hoover, K. L., Lim, S., & Maus, K. C. (2006). A comparison of breastfeeding rates in an urban birth cohort among women delivering infants at hospitals that employ and do not employ lactation consultants. *Journal of Public Health Management and Practice, 12*(6), 578-585.

Centers for Disease Control and Prevention (CDC). (2013). Progress in increasing breastfeeding and reducing racial/ethnic differences – United States, 2000-2008 births. *Morbidity and Mortality Weekly Report; 62*(5), 77-80. Retrieved from http://www.cdc.gov/mmwr/preview/mmwrhtml/mm6205a1.htm.

Centers for Disease Control and Prevention (CDC). (2014a). Racial disparities in access to maternity care practices that support breastfeeding – United States, 2011. *Morbidity and Mortality Weekly Report; 63*(33), 725-728. Retrieved from http://www.cdc.gov/mmwr/preview/mmwrhtml/mm6333a2.htm.

Centers for Disease Control and Prevention (CDC). (2014b). *Breastfeeding Report Card -- United States, 2014.* Retrieved from http://www.cdc.gov/breastfeeding/pdf/2014breastfeedingreportcard.pdf.

Centers for Disease Control and Prevention (CDC). (2015). *Nutrition, physical activity and obesity data, trends and maps website.* Atlanta, GA. Retrieved from http://www.cdc.gov/nccdphp/DNPAO/index.html.

DiGirolamo, A. M., Grummer-Strawn, L. M., & Fein, S. B. (2008). Effect of maternity-care practices on breastfeeding. *Pediatrics, 122*(Suppl 2), S43-49.

Grummer-Strawn, L. M., Shealy, K. R., Perrine, C. G., MacGowan, C., Grossniklaus, D. A., Scanlon, K. S., & Murphy, P.E. (2013). Maternity care practices that support breastfeeding CDC efforts to encourage quality improvement. *Journal of Women's Health, 22*(2), 107-112.

International Board of Lactation Consultant Examiners. (2012). *Preparing for IBCLC certification.* Retrieved from http://www.iblce.org/preparing-for-ibclc-certification.

Rishel, P. E., & Sweeney, P. (2005). Comparison of breastfeeding rates among women delivering infants in military treatment facilities with and without lactation consultants. *Military Medicine, 170*(5), 435-438.

U.S. Department of Health and Human Services. (2011). *The Surgeon General's Call to Action to Support Breastfeeding.* Washington, DC: U.S. Department of Health and Human Services, Office of the Surgeon General. Retrieved from http://www.surgeongeneral.gov/library/calls/breastfeeding/calltoactiontosupportbreastfeeding.pdf.

Yun, S., Liu, Q., Mertzlufft, K., Kruse, C., White, M., Fuller, P., & Zhu, B. P. (2010). Evaluation of the Missouri WIC (Special Supplemental Nutrition Program for Women, Infants, and Children) breast-feeding peer counselling programme. *Public Health Nutrition, 13*(2), 229-237.

Advocacy for IBCLC Care: A Toolkit for Action Based on Cost/Benefit Analysis and GIS Mapping in North Carolina

Kathryn Houk, Ellen Chetwynd,
and Catherine Sullivan

In 2012, Section 2713 of the Patient Protection and Affordable Care Act (ACA) stipulated that new insurance plans cover the cost of "Comprehensive lactation support and counseling, by a trained provider during pregnancy and/or in the postpartum period" (U.S. Department of Health and Human Services, 2012). Numerous trained providers offer lactation services, including peer counselors, physicians, nurses, and International Board Certified Lactation Consultants (IBCLCs). Since the ACA fails to define a specific provider of lactation support, interpretation of this provision differs by insurance provider, and Medicaid coverage varies based on each state's individual policies and acceptance of expansion funding. Breastfeeding advocates have been working across the country to help insurance providers understand the landscape of breastfeeding support to enable ACA policy to create consistency in the provision of optimal care.

As individual states take steps to improve equity in access to lactation services through Medicaid reimbursement, research is needed to explore the availability of lactation support services, their association with improved breastfeeding outcomes, and the cost-effectiveness of the delivery model. We conducted three integrated analyses to build the case for Medicaid reimbursement of IBCLCs, providing a model for adoption by other states seeking a consistent interpretation of the ACA to improve affordable and accessible lactation services.

Using North Carolina (NC) as a case study, we present geospatial data of IBCLC, WIC agency, and maternity center locations along with breastfeeding rates for low-income infants to explore geographic variation and workforce availability. Next, we analyze the association between these breastfeeding rates and county-level IBCLC density. Finally, we calculate a cost-benefit analysis to highlight the economic value of Medicaid reimbursement of medical lactation support services delivered by IBCLCs. While NC specifically targeted IBCLC reimbursement, this toolkit illustrates steps that can be replicated by advocacy groups across the country working to interpret the ACA lactation guidelines for any type of lactation support and counseling.

Method

Breastfeeding data from the Pediatric Nutrition Surveillance System (PedNSS) were requested from the NC Nutrition Services Branch of DPH. PedNSS is a cross-sectional study that compiles surveillance data from public health clinic visits of low-income infants and children, allowing us to explore variations in breastfeeding practices of low-income infants across the state. We used ArcMap 10.1 to map both county-level breastfeeding rates and lactation support resources in NC. We obtained de-identified zip code locations of credentialed IBCLCs from the International Board of Lactation Consultant Examiners (IBLCE). We also used publicly available 2010 county-level data from the NC State Center for Health Statistics (SCHS) (2010) to adjust the absolute number of IBCLCs to a measure of the local demand for services. Figure 1 indicates both "IBCLC hotspots," of concentrated IBCLC density and locations of maternity centers and WIC agencies across the state. Figure 2 shows regional variation in breastfeeding rates at 6 weeks, and the number of IBCLCs per 1,000 live births.

To further build the case for the inclusion of IBCLCs in the medical lactation support services reimbursement structure, we estimated the association between county-level IBCLC density and breastfeeding at 6 weeks among a population at high-risk for early breastfeeding cessation using the PedNSS and IBLCE data. Using SAS 9.4, we conducted a logistic regression to examine the association between IBCLC availability and any breastfeeding at 6 weeks among PEDNSS infants. Median IBCLC density across all counties included in this dataset was 3.7 IBCLCs per 1000 live births, so we stratified the exposure across counties with 0 IBCLCs, counties with >0 and ≤3.7 IBCLCs per 1000 live births, and counties with >3.7 per 1000.

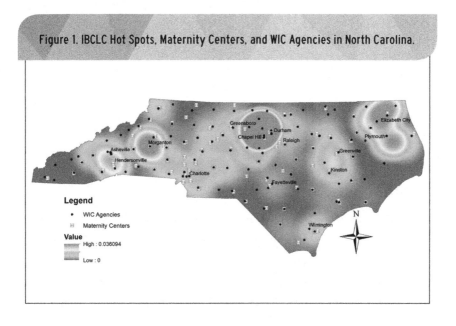

Figure 1. IBCLC Hot Spots, Maternity Centers, and WIC Agencies in North Carolina.

Finally, we performed a cost-benefit analysis to demonstrate the potential cost savings associated with reduced infant illness should the breastfeeding rates increase as might be anticipated from increasing availability of lactation support. We used the breastfeeding cost benefit methodology of Bartick and Reinhold (2010), which has also been used in Louisiana (Ma, Brewer-Asling, & Magnus, 2013), as a guide for estimating the savings associated with the impact of increased breastfeeding rates on three infant illnesses. NC birth rates, disease rates, and breastfeeding rates from the Medicaid population were used to calculate state-specific cost savings for providing lactation services.

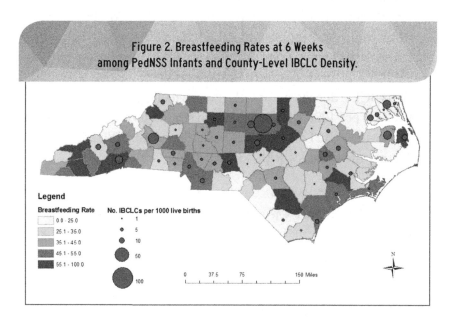

Figure 2. Breastfeeding Rates at 6 Weeks among PedNSS Infants and County-Level IBCLC Density.

Results

Figure 1 shows the distribution of "IBCLC hotspots" across the state. While hotspots appear to be most concentrated in about five regions, the distribution of warmer tones indicates that the regional availability of IBCLC services is relatively well-aligned with maternity center locations. Maternity centers and WIC agencies in regions farther from

IBCLC hotspots highlight locations where future IBCLC training should be prioritized and where other existing providers need to be included in Medicaid reimbursement policy, such as physicians and physician extenders.

Figure 2 illustrates 6-week county-level breastfeeding rates of low-income infants, and the spatial relationship between IBCLCs and other breastfeeding support services across NC. The percentage of PedNSS infants' breastfeeding at 6 weeks was lower in the eastern coastal plain and southern Piedmont counties than in the highly populated central and western counties of the state. There is a total of 574 IBCLCs available across the state, with the majority located in Orange, Mecklenberg, and Wake counties, which are the most populous in the state. Once adjusted for the number of annual births, the relationship between county-level IBCLC density and breastfeeding rates appeared most dramatic in Orange, Burke, in some of the coastal counties like Camden and Tyrrell, and in some western counties like Henderson and Haywood. While gaps in availability were observed in 47 counties, the distribution of IBCLCs indicates that these providers are generally available regionally to provide coverage across the state, supporting their inclusion in Medicaid reimbursement policy.

Table 1 presents the results of the logistic regression analysis, showing that county-level density of IBCLC services appears to be associated with increased breastfeeding prevalence at 6 weeks. As the density of IBCLCs increases, the prevalence of any breastfeeding at 6 weeks also increases. When we stratified by county urbanity, we see a trend of increasing breastfeeding rates with increasing urbanity, likely associated with more access to available IBCLC resources.

Table 1. Comparison of Crude and Stratified Prevalence Ratios of Any Breastfeeding at 6 Weeks Among North Carolina Pediatric Nutrition Surveillance System (PedNSS) Infants by County-level International Board Certified Lactation Consultant (IBCLC) Density.

		County-Level IBCLC Density*	
	0	>0 and 3.7	>3.7
Crude Prevalence Ratio (95% CI)	1.00	1.16 (1.08, 1.24)	1.20 (1.12, 1.28)
Prevalence Ratio Stratified by Percentage of County Urban (95% CI)			
52%	1.00	0.97 (0.89, 1.06)	1.10 (1.01, 1.21)
72%	1.00	1.17 (1.04, 1.31)	1.15 (1.02, 1.29)
94%	1.00	1.44 (1.22, 1.70)	1.20 (1.02, 1.41)

Finally, Table 2 presents the results of the cost-benefit analysis. Coverage of lactation support services by NC Medicaid was calculated to cost approximately $4.77 million annually. While this represents a significant expenditure, the cost savings for the three identified diseases alone would be $7.1 million, were NC breastfeeding rates to reach Healthy People 2020 targets. The overall estimated cost savings was $2.33 million.

Table 2. Results of cost/benefit analysis for coverage of lactation care by North Carolina Medicaid.

Births	n	%	Cost
North Carolina live births	119,767	--	--
Births covered by Medicaid	61,200	0.51	--
Cost: Medical Lactation Therapy			
Women on Medicaid initiating breastfeeding	48,960	0.80[1]	--
Breastfeeding women on Medicaid receiving a lactation consult	36,720	0.75[2]	--
Estimated number of lactation visits needed (Average 1.3 per woman)[3]	47,736	--	
Medicaid expenditure per visit	--	--	$100
Total Cost to NC Medicaid of Providing Lactation Care			**$4.77 Million**

Benefit: Averted Disease Cases when Breastfeeding Rates Increased from Baseline to 2020 Goals	n		Cost $ Million
Averted lower respiratory tract infections	500	--	$2.5
Averted cases of gastroenteritis	6,000	--	$2.5
Averted necrotizing enterocolitis	10	--	$2.1
Averted cases of Sudden Infant Death Syndrome	14-18	--	Negligible
Total Savings to NC Medicaid of Providing Lactation Care			**$7.10 Million**
Overall Cost Savings			**$2.33 Million**

Discussion

Our integrated analyses provide a roadmap for advocates and other state leaders to accomplish a data-informed approach to consistent implementation of the ACA lactation policy. We found that North Carolina has a good distribution of IBCLCs across the state to support Medicaid reimbursement advocacy. However, identifying some gaps in coverage led us to expand the provider list for medical lactation services and helped us to identify locations for future IBCLC recruitment targeting.

We found that breastfeeding rates among low-income infants increased as the density of IBCLC coverage increased, especially when stratified by county urbanity, supporting the importance of the availability of IBCLC services. Finally, we showed that IBCLC services are cost-effective for the Medicaid budget. The economic argument for reimbursement is an issue that we recommend all breastfeeding support advocates address in making their case to insurance providers in their respective states.

This stepwise action plan for medical lactation support service reimbursement provides a framework for states to organize resources and align interinstitutional partners toward a consistent interpretation of the lactation reimbursement stipulations of the ACA. In conclusion, we used North Carolina as a model to present a number of analyses in support of advocacy for Medicaid reimbursement of IBCLCs. While NC specifically targeted IBCLC reimbursement, these analyses can be replicated by advocacy groups across the country working toward any kind of insurance reimbursement for any type of lactation support and counseling.

References

Bartick, M., & Reinhold, A. (2010). The burden of suboptimal breastfeeding in the United States: A pediatric cost analysis. *Pediatrics, 125*(5), e1048-e1056.

Ma, P., Brewer-Asling, M., & Magnus, J.H. (2013). A case study on the economic impact of optimal breastfeeding. *Maternal and Child Health Journal, 17*(1), 9-13.

North Carolina State Center for Health Statistics. (2010). *North Carolina Vital Statistics, Volume 1.* Retrieved from http://www.schs.state.nc.us/schs/vitalstats/volume1/2010/.

U.S. Department of Health and Human Services. (2012). *Women's preventive services: required health plan coverage guidelines.* Retrieved from http://www.hrsa.gov/womensguidelines/.

CHAPTER 39

Lions, and Bottles, and Teats, Oh My! Legal Analysis: International-Code-Supportive Teaching about Bottle and Teat Use

Elizabeth C. Brooks

In 2015, the field of lactation and breastfeeding support suffers from a bit of "halo adjusting" by a vocal few who, in the name of upholding the anti-predatory-marketing mandate of the International Code of Marketing of Breastmilk Substitutes (IBFAN, n.d.), publicly and privately scold their colleagues for not sufficiently following the Code. Rather than generate better understanding of the Code, and how health workers can support breastfeeding families to meet optimal infant feeding goals, this "shame-and-blame" tactic drives health workers *away* from learning how better to uphold the Code (lest they suffer the slings and arrows of colleagues). Consider:

1. An International Board Certified Lactation Consultant (IBCLC) wrote the seminal article in 2002, "Bottle-feeding as a tool to reinforce breastfeeding" (Kassing, 2002), which was designated the *Journal of Human Lactation's* most useful article

of 2002. The author withstood several negative interactions when she taught the topic at breastfeeding conferences.

> The "nasty-grams" on conference evaluation forms were a bit hard to take. Conference attendees asked questions, and even made accusations that were definitely negative. One woman ... even accused me of killing babies (D. Kassing, personal communication, February 22, 2015).

2. Another IBCLC wrote a blog post intended for her breastfeeding family audience describing how to offer a supplement using a bottle-and-teat in a breastfeeding-supportive, baby-respecting manner (Bickford, n.d.) It was a very popular article, receiving over 4,000 hits a month (at the time of this publication) ... And yet, she notes that she "received a fair amount of flak from the lactation community when I posted my baby-led bottle-feeding article, and I was told that it's not WHO Code compliant" (F. Bickford, personal communication, February 16, 2015).

3. One IBCLC teamed with a speech language pathologist to write the first book (completed without commercial funding) exploring, from a clinical perspective, the different ways babies suck on breast versus bottle (Peterson & Harmer, 2009). The IBCLC author wrote,

> I have been told that my own website [for the book] is a Code violation. [Code section] 4.2 [says] "Such materials should not use any pictures or text which might idealize the use of breastmilk substitutes." This statement has been explained to me by people-in-the-know that any pictures of a baby on a bottle are idealizing bottle use. I have been specifically told by someone who attended one of the WHO Code trainings that they interpret online educa-

tion as both public and promotional (A. Peterson, personal communication, February 16, 2015).

The noble motives for the Code are undermined when skilled clinicians, who aim to respect a family's need or desire to use a bottle-and-teat to offer a supplement (of any kind), fear (or are) being vilified in the name of the Code. If we are to uphold breastfeeding and breast-milk-feeding as a public health imperative (IBFAN & ICDC, 2008, annotating Code's Preamble), then a discussion of how *all* members of the public may realistically and safely discuss human milk acquisition and use is warranted; this includes discussion of evidence-based information about the risks and benefits of using any breastfeeding equipment. Yet, the foregoing examples demonstrate that generally accepted professional guidance about Code-supportive teaching of bottle-and-teat use (assuming there is no actual marketing of brands or logos) has led to polarization of caregivers who seek to offer excellent evidence-based practice. My legal analysis of pertinent documents suggests that this oppositional stance is unwarranted.

Legislative History of the International Code

The International Code, adopted by resolution of the World Health Assembly in 1981, despite intense lobbying by the formula industry, was hailed as, "Perhaps the most significant international consumer protection standard of modern time" (Baumslag & Michels, 1995, p. 164). The International Code calls upon the governments of nations around the world to enact the Code, to restrict predatory marketing of bottles, teats, and breastmilk substitutes (formula or artificial baby milks, and weaning foods and juices intended to supplant breastfeeding-at-breast). Code sections and interpretation are "clarified" by World Health Assembly Resolutions approximately every two years (Sokol, 2005). The Code's underlying premise recognizes the:

> Right of every child and every pregnant and lactating woman to be adequately nourished as a means of attain-

ing and maintaining health. [B]reastfeeding forms a
unique biological and emotional basis for the health of
both mother and children [and] in view of the vulnerability of infants in the early months of life, and the risks
involved in inappropriate feeding practices [the] marketing of breastmilk substitutes requires special treatment,
which makes usual marketing practices unsuitable for
these products (IBFAN & ICDC, 2008, p. 4).

Each country must pass legislation to effectuate the Code within its
borders. Of 199 countries reporting in 2011, all elements of the International Code had been passed into law in 37 nation states; 47 had
passed many elements; 21 had passed a few elements (WHO, 2013, p.
6). The United States has *not* passed any Code-related legislation, due
in no small part to our multi-payer system of health care lacking a
centralized mandatory health care system administered and enforced
by a national public health ministry.

Nonetheless, support for the International Code is made manifest
by professional association policies and bylaws, such as those for the
International Lactation Consultant Association (ILCA; Akers, 2015),
by individual health care provider commitment, and—significantly—
by hospitals in the USA seeking designation under the Baby-Friendly
Hospital Initiative, which requires support for the breastfeeding-pro-
tective concepts underpinning the Code (Baby-Friendly USA, 2012),
and for good reason. Breastfeeding has been hailed as a public health
imperative, the biologic norm, the way simply that mammals feed their
young (IBFAN/Asia & BPNI, 2012; IBFAN & ICDC, 2012; WHO &
UNICEF, 2003).

Breastfeeding is Not Just for Breastfeeders

It offers some perspective to consider that the Code was written in
1981, before the advent of the Internet, with its websites and social
media sites that undeniably offer the preferred means of sharing and
collecting information by today's childbearing population. In 1981,

offering a bottle meant offering formula. Babies were assumed to be carried and borne by their genetic mothers, to master breastfeeding-at-breast, and to be separated for short periods (perhaps part of a day, for work or school outside the home by the mother), and to be reunited within hours to resume breastfeeding-at-breast.

But 2015 is a world where blended families, same-sex unions, adoption, surrogacy, and assisted reproductive technology mean children are being raised in families where breastfeeding is not just for breastfeeders anymore. Lactating parents may have jobs that require them to be separated for days or weeks from their children. It is paternalistic by the health care providers (HCPs), and disempowering to the parents and caregivers looking after these children, for HCPs to gate-keep information about safe and baby-respective bottle-and-teat use. To deny families access to pertinent information means they will turn to commercial marketers for their teaching—precisely what the Code hoped to curtail. It denies families the dignity of making a fully informed decision on all aspects of childcare, including how best to offer supplements to a young child.

Interpreting and Enforcing the Code

To reiterate: there is no ultimate international legal authority empowered to enforce the model document as passed in 1981. In the absence of legislation or regulation within a country, and precedent-setting interpretation of such legal authority, Code supporters are left to interpret the Code's language and intent on their own, and to so interpret with no sanction for failure to do so accurately.

Alternatively, they can seek guidance from the recognized Code-monitoring and reporting organizations, such as the International Code Documentation Centre (ICDC), International Baby Food Action Network (IBFAN), the National Alliance for Breastfeeding Advocacy (NABA) in the USA, and Baby Milk Action in the UK. But these are the very organizations whose mission it is to promote, support, and help enact the Code. That mission seeks as broad an application and interpretation of the Code's language as possible. The groups wear their advocacy on their sleeves, and serve an enormously important role in doing so. But it does raise a legitimate query as to whether these same organizations can *impartially* interpret elements of the Code. Unlike a traditional court of law with no vested outcome in a case, the triers-of-fact here are incredibly invested in the outcome—that is, in how the Code is held out, and upheld, worldwide. The following points about Code interpretation are important areas for discussion.

(1) Teaching about Bottle Use: One-to-One is Preferred, But Not Required.

The Code itself is vague about one-on-one teaching. Article 6 covers "health care systems," but clearly Article 6.5 is referring to the use of formula:

> 6.5 *Feeding with infant formula*, whether manufactured or home prepared, should be *demonstrated only by health workers*, or other community workers if necessary; and *only to the mothers or family members who need to use it*; and the information given should include a clear explanation of the hazards of improper use (IBFAN, n.d., emphasis added).

Even ICDC concedes that Article 6.5 does not clearly cover (or curtail) the teaching of bottle use, saying:

> [We have] discussed your question regarding the interpretation of Art 6.5 with ... our legal advisor and we agreed that ... there ARE no clear answers. Of course, the article was principally written to stop [formula] companies from teaching groups of mothers, which was a regular occurrence before the Code. Ideally, any teaching about formula feeding should be done

one-to-one. [Art 6.5] does not say anything about bottle- feeding ... So, I see no legal problem for teaching about safe use of a bottle-and-teat (A. Allain, personal communication, February 25, 2015, emphasis in bold added).

(2) Use of "Idealized Images" Does Not Automatically Exclude Babies with Bottles.

The Code refers to "idealized images" in just two sections: Article 4, which covers "information and education," and Article 9, about "labelling." Specifically:

4.2 Informational and educational materials, whether written, audio, or visual, dealing with the feeding of infants and intended to reach pregnant women and mothers of infants and young children, should include clear information on all the following points:

1. the benefits and superiority of breastfeeding;

2. maternal nutrition, and the preparation for and maintenance of breastfeeding;

3. the negative effect on breastfeeding of introducing partial bottle-feeding;

4. the difficulty of reversing the decision not to breastfeed; and

5. where needed, the proper use of infant formula, whether manufactured industrially or home prepared.

When such materials contain information about the use of infant formula, they should include the social and financial implications of its use; the health hazards of inappropriate foods or feeding methods; and, in particular, the health hazards of unnecessary or improper use of infant formula and other breastmilk substitutes. *Such materials should not use any pictures or text which may idealise the use of breastmilk substitutes.* (IBFAN, n.d., emphasis added).

9.2 Manufacturers and distributors of *infant formula* ... *Neither the container nor the label should have pictures of infants, nor should they have other pictures or text which may idealise the use of infant formula.* They may, however, have graphics for easy identification of the product as a breastmilk substitute, and for illustrating methods of preparation... (IBFAN, n.d., emphasis added).

Again, the language here is focused on images and teaching associated with *formula use*. And again, ICDC agrees:

Article 9.2 applies only to infant formula. [T]he phrase "should not contain pictures or text which may idealise the use of infant formula" in Article 9.2 is intended to prevent consumers from being misled into believing that bottle-feeding may be equivalent or superior to breastmilk (IBFAN & ICDC, 2008, pp. 23-24, emphasis added).

(3) Return to the underlying legal premise.

Thus, we have no clear direction from the model Code language about bottle teaching and images. There is no legislation or case law to provide legal interpretation here in the USA, and we have ambiguous guidance from the international organizations vested with authority to interpret, monitor, and promote the International Code. Perhaps it is no wonder that some self-taught Code experts have taken it upon themselves to pass judgment on their colleagues; it is simply their wont. It is unfortunate that the end result is to make HCPs leery of being shamed-and-blamed should they seek to teach a family, or offer a website article with lots of images, about safe and baby-respective bottle-and-teat use.

This writer, admittedly also self-taught on Code matters, suggests another analytical approach, and one long-revered by courts under the rule of law, when they are asked to interpret legislative text and intent. When there is ambiguity in legal language, insight is found by examining the legislators' original objectives when passing the law. What were the lawmakers trying to do?

Thus, we know, "The *intent of the Code is to protect babies, mothers and health professionals from inappropriate marketing* of breastmilk substitutes, feeding bottles and teats. It seeks to eliminate man-made obstacles to breastfeeding which result from *direct and indirect promotion of these products*" (IBFAN & ICDC, 2009, p. 6, emphasis added) and "aims to ensure that unbiased information about infant feeding is available *so that parents can make infant feeding decisions free of commercial influence*" (IBFAN & ICDC, 2008, p. 8, emphasis added).

We know the 2003 *Global Strategy on Infant and Young Child Feeding* continues the theme of breastfeeding as a public health imperative, stating "35. Governments, international organizations and other concerned parties share responsibility for ensuring the fulfillment of *the right of children to the highest attainable standard of health and the right of women to full and unbiased information*" (WHO & UNICEF, 2003, p. 19, emphasis added).

Thus,

- If breastfeeding/breastmilk-feeding are a universal public health imperative, and

- If the Code is intended to prevent predatory marketing of certain products to vulnerable families, and

- If the Code is intended to prevent commercial conflicts-of-interest by health workers and health care providers, and

- If an important public health objective is to avoid use of breast-milk substitutes (formula, or too-soon-complements) using delivery systems that can be unsanitary (bottles-and-teats), and

- If family-centric support improves breastfeeding self-efficacy, and

- Families are entitled, by right, to fully informed decision-making about feeding decisions and health care,

Then,

- We need to stop nit-picking elements of the Code, read in isolation of its larger intent to prevent predatory marketing,

- Especially when the Code is being discussed by proponents and HCPs as a model document, and not being interpreted by the legal system in a country that has passed Code-related legislation.

It is simply not in keeping with the needs and questions of 21st century families to assume that any-and-all bottle-and-teat use is equivalent to formula use. Even if formula is being used, families are entitled to a fully informed discussion, with a trusted HCP, about the use of all feeding equipment, including safe and sanitary use of bottles-and-teats. So long as brands as logos of Code-covered products are not displayed (offering implied endorsement of the product), HCPs should feel comfortable teaching about baby-led bottle use to any family, even on Internet-based venues, and even using images of babies sucking from bottles.

References

Akers, L. (2015, March 31). *Ethical leadership: Meeting obligations under the international code* [Blog post]. Retrieved from http://lactationmatters.org/2015/03/31/ethical-leadership-meeting-obligations-under-the-international-code/

Baby-Friendly USA. (2012). *Baby-friendly hospital initiative.* Retrieved from https://www.babyfriendlyusa.org/about-us/baby-friendly-hospital-initiative

Baumslag, N., & Michels, D. (1995). *Milk, money and madness: The culture and politics of breastfeeding.* Westport, CT: Bergin & Garvey.

Bickford, F. (n.d.). *Baby-led bottle feeding.* Retrieved from http://blog.nurturedchild.ca/index.php/pumping-bottle-feeding/bottle-feeding/

International Baby Food Action Network. (n.d.). *The full Code and WHA resolutions.* Retrieved from http://ibfan.org/the-full-code

International Baby Food Action Network, & International Code Documentation Centre. (2008). *Code essentials 1: Annotated International Code of Marketing of Breastmilk Substitutes and subsequent WHA resolutions* (Report No. 1). Penang, Malaysia: International Baby Food Action Network and International Code Documentation Centre. Available at http://www.ibfan-icdc.org/index.php/publications/publications-for-sale.

International Baby Food Action Network, & International Code Documentation Centre. (2009). *Code essentials 3: Responsibilities of health workers under the International Code of Marketing of Breastmilk Substitutes and subsequent WHA resolutions* (Report No. 3). Penang, Malaysia: International Baby Food Action Network and International Code Documentation Centre. Available at http://www.ibfan-icdc.org/index.php/publications/publications-for-sale.

International Baby Food Action Network, & International Code Documentation Centre. (2012). *Code essentials 4: Complying with the International Code of Marketing of Breastmilk Substitutes and subsequent WHA resolutions* (Report No. 4). Penang, Malaysia: International Baby Food Action Network and International Code Documentation Centre. Available at http://www.ibfan-icdc.org/index.php/publications/publications-for-sale.

International Baby Food Action Network (IBFAN)-Asia, & Breastfeeding Promotion Network of India (BPNI). (2012, December). *Babies need mom-made not man-made.* Paper presented at The 2012 World Breastfeeding Conference Declaration and Call to Action, New Delhi, India. Retrieved from http://International Baby Food Action Network (IBFAN)-Asia/ Breastfeeding Promotion Network of India (BPNI).

Kassing, D. (2002). Bottle-feeding as a tool to reinforce breastfeeding. *Journal of Human Lactation, 18*(1), 56-60.

Peterson, A., & Harmer, M. (2009). *Balancing breast & bottle: Reaching your breastfeeding goals.* Amarillo, TX: Hale Publishing.

Sokol, E. (2005). *The Code handbook: A guide to implementing the International Code of Marketing of Breastmilk Substitutes* (2d Ed.). Penang, Malaysia: International Code Documentation Centre.

World Health Organization. (n.d.). *The full Code and subsequent WHA resolutions.* Retrieved from http://ibfan.org/the-full-code

World Health Organization. (2013). *Country implementation of the International Code of Marketing of Breastmilk Substitutes: Status report 2011.* Retrieved from http://apps.who.int/iris/bitstream/10665/85621/1/9789241505987_eng.pdf

World Health Organization, & UNICEF. (2003). *Global strategy for infant and young child feeding.* Geneva, Switzerland: World Health Organization. Retrieved from http://www.who.int/nutrition/publications/infantfeeding/9241562218/en/

Opening More than a Cervix: Viewing Childbirth from Multiple Perspectives

Deborah McCarter-Spaulding

A liberal arts education is considered to be foundational for the development of critical thinking and sensitivity to the complex cultural, political, and socioeconomic influences on contemporary life and work. As a nursing professor, the value of interdisciplinary discourse became ever more vivid to me by my experience in participating in several Breastfeeding and Feminism International Conferences, including writing a chapter for the text, *Beyond health, beyond choice: Breastfeeding constraints and realities* (Smith, Hausman, & Labbok, 2012), which grew out of such conversation. The intellectual stimulation, joy of discovery, and expanding understanding of breastfeeding from many perspectives inspired me to offer an elective course on childbirth, known as *Born in the USA: Childbirth from multiple perspectives.* The purpose of this presentation is to share experiences, and reflect on the value of a course such as this for undergraduates of varied disciplines.

Childbirth is a universal life event, and many diverse factors influence perceptions, experiences and birth outcomes. In the maternity course for nursing students, there is little opportunity to consider how ideas about birth have been shaped and formed from a social, cultural and family context, and no opportunity to consider influences or assumptions with students from other majors. My goal for the course was to provide an opportunity for students from any discipline to explore the phenomenon of childbirth as it is situated and experienced in the United States today. I was particularly eager to give space for them to recognize and perhaps challenge assumptions, and to begin to articulate their own values and opinions.

Course Learning Objectives

- Identify the most significant areas of reading and discussion.
- Identify the historical framework in which birth is situated today.
- Describe health policy issues related to birth (e.g., access to care, racial/ethnic disparities, political influences).
- Describe health care issues related to birth (e.g., care providers and place of birth, birth- related interventions, anesthesia, use of technology).
- Identify influences of the women's health movement and feminist thinking on current thought about childbirth.
- Articulate values and assumptions related to childbirth (e.g., importance of fertility, meaning of family and parenthood, management of pain in birth, autonomy/control in health care, infant feeding choice).
- Identify what values are expressed in media portrayal of childbirth.
- Describe how childbirth is viewed in the theological context of the Bible.
- Engage in written and oral discussion about their own thoughts, feelings, and values related to birth, and their re-

sponse to varying perspectives from the material presented in class and assigned readings.

- Identify a topic of interest related to childbearing, and present a written and oral synthesis of differing viewpoints or perspectives, as well as personal opinion. (Note: This ended up being a book review of a text about birth.)

Based on journals and course evaluations, students were challenged by the format of the course, which minimized lecture, and encouraged reading, discussion with peers online, and in the classroom, and readings outside of their own discipline. Although designed to be interdisciplinary in nature, only one student from a major outside of nursing enrolled. Most likely, no prior elective taught by a nursing professor had ever been open to other students, and all identified as women. Some students had studied maternity nursing, and others had not. Only one assignment (the final exam) gave a grade based on a "correct" answer; all others were assessed based on evidence of interacting with and articulating diverse ideas in the literature, and active, thoughtful participation in discussion both online and in class.

Through initial reflective journals, it became clear that one common assumption about birth was that it was frequently scary and painful, but also something miraculous, valuable, and personally fulfilling. These views led many students to see hospital birth, and technological interventions as vital to safe birth. Midwifery, home births, and Caesarean section rates in the United States were new concepts for them, and attitudes changed over the semester about pain management and the possible role of a midwife in low-risk births. Historical perspectives on anesthesia, place of birth, role of health care providers, science and technology, and motherhood/fertility, in general, allowed students to see the development of current thoughts and values about birth.

Various feminist perspectives were addressed, and how ideas such as motherhood, fertility, sexuality, birth options, science, and technology might be viewed through a feminist lens were topics of discussion. All students felt the class met the learning objective of understanding how the women's health movement and feminism influence current thought about birth, and many reported gaining new insights and perspectives.

Overwhelmingly, students found guest panel presentations to be enjoyable and thought provoking. The first panel consisted of health care providers (midwives and physicians), and students developed questions for the panel to address. The second panel included three couples with experiences related to fertility, including a lesbian couples' path to parenthood, and a gestational carrier and her husband's experience of carrying a child for close friends who could not conceive. Students reported that they wished they had been able to spend more time in these classes.

Other classes that inspired students included a guest lecture from the psychology department on gender and parenting, and another from the politics department on health policy related to pregnancy, maternity health care coverage, and maternity leave. Readings before the guest lectures and time for discussion in the class following the guests allowed students to explore topics in greater depth, and gain insight into how different disciplines address the topic of birth and parenthood (see Table 1 for list of course readings and materials).

Discussion posts online provided opportunity/motivation for students who were reticent to share their thoughts in class to engage in discussion with peers. Reflective journals were also used to allow students to consider how their thinking was evolving during class, and to explore any issues that raised questions or concerns. These journals were extremely helpful in monitoring student understanding of concepts presented, allowing for modification of content to clarify concepts. For example, the complex relationship of education to socioeconomic status, and to health outcomes.

Students worked in groups to read and present summaries of four books related to birth, which gave them the opportunity to learn about ecology, economics, racial history, and pain in childbirth and to share their thoughts in a class presentation, and to connect ideas from the book with class content through an individually written book review.

Table 1. Readings and Materials for Class

- Amnesty International. (2010). *Deadly delivery: The maternal health care crisis in the USA Summary.* New York.
- Apple, R. D. (1995). Constructing mothers: Scientific motherhood in the nineteenth and twentieth centuries. *Social History of Medicine, 8*(2), 161-178. doi: 10.1093/shm/8.2.161
- Arbour, M. W., Corwin, E. J., Salsberry, P. J., & Atkins, M. (2012). Racial differences in the health of childbearing-aged women. *MCN: The American Journal of Maternal Child Nursing, 37*(4), 13-20. doi: 10.1097/NMC.0b013e31824b544e
- Chabat, A. (Producer). (2010). *Babies.* [Documentary]
- Davis-Floyd, R. (1986). Belief systems about birth: The technocratic, wholistic, and natural models. In *Birth as an American rite of passage* (pp.154-186). Berkeley,CA: University of California Press.
- Epstein, A. (2008). *The business of being born* [Film]. USA: Barranca Productions.
- Ford, L. E. (2011). Two paths to equality. In *Women and politics: The pursuit of equality* (pp. 1-29). Boston: Wadsworth.
- Foss, K.A. (2013). "That's not a beer bong, It's a breast pump!" Representations of breastfeeding in prime-time fictional television. *Health Communication, 28*(4), 329-340. doi: 10.1080/10410236.2012.685692
- Lucas, J. C., & McCarter-Spaulding, D. (2012). Working out work: Race, employment and public policy (pp. 144-156). In P. H. Smith, B. L. Hausman, & M. Labbok (Eds.), *Beyond health: Beyond choice.* New Brunswick, NJ: Rutgers University Press.
- Malacrida, C., & Boulton, T. (2012). Women's perceptions of childbirth "choices": Competing discourses of motherhood, sexuality, and selflessness. *Gender and Society, 26,* 748-772. doi: 10.1177/0891243212452630
- Martin, K. A. (2003). Giving birth like a girl. *Gender and Society, 17*(1), 54-72. doi: 10.1177/0891243202238978
- Rothman, B. K. (2000). Recreating motherhood: Toward feminist social policy. In *Recreating motherhood* (pp. 193-205). New Brunswick, New Jersey: Rutgers University Press.
- Scholten, C. M. (1985). *Childbearing in American society, 1650-1850.* New York: New York University Press.
- Schwartz, M. J. (2006). *Birthing a slave: Motherhood and medicine in the antebellum South.* Cambridge: Harvard University Press.
- Smith, P. H., Hausman, B. L., & Labbok, M. (Eds.). (2012). *Beyond health, beyond choice: Breastfeeding constraints and realities.* New Brunswick, NJ: Rutgers University Press.
- Spar, D. (2006). *The baby business: How money, science and politics drive the commerce of conception.* Boston: Harvard Business School Publishing.
- Steingraber, S. (2001). *Having Faith: An ecologist's journey to motherhood.* New York: The Berkeley Publishing Group.
- Wolf, J. H. (2009). *Deliver me from pain: Anesthesia and birth in America.* Baltimore: The Johns Hopkins University Press.

All students reported that they would recommend the course be offered again, and that it would be of value to students from all majors. Participants at Breastfeeding and Feminism 2015 agreed and made suggestions for content and resources.

References

Amnesty International. (2010). *Deadly delivery: The maternal health care crisis in the USA Summary*. New York.

Apple, R.D. (1995). Constructing mothers: Scientific motherhood in the nineteenth and twentieth centuries. *Social History of Medicine, 8*(2), 161-178. doi: 10.1093/shm/8.2.161.

Arbour, M. W., Corwin, E. J., Salsberry, P. J., & Atkins, M. (2012). Racial differences in the health of childbearing-aged women. *MCN: The American Journal of Maternal Child Nursing, 37*(4), 13-20. doi: 10.1097/NMC.0b013e31824b544e.

Chabat, A. (Producer). (2010). *Babies*. [Documentary].

Davis-Floyd, R. (1986). Belief systems about birth: The technocratic, wholistic, and natural models. In *Birth as an American rite of passage* (pp.154-186). Berkeley, CA: University of California Press.

Epstein, A. (2008). *The business of being born* [Film]. USA: Barranca Productions.

Ford, L. E. (2011). Two paths to equality. In *Women and politics: The pursuit of equality* (pp. 1-29). Boston: Wadsworth.

Foss, K. A. (2013). "That's not a beer bong, It's a breast pump!" Representations of breastfeeding in prime-time fictional television. *Health Communication, 28*(4), 329-340. doi: 10.1080/10410236.2012.685692.

Lucas, J. C., & McCarter-Spaulding, D. (2012). Working out work: Race, employment and public policy (pp. 144-156). In P. H. Smith, B. L. Hausman, & M. Labbok (Eds.), *Beyond health: Beyond choice*. New Brunswick, NJ: Rutgers University Press.

Malacrida, C., & Boulton, T. (2012). Women's perceptions of childbirth "choices": Competing discourses of motherhood, sexuality, and selflessness. *Gender and Society, 26*, 748-772. doi: 10.1177/0891243212452630.

Martin, K. A. (2003). Giving birth like a girl. *Gender and Society, 17*(1), 54-72. doi: 10.1177/0891243202238978.

Rothman, B. K. (2000). Recreating motherhood: Toward feminist social policy. In *Recreating Motherhood* (pp. 193-205). New Brunswick, New Jersey: Rutgers University Press.

Scholten, C. M. (1985). *Childbearing in American society 1650-1850.* New York: New York University Press.

Schwartz, M. J. (2006). *Birthing a slave: Motherhood and medicine in the antebellum South.* Cambridge, MA: Harvard University Press.

Smith, P. H., Hausman, B. L., & Labbok, M. (Eds.). (2012). *Beyond health, beyond choice: Breastfeeding constraints and realities.* New Brunswick, NJ: Rutgers University Press.

Spar, D. (2006). *The baby business: How money, science and politics drive the commerce of conception.* Boston: Harvard Business School Publishing.

Steingraber, S. (2001). *Having Faith: An ecologist's journey to motherhood.* New York: The Berkeley Publishing Group.

Wolf, J. H. (2009). *Deliver me from pain: Anesthesia and birth in America.* Baltimore: The Johns Hopkins University Press.

CHAPTER 41

Knowledge and Use of Herbal Galactagogues among Health Care Providers and Breastfeeding Mothers in the U.S.

Catherine Palmer and Aunchalee Palmquist

Herbal galactagogues are plants that are used for the purpose of increasing the production of breastmilk. They are among the many plant-based medicines used to support peripartum health found cross-culturally, historically, and in the present day. Such practices reflect the biocultural context of lactation in human evolution, and provide a foundation for understanding their importance in contemporary breastfeeding practices. The nearly universal presence of herbal galactagogues in medical systems practiced around the world reflects a shared concern with breastmilk production, as well as the wide variation in lactation between individuals, even in contexts where breastfeeding is a cultural norm.

Breastfeeding mothers across the world use plant-based galactagogues. In industrialized societies, they are typically purchased over the counter in the form of dried herbal capsules, teas, and tinctures, and have grown popular among breastfeeding mothers attempting to increase the volume of milk they can produce. Sim Hattingh, Sherriff, and Tee (2014) conducted semi-structured, in-depth interviews with 20 breastfeeding women in Australia, and found that most women used herbal galactagogues due to a perceived insufficient milk supply. Additionally, the researchers found that their participants displayed a great determination to breastfeed, and asserted that they would be willing to try anything that could help them breastfeeding. The ability to breastfeed with the use of herbal galactagogues produced a sense of self-empowerment, and an increase in confidence for many women. Similar findings were recorded for the United States, where use of plant-based therapies, and other complementary and alternative medicines during pregnancy and lactation were associated with women's desire to have greater personal control over their own health and well-being (Low Dog, 2009).

The specialized knowledge and use of plant-based lactogens has historically been the domain of women, particularly midwives and experienced breastfeeding mothers. Increasingly, however, use of herbal galactagogues to influence lactation is conceptualized as a "risk behavior" in biomedicine (Academy Of Breastfeeding Medicine Protocol Committee, 2011; Amer, Cipriano, Venci, & Gandhi, 2015; Budzynska, Gardner, Low Dog, & Gardiner, 2013; Sachs et al., 2013; Zuppa et al., 2010). Taking an over the counter herbal supplement is a contraindication to donating milk to a Human Milk Banking Association of North American milk bank (Updegrove, 2013). A major reason for biomedical anxieties around herbal galactagogue use is that the physiological mechanisms by which plants influence human lactation, and their impact on infant health, are not well-described in the biomedical literature (Budzynska, Gardner, Dugoua, Low Dog, & Gardiner, 2012; Forinash, Yancey, Barnes, & Myles, 2012; Mortel & Mehta, 2013; Sim et al., 2014).

The purpose of this exploratory study was to collect information on the perceptions and use of plant-based galactagogues among breastfeeding mothers and perspectives of health providers who oversee lactation support as well as lay community breastfeeding support persons.

Method

Following ethics approval from the Elon University Institutional Review Board, a link to an anonymous self-selecting open-access online survey was distributed via email, public Facebook pages, private breastfeeding Facebook groups, and Twitter. An incentive for completing the survey was offered. Respondents were eligible for the survey if they were at least 18 years of age or older, had personal breastfeeding experience, and/or were a health care professional (HCP) or other lay community breastfeeding support (CBS) person. Data were collected between February-May 2015 and were analyzed in Microsoft Excel.

Preliminary Results

Respondents included 130 breastfeeding mothers, and 106 HCP or lay CBS persons. Respondents primarily self-identified as Caucasian, reported an average income bracket of $100,001-$150,000, and had at least a college degree.

A majority of breastfeeding mothers (68%, 87/128) reported experiencing low milk supply. Of those who reported low milk supply, only 57% (50/87) indicated that they were told they had low milk supply by a HCP. Seventy-four percent (95/128) of breastfeeding mothers reported having ever used herbal galactagogues while breastfeeding. Seventy-seven percent (92/199) indicated they knew someone who was using herbal galactagogues while breastfeeding. The frequency of herbal galactagogues use was always (21%, 20/94), quite often (28%, 26/94), and sometimes (33%, 35/94) and rarely (16%, 15/94). However, only 49% (46/94) of these respondents indicated that herbal galactagogues significantly increased their milk supply. Of the respondents who reported using herbal galactagogues, 62% (59/95) agreed that using galactagogues while breastfeeding made them feel more confident in their breastmilk supply.

The most common sign of low milk supply that mothers identified was a failure to express as much milk as they perceived their babies needed. Respondents also commonly selected the following options as important signs that they used to determine that they had low milk supply: the "baby had slow weight gain," "I did not make as much milk as I expected," and the "baby was fussy at the breast." Fenugreek was by far the most commonly used herbal galactagogue, followed by Mother's Milk brand teas, and blessed thistle. Breastfeeding mothers rated doulas, lactation consultants, midwives, and peer breastfeeding counselors as the most knowledgeable about the proper use, safety, and effectiveness of galactagogues, while they rated family practice physicians, nurses, OB/GYN, and pediatricians as the least knowledgeable. They reported relatively higher rates of a HCP encouraging them to use a galactaogue than rates of HCP discouraging galactagogue use. Thirty-six percent (44/121) respondents agreed with the statement herbal galactagogues were safer then pharmaceutical ones, compared with 9% (11/21) who disagreed, and 55% (66/121) who neither agreed nor disagreed.

Respondents who were HCP were primarily doulas, lactation consultants, a family practice physician, midwives, nurses, and pediatricians. No obstetricians/gynecologists completed the survey. CBS persons included La Leche League leaders, peer breastfeeding counselors, and other types of lay CBS persons. Seventy-five percent (78/104) of HCP/CBS indicated that they recommended herbal galactagogues as a response to low milk supply. Sixty-three percent of HCP/CBS (56/89) reported ever using herbal galactagogues themselves. A majority (67%, 67/100) of HCP/CBS believed they were knowledgeable about herbal galactagogues. Seventy-seven percent of HCP/CBS felt confident about their ability to effectively manage low milk supply in a breastfeeding dyad. Seventy-eight percent (78/100) of HCP/CBS indicated they agreed that herbal galactagogues may help to increase milk supply. Forty-four percent (44/100) agreed that herbal galactagogues were safer than pharmaceutical ones, compared with 17% (17/100) who disagreed, and 39% (39/100) who neither agreed or disagreed.

All health care providers expressed concern regarding potential negative side effects of herbal galactagogues. The most common concern was regarding the quality of the herbs used. A total of 94% of health care providers and lay breastfeeding support persons indicated that they would support greater use of herbal galactagogues in breastfeeding if there were a greater evidence-base supporting their safety. Health care providers did not have a unanimous opinion on the efficacy of herbal galactagogues. In their open-ended responses, many expressed that a "cookie cutter approach" to use galactagogues often does not reflect women's individual needs. Many providers stated that the efficacy of a galactagogue depends on the individual mother and her medical background, and that they could not draw general conclusions about herbal galactagogues. HCP/CBS indicated that they were asked to provide information about herbal galactagogues relatively more frequently (82%, 81/99) than rarely/never (18%, 18/99).

Discussion

Our preliminary findings show that low milk supply is a common breastfeeding concern, and that herbal galactagogues are widely used to support lactation by breastfeeding mothers and HCP/CBS. There is discordance between mothers' perceptions of low milk supply and diagnosis of low milk supply by a health care provider. The signs that mothers interpret low milk production are informative, and they illustrate that perceived lactation difficulties are not simply constructed based on volume of milk, but also on infant responses to breastfeeding. Mothers' expectations regarding typical milk production, and measures of expressed breastmilk, may play a significant role in perceived low milk supply and mothers' decision to use herbal galactagogues.

Both breastfeeding mothers and health care providers perceive that herbal galactagogues may increase lactation. Most HCP are confident in their ability to manage low milk supply, and feel knowledgeable about herbal galactagogues. However, breastfeeding mothers' perceptions about HCP knowledge indicates that there are biases in the type of HCP they perceive to have such knowledge. These perceptions may influence the extent to which mothers seek out professional advice when considering the use of herbal galactagogues.

Breastfeeding mothers and HCP/CBS shared concern about possible side effects, and concern about the quality of commercially available herbal galactagogues, yet these were perceived as relatively safe as compared to prescription pharmaceuticals. HCP/CBS are concerned about how to prescribe and use galactagogues. This study highlights the importance for further research on galactagogue use and their bioactive ingredients, as well as the everyday circumstances and experiences with breastfeeding that shape decisions to use herbal galactagogues.

References

Academy of Breastfeeding Medicine Protocol Committee. (2011). ABM Clinical Protocol #9: Use of galactogogues in initiating or augmenting the rate of maternal milk secretion (First Revision January 2011). *Breastfeeding Medicine, 6*(1), 41–49.

Amer, M. R., Cipriano, G. C., Venci, J. V., & Gandhi, M. A. (2015). Safety of popular herbal supplements in lactating women. *Journal of Human Lactation,* [epub ahead of print] http://doi.org/10.1177/0890334415580580.

Budzynska, K., Gardner, Z. E., Dugoua, J.-J., Low Dog, T., & Gardiner, P. (2012). Systematic review of breastfeeding and herbs. *Breastfeeding Medicine, 7*(6), 489–503.

Budzynska, K., Gardner, Z. E., Low Dog, T., & Gardiner, P. (2013). Complementary, holistic, and integrative medicine: advice for clinicians on herbs and breastfeeding. *Pediatrics in Review, 34*(8), 343–352; quiz 352–353.

Forinash, A. B., Yancey, A. M., Barnes, K. N., & Myles, T. D. (2012). The use of galactogogues in the breastfeeding mother. *The Annals of Pharmacotherapy, 46*(10), 1392–1404.

Low Dog, T. (2009). The use of botanicals during pregnancy and lactation. *Alternative Therapies in Health and Medicine, 15*(1), 54–58.

Mortel, M., & Mehta, S. D. (2013). Systematic review of the efficacy of herbal galactogogues. *Journal of Human Lactation, 29*(2), 154–162

Sachs, H. C., Frattarelli, D. A. C., Galinkin, J. L., Green, T. P., Johnson, T., Neville, K., … & Anker, J. V. (2013). The transfer of drugs and therapeutics into human breastmilk: An update on selected topics. *Pediatrics, 132*(3), e796–e809.

Sim, T. F., Hattingh, H. L., Sherriff, J., & Tee, L. B. (2014). Perspectives and attitudes of breastfeeding women using herbal galactagogues during breastfeeding: A qualitative study. *BMC Complementary and Alternative Medicine, 14*(1), 216.

Updegrove, K. H. (2013). Nonprofit human milk banking in the United States. *Journal of Midwifery & Women's Health, 58*(5), 1542–2011.

Zuppa, A. A., Sindico, P., Orchi, C., Carducci, C., Cardiello, V., & Romagnoli, C. (2010). Safety and efficacy of galactogogues: Substances that induce, maintain, and increase breastmilk production. *Journal of Pharmacy & Pharmaceutical Sciences: A Publication of the Canadian Society for Pharmaceutical Sciences, 13*(2), 162–174.

CHAPTER 42

The Breastfeeding Woman: Who Are Breastfeeding Books Really For?

Hannah Luedtke

Breastfeeding education takes place in a variety of venues. Through books, workshops, classes, one-on-one discussions, and websites, women are told why and how to breastfeed. One of the most long-standing and slow-changing educational venues are books on breastfeeding. Written by a variety of individuals and organizations, each book on breastfeeding takes a slightly different approach to the topic. Although they all have a similar goal in convincing the reader that breastfeeding is the best choice, and assisting the readers to successfully breastfeed, the differing approaches the authors bring to the topics may provide women with the option of deciding which book would best suit their needs.

Analysis of the content of a few specific books may provide an idea of which women may be highlighted or excluded from breastfeeding education and conversations can be gained. The groups that may be highlighted or excluded, in turn, affect the social perceptions of breastfeeding. How do these books directly and indirectly exclude certain populations from breastfeeding education? In order to look more closely at this question, I looked at the infant feeding practices, discussions of biology, and personal/social contexts presented in these books.

The books chosen for this project are *The Womanly Art of Breastfeeding* 8th ed. by Diane Wiessinger, Diana West, and Teresa Pitman, *Breastfeeding Made Simple* 2nd ed. by Nancy Mohrbacher and Kathleen Kendall-Tackett, *The Nursing Mother's Companion* 6th ed. by Kathleen Huggins, and *Ina May's Guide to Breastfeeding* by Ina May Gaskin.

Are these books reaching the mothers the authors had hoped they would? The sections will all come together to create a picture of who is assumed to be the breastfeeding mother. What changes could be made to any of these books or to breastfeeding education strategies to make breastfeeding education more accessible to all mothers? How inclusive are these four breastfeeding books in addressing all mothers interested in reading about breastfeeding? Moreover, what does this image of the breastfeeding mother say about the social messages of breastfeeding education? What are the consequences of excluding certain mothers from who is valued enough to receive breastfeeding assistance? What does this, in turn, say about how the children of those women are valued?

In addition, how does (the lack of) addressing contextual issues in breastfeeding education affect larger issues of women's status? Why does it matter if these books address pumping, being away from your baby, partner involvement, or societal response? Helping mothers have success breastfeeding has motivation beyond the individual breastfeeding relationships. Breastfeeding can be used as a reason to deny women certain opportunities or to place certain judgments on them unless these issues are addressed more largely in society. Educating mothers about breastfeeding includes educating them about how society might react to their breastfeeding and how they can be prepared for certain reactions.

The Breastfeeding Woman

Gaskin et al. (2009), and Wiessinger et al. (2010) present different ideas of who the breastfeeding women may be. How can their ideas be put together so that a clearer picture of who their audience is can be framed? Essentially, who is the breastfeeding woman? Who is left out of the conversation? From the analysis conducted here, it seems that the "Breastfeeding Woman" would be a heterosexual, cisgender, economically stable woman in a committed relationship. Racial qualities could be deduced by looking at very specific details. Racial disparities are evident in studies of breastfeeding rates (Center for Disease Control and Prevention [CDC], 2014; United States Department of Health and Human Services, 2011). While the books do not address racial differences, inferences can be made about what racial groups are expected as readers by the other demographic markers.

The main groups of potential readers that are excluded are economically lower-class readers, readers who are employed in positions where they have little control over scheduling, breaks, or time off, single mothers, non-cisgender readers, and non-heterosexual readers. There could be improvement in the treatment of these groups in many cases by simply offering additional resources. While this is merely a first step, by addressing that these groups too are important in conversations on breastfeeding, there can continue to be more attention paid to being inclusive.

Economically lower-class readers and those in low-control employment positions are glanced over at multiple points in these books. There are few resources provided for readers who may be looking for financial help. Whether it be more information on WIC programs, information on how to apply for food stamps, or a way that child care expenses can be reduced, there is an opportunity to direct families to resources in these books that is not being taken advantage of. By addressing employment, but leaving out many of those who have little choice in their employment, these individuals are ignored once again. According to the National Poverty Center (2015), families headed by single mothers have the highest poverty rates. With this data widely available, it is amazing that not one of these books tries to address additional support options. The authors each tout the economic savings of breastfeeding and how this can help families. But without providing information on how breastfeeding can work in situations where employment or childcare arrangements are not flexible, many readers or potential readers are, once again, left without support.

Not only are the readers referred to using female pronouns, but partners are almost exclusively referred to with male pronouns. Not only does this create the assumption that the reader will have some sort of partner to help with childcare and household responsibilities, but it also implies that the reader is in a heterosexual relationship. This again excludes multiple groups of readers. Wiessinger et al. (2010) can be an example of how to better include readers. They not only use the term "partner" reliably and without associating it with male pronouns, but they explain that "partner" can be any support person. There is still room for improvement in *The Womanly Art of Breastfeeding*, but these authors do a far better job of not excluding readers based on sexuality. One good next step for any of the authors would be to include personal anecdotes from one of these groups. Maybe include the experience of a female partner who decided to breastfeed, even if she did not carry the child. Or include the story of a trans* parent who is breastfeeding. The personal anecdotes, already a part of all of these books, would be a simple and influential way to welcome experiences from a wider group of individuals.

Conclusion

Each of these books has a unique tone and style that will appeal to a different personality group. This type of differentiation is important in breastfeeding books to be able to reach a large audience. Now is the time for these books to continue this effort and not only appeal to different personality groups, but different demographics as well. Breastfeeding rates are on the rise in the U.S. (CDC, 2013; United

States Department of Health and Human Services, 2011), but this will only continue if the conversations regarding breastfeeding are open to all who are interested. While social change is often slow, it can speed up with different groups working toward common goals together. By addressing larger groups of lactating individuals, not only will breastfeeding rates and support rise, but so will the members of these groups.

References

Gaskin, I. M. (2009). *Ina May's guide to breastfeeding.* New York: Bantam Books.

Heymann, J., Raub, A., & Earle, A. (2013). Breastfeeding policy: A globally comparative analysis. *Bulletin of the World Health Organization,* 91, 398-406.

Huggins, K. (2010). *The nursing mother's companion.* 6th Ed. Boston, MA: The Harvard Common Press.

Mohrbacher, N., & Kendall-Tackett, K. (2010). *Breastfeeding made simple: Seven natural laws for nursing mothers,* 2nd Ed. Oakland, CA: New Harbinger Publications.

Smith, P. H., Hausman, B.L., & Labbok, M. (2012). *Beyond health, beyond choice: Breastfeeding constraints and realities.* New Brunswick, NJ: Rutgers University Press.

Center for Disease Control and Prevention. (2014). *Infant feeding practices study ii and its year six follow-up.* Retrieved from http://www.cdc.gov/breastfeeding/data/ifps/index.htm.

Center for Disease Control and Prevention. (2013). *Breastfeeding report card.* Retrieved from http://www.cdc.gov/breastfeeding/data/reportcard.htm.

National Poverty Center (2015). *Poverty facts.* Retrieved from http://www.npc.umich.edu/poverty/.

United States Department of Health and Human Services. (2011). *The Surgeon General's Call to Action to Support Breastfeeding.* Retrieved from http://www.surgeongeneral.gov/library/calls/breastfeeding/calltoactiontosupportbreastfeeding.pdf.

Wiessinger, D., West, D., & Pitman, T. (2010). *The womanly art of breastfeeding,* 8th Ed. New York: Ballantine Books.

Sabotaging Breast is Best: Media's Role in Shifting Infant Feeding Ideologies in the 19th Century

Katherine A. Foss

In May of 1867, an early advertisement for commercial formula appeared in the *New York Times* classified section, with the text "Breastmilk for infants (a perfect substitute) and nourishments for invalids is Comstock's Rational Food (Liebig's formula)." Aside from the outdated language regarding disability, the message was not too distant from contemporary commercial formula marketing. Although breastfeeding rates have dramatically fluctuated over the last 150 years, the commercialization of infant feeding, and the impact of its marketing have remained a constant.

It has been well-established that media representations play a significant role in shaping perceptions of breastfeeding, especially for those who lack breastfeeding education from other sources. Media provide health information, define what is considered "normal," and enact changes in health behavior (Conrad, 2007; Soumerai, Ross-Degnan, & Kahn, 2002). Indeed, past health campaigns on breastfeeding have demonstrated media's impact by improving awareness, increasing initiation rates, and producing positive attitudes toward breastfeeding (Kim, 1998; McDivitt et al., 1993). Scholarly studies of media coverage suggest that media have contributed to lower breastfeeding rates by normalizing bottle-feeding, and perpetuating the difficulty of breast-feeding (Brown & Peuchaud, 2008; Foss & Southwell, 2006).

Even more disturbing, Hausman (2003) explained how media mes-sages have framed breastfeeding as harmful, even dangerous, to infants, with stories of "dead babies" saturating media. Breastfeeding trends in magazines and parenting manuals have depicted breastfeeding as generally positive, but difficult (Foss, 2010; Frerichs et al., 2006; Potter, Sheeshka, & Valaitis, 2000; Young, 1990). Moreover, Wolf (2006) described how risk campaigns promoting breastfeeding have been stra-tegically silenced by commercial formula companies. Media has likely influenced breastfeeding in other ways, by sexualizing breasts, defining appropriate ages and places for breastfeeding (that contradict public health recommendations), fulfilling an agenda-setting function for health care providers (by prescribing what is "normal"), and commodi-fying infant feeding so that breastfeeding is perceived as "less valuable" in our monetary-driven society.

Media messages about breastfeeding can also be used as a cultural marker, denoting both ideological shifts and fixtures over time, which draw from hegemonic structures of the moment. Exploring media from an earlier time can provide insight into shifts in cultural perception. In this project, I use magazine articles and advertisements to demonstrate how breastfeeding shifted from the only way to feed babies to be con-sidered outdated and abnormal over a relatively short period of time.

Until the 19th century, it was common sense that babies needed breastmilk to survive. Therefore, the extent to which a woman was successful at breastfeeding would determine whether her baby would live or die. An infant needed to either suckle at their mother's breasts or at the breasts of another woman (Golden, 1996). Abandoned babies had very little chance of survival, even if adopted by well-meaning caregivers, unless a wet nurse could be found (Golden, 1996). Yet, by the early 1900s, many women did not breastfeed and instead used artificial food, often with dire results. Considering that women had been taught for generations that breastmilk was the *only* suitable food for babies, how did the tides turn? How do you move from a breastfed population to an artificially fed one, particularly when the consequences were often fatal?

Scholars have speculated about the timing and primary causes of this shift. According to Janet Golden (1996), the popularity of wet nursing in the 1700s and 1800s started the trend of women not breastfeeding their babies. By the mid-19th century, this arrangement between wealthy families and wet nurses (working women usually of a lower socioeconomic status) had become so popular that people began to associate class with a lower milk supply, falsely believing that high-society women simply did not produce like those of the lower classes (Golden, 1996; Wolf, 2001). Historian Jacqueline Wolf (2001) has demonstrated that women stopped breastfeeding their children long before the medical profession began endorsing artificial feeding. False perceptions of insufficient milk and changing conceptions of motherhood altered the infant feeding relationship, which occurred during drastic cultural shifts in the 1800s, including moral reform, immigration, and urbanization (Golden, 1996; Wolf; 2001).

Furthermore, the rise of the scientific paradigm in the late 1800s prompted the medicalization of many aspects of American life, including infant feeding. Initially, the heightened prominence of doctors in this area meant that physicians started to oversee the practice of wet nursing, as breastmilk was still highly recommended as the food for babies (Golden, 1996). However, wet nursing went out of favor, as artificial food became its own "science," produced and studied in laboratories so that the perfect concoction or "formula" could be determined for each child (Apple, 1987). As part of this era of "modernity" in which science trumped nature, physicians started advising early weaning for almost any difficulty, advocating the switch to artificial food, whether homemade or factory-produced (Apple, 2006). Babies died at an alarming rate from these substitutes, as breastfeeding rates continued to decline for the next 70 years (Apple, 1987, 2006; Golden, 1996; Wolf, 2001).

Throughout this shift, media played a critical role in convincing women not to nurse their babies. The marketing of wet nursing through newspaper advertisements first established milk as a commodity (Golden, 1996). But it was the extensive and relentless marketing of commercially produced substitutes that cemented the decline of breastfeeding. In an era without regulation, artificial food companies could make any claims about their products' effectiveness without fear of litigation, with a persistence that could easily counter recommendations for infant feeding from the medical profession. A case study of *Ladies' Home Journal*, 1884 to 1907, demonstrates the shift in perceptions of infant feeding, couched in a sea of milk-substitute advertising.

Articles in the early years of the magazine consistently promote extended breastfeeding, encouraging women to nurse until 18 months or so. Writers warn women of the risks of not breastfeeding, using cautionary tales of children who had died from artificial food. Practical advice on overcoming common breastfeeding obstacles is given, including tips on relieving clogged ducts and sore nipples. Most of the authors appear to be "regular" women, with bylines that often used "Mrs.," suggesting the credibility of mother-to-mother advice in this era.

Yet, advertisements from 1884 to 1889 tell a different story. While the articles convey the danger of weaning before the "Second Summer" due to the danger of mortality from diarrhea (called *cholera infantum* or "Summer Complaint"), the milk substitute companies repeatedly reassure readers that their products alone could protect babies from succumbing to this condition. Testimonies of healthy children raised on their products, mixed with scientific-sounding language, and a physician's recommendation bolster these claims. Milk-substitute companies even offered free brochures, pamphlets, and books on infant feeding advice, presenting themselves as "qualified" resources for new parents. The messages and images in these ads (a novelty at this time) were highly persuasive, straight-forward, and convincing, so much so that the articles in the following years would begin to match their tone.

In the 1890s, magazine writers did not assume breastfeeding as the only way to feed babies. While articles on infant feeding mentioned the preference for breastfeeding, increasingly, authors noted its difficulty and acknowledged a growing population of bottle-feeders (even if statistics may not have confirmed its prevalence). Messages detailing the careful and scientific preparation of homemade concoctions for babies frequently appeared throughout this era.

Advice for appropriate weaning ages also shifted, recommending weaning by 12 months, except in hot weather. By the early 1900s, *Ladies' Home Journal* messages suggest that breastfeeding might be better for infants, but only when adhering to rigid rules and schedules that would have likely destroyed milk supplies. Physicians regularly contributed columns about infant feeding, recommending supplementing or weaning for almost any, what would be considered, minor challenge (i.e., a tired mother, a crying baby, a baby that wakes at night, etc.). Stories on the dangers of hot weather no longer promote breastfeeding, instead, address modifying the artificial food mixture. Furthermore, if a woman can breastfeed, the "experts" strongly encourage weaning by 9 to 12 months, claiming that nursing longer than a year heightens the baby's risk of rickets, anemia, rheumatism, and other ailments. Advertisements for milk substitutes and, increasingly, for artificial-feeding supplies, flourished, continuing many of the tactics of earlier years, with outrageous claims, the use of "experts," and testimonies that attempted to validate the bold declarations of the products' effectiveness.

Overall, the articles and advertisements in *Ladies' Home Journal* illustrate the shift in infant feeding discourse. Even if women were breastfeeding by the end of the 19th century (and we know that some obviously were), this magazine, like many others, told them they were abnormal, doomed to fail, and possibly putting their babies at risk for illness, or even death. In other words, media strongly contributed to declining breastfeeding, undermining even positive messages about nursing with the heavy advertising of milk substitutes, firmly establishing artificial feeding as the norm, despite its often fatal consequences.

References

Apple, R. (2006). *Perfect motherhood: Science and childrearing in America.* New Brunswick, NJ: Rutgers University Press.

Apple, R. D. (1987). *Mothers and medicine: A social history of infant feeding, 1890–1950* (Vol. 7). Madison, WI: University of Wisconsin Press.

New York Times. (30 May 1867). *"Breastmilk is for infants."* p. 5.

Brown, J., & Peuchaud, S. (2008). Media and breastfeeding: Friend or foe? *International Journal of Breastfeeding. 3*(15). Retrieved from http://internationalbreastfeedingjournal.com/content/3/1/15.

Conrad, P. (2007). *The medicalization of society: The transformation of human conditions into treatable disorders.* Baltimore: The Johns Hopkins University Press.

Foss, K., & Southwell, B. (2006). Infant feeding and the media: The relationship between *Parents* content and breastfeeding, 1972-2000. *International Breastfeeding Journal, 1*(10) Retrieved from http://www.biomedcentral.com/content/pdf/1746-4358-1-10.pdf.

Foss, K. (2010). Perpetuating scientific motherhood: Infant feeding discourse in *Parents* magazine, 1930-2007. *Women & Health, 50*(3), 297-311.

Frerichs, L., Andsager, J.L., Campo, S., Aquilino, M., & Dyer, C.S. (2006). Framing breastfeeding and formula-feeding messages in popular U.S. magazines. *Women & Health, 44*(1), 95-118.

Golden, J. (1996). *A social history of wet nursing in America: From breast to bottle.* Cambridge, UK: Cambridge University Press.

Hausman, B. (2003). *Mother's milk: Breastfeeding controversies in American culture.* New York: Routledge.

Kim, Y. (1998). The effects of a breastfeeding campaign on adolescent Korean women. *Pediatric Nursing, 24*(3), 235-240.

McDivitt, J., Zimicki, S., Hornik, R., & Abulaban, A. (1993). The impact of the healthcom mass media campaign on timely initiation of breastfeeding in Jordan. *Studies in Family Planning, 24*(5), 295-309.

Potter, B., Sheeshka, J., & Valaitis, R. (2000). Content analysis of infant feeding messages in a Canadian women's magazine, 1945 to 1995. *Journal of Nutrition Education, 32*, 196-203.

Soumerai, S., Ross-Degnan, D., & Kahn, J. (2002). The effects of professional and media warnings about the association between aspirin use in children and Reye's Syndrome. In R. Hornik (Ed.) *Public health communication: Evidence for behavior change* (pp. 265-288). New Jersey: Lawrence Erlbaum Associates.

Wolf, J. H. (2006). What feminists can do for breastfeeding and what breastfeeding can do for feminists. *Signs, 31*(2), 397-424.

Wolf, J. H. (2001). *Don't kill your baby: Public health and the decline of breastfeeding in the nineteenth and twentieth centuries.* Dayton, OH: Ohio State University Press.

Young, K. (1990). American conceptions of infant development from 1955 to 1984: What the experts are telling parents? *Child Development. 61*, 17-28.

CHAPTER 44

A Mobile Application to Promote Breastfeeding Among Low-income African American Women

Anise Gold-Watts, Jennifer Lawall,
Marielle Matthews, Jewels Rhode, David Potenziani,
Dykki Settle, Girdhari Bora,
and Kathryn E. Muessig

In the United States, African American women are significantly less likely to breastfeed, and more likely to report barriers to breast-feeding, than their White or Hispanic counterparts (U.S. Department of Health and Human Services, 2011; McCann et al., 2007). Moreover, they often do not receive the necessary support to start or maintain exclusive breastfeeding habits (Evans et al., 2011). In addition, North Carolina has lower breastfeeding rates than the national average, which supports the need for additional breastfeeding interventions in the state (Gazmararian et al., 2014).

Mobile health (mhealth) interventions have potential to address factors that contribute to breastfeeding disparities. Recent studies found that among smartphone owners, 19% had mobile applications (apps) that tracked or managed their health, and African Americans were more likely than others to use their phones to look for health information (Baker et al., 2003; Fox et al., 2012; Ohlendorf et al., 2012; Shieh et al., 2009). An mhealth app specifically tailored for low-income African American families has potential to support breast-feeding and reduce negative physical health outcomes (Tirado, 2011).

This paper describes and adaptation to an existing app in order to create an app that promotes breastfeeding, and is tailored to the needs of low-income African American families. The researchers involved in this project were part of a Capstone team in the Department of Health Behavior at the University of North Carolina, Chapel Hill. Capstone is a year-long project in which second year Public Health Masters' students work with an organization, applying public health methods to solve an identified community need. The Capstone team consisted of four student researchers, and two faculty advisors, who were paired with IntraHealth International, and tasked with adapting a mobile app from India called mSakhi to an American context.

MSakhi Breastfeeding Mobile Application

MSakhi was originally developed to promote maternal and child health in India, and is currently used by community health workers (CHWs) to collect and store data, as well as to supplement health lessons that are traditionally verbally delivered with pictures, audio, and videos. MSakhi has one end user, the CHW, and the content was developed for a cross-cultural population with low literacy. The structure of mSakhi provided an opportunity for adaptation due to its ability to collect and store health data, provide responsive curriculum while tracking, end-user progress through the curriculum, and be used with low-literacy audiences. The IntraHealth Capstone team's proposed adaptation of mSakhi aims to increase breastfeeding among low-income African American women by focusing on increasing knowledge and self-efficacy, and strengthening peer networks.

Method

In order to determine the potential scope of the app and understand common barriers to breastfeeding, the Capstone team reviewed peer reviewed literature on breastfeeding interventions for low-income African American women. This review informed the design of interview guides for primary data collection.

Interviews were conducted over the period of 7 months. The goals of the interviews were to: 1) gain the opinions of experts regarding the local relevancy of breastfeeding barriers identified in the literature, 2) understand the personal histories of potential end users, 3) identify who should be the intended end users of the app (i.e., pregnant mothers, mothers who gave birth within the past year, grandmothers, fathers, lactation counselors, other health workers, among other options), and 4) identify potential features of the adapted app. Two interviews were completed with Women, Infants, and Children (WIC) program participants. Sixteen interviews were completed with breastfeeding researchers and experts. Experts and researchers were identified by online research, recommendations from UNC Gillings School of Global Public Health faculty, and by snowball sampling. Interviews were transcribed, coded, and analyzed to identify overarching themes.

Interview data was supplemented with an analysis of publicly available data from the Facebook group Black Women Do Breastfeed (BWDBF). Data collected from this page consisted of posts by the page moderator and comments on those posts from Facebook users. Posts typically included a question submitted to the moderator by a Facebook user about breastfeeding, or an encouraging statement accompanied by a photo submitted by a Facebook user of the user breastfeeding.

Themes from the interviews and Facebook data analyses were compared and combined to create a list of possible tailored features for the adapted mSakhi app that could address the needs of low-income African American women. The team then created a summary of functional gaps that would need to be reconciled by mSakhi's developers in order to implement the adapted app.

Results

Literature review results revealed that interventions designed to improve breastfeeding often applied the construct of self-efficacy from the Health Belief Model, as well as concepts from Social Support Theory. Several interventions were identified in the literature review that met one of these criteria: 1) targeted increased breastfeeding as the intended outcome, 2) used a mobile application to deliver the intervention, 3) focused on African American women, or 4) focused on low-income women. However, no interventions were found that used mobile applications to increase breastfeeding specifically among low-income African American women.

Three major topics were identified that could be addressed by a mobile app: 1) lack of social support, 2) low self-efficacy to breastfeed, and 3) lack of informational support. Formative research also identified resources that low-income breastfeeding mothers used, which were not represented in the current literature, including online forums, such as the BWDBF Facebook page, as well as growth and development apps, such as *What to Expect When You're Expecting*. The following comment on the BWDBF page was typical of many of the encouraging posts on the page:

> This is my 3-week-old daughter that I've been breast-feeding since birth. This last week I've had to switch to combination bottle-feeding because her mouth is too small, and she isn't latched well. If it wasn't for finding this page, I would have quit breastfeeding all together. All of the tips and pictures are pure motivation for me! I tried to breastfeed my three-year-old, but he wouldn't latch when he was born, and it was so frustrating I gave up his first week home. This time I am thankful

to make it 3 weeks, even if it is combination, thank you for having such a wonderful page!

—Data from BWDBF Facebook page

Data from interviews with breastfeeding experts confirmed some of the barriers identified in the literature among low-income African American women. These barriers included environmental factors, such as need to return to work, and lack of appropriate breastfeeding or pumping facilities available at workplaces, as well as social factors, such as lack of social support, stigma, and lack of breastfeeding role models. One expert spoke to the importance of social support within mothers' peer networks:

> We're constantly bombarded by experts telling us the things we should do. And the chances of us doing some of those things are extremely small, especially if we don't see those things fitting into our current lifestyle. When we have people who are our peers, or are in our social network, when they say "This is what I'm doing, you should do this," usually it's followed up with, "and this is how I do it, in my world." And because they're part of our social network, chances are that we have some sort of connection with them that makes us somewhat similar to us ... You know I think it's just a different kind of credibility when it comes from someone in your network versus the doctor or the nurse, who you obviously don't see very often, tells you should do that.

—Participant 6, Breastfeeding Interventionist

Social support was indicated in data analysis as a major influence on breastfeeding behavior and acceptance. In particular, informants mentioned the influence of their babies' fathers on the decision to breastfeed. Another important social factor was having another woman in the family, or within a mother's close friend group who had breastfed, or was currently breastfeeding. One mother also described social support she received through photos of African American women breastfeeding on social media:

> I love seeing those pictures. I mean, the babies are always so cute. And just knowing that I am not the only Black breastfeeding mother, and you know not having to cover up and hide yourself, feeling ashamed. Or that your family may not be encouraging you or be supportive of you ... well we can be a network that is supportive of each other. And those pictures kind of help other people see we are moms too. We breastfeed too. It's not just a certain type of people that do that.
>
> *−Participant 1, mother and WIC participant*

Limitations

Due to time constraints and difficulty with recruiting members of the target population, the voices of low-income African American women in North Carolina are underrepresented in this report. The Capstone Team addressed this shortcoming by collecting women's voices from the BWDBF Facebook page and from experts who work closely with this community. Although the BWDBF Facebook page is national, and not specifically low-income, this page informed our understanding of general challenges to breastfeeding that African American women face.

Discussion

Preliminary formative research with breastfeeding experts supported the importance of focusing on social support as a key theoretical construct for increasing breastfeeding. This focus was reinforced by subsequent research with low-income African American mothers (interviews and Facebook data), additional interviews with breast-feeding experts, and contacts at the Breastfeeding and Feminism

International Conference. In an effort to increase social support, the Capstone team recommended that the adapted version of the mSakhi app have multiple end users, including mother, grandmother, father, partner, and friend. Engaging these multiple end users may increase support for and knowledge of breastfeeding practices within the mother's social circle (see Figure 1 for a guide to the features of the adapted app).

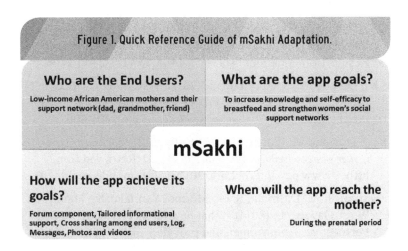

Figure 1. Quick Reference Guide of mSakhi Adaptation.

Who are the End Users?

Low-income African American mothers and their support network (dad, grandmother, friend)

What are the app goals?

To increase knowledge and self-efficacy to breastfeed and strengthen women's social support networks

mSakhi

How will the app achieve its goals?

Forum component, Tailored informational support, Cross sharing among end users, Log, Messages, Photos and videos

When will the app reach the mother?

During the prenatal period

The Capstone team also recommended that the app contain a forum, where mothers can post questions to other users. Forums should be specific to the end user, so that mothers can communicate with other mothers, fathers with other fathers, and so on. Research by Mwamba (2015) and Spencer (2015) reinforced the need for specific and tailored communication channels for breastfeeding supporters within a mothers' network. The goal of the forum would be to engage those supporters in a solution-oriented dialogue with each other.

The near ubiquity of mobile technologies provides a unique platform to deliver behavioral interventions when people need them via a familiar medium. A breastfeeding support app has the potential to have significant positive health impact among low-income African American mothers and their families. Adapting an existing app for this purpose saves development costs, and models the types of creative cross-cultural, cross-health topic solutions that are needed amidst continued budget constraints and increasingly complex technologies.

References

Baker, L., Wagner, T. H., Singer, S., & Bundorf, M. K. (2003). Use of the Internet and e-mail for health care information: Results from a national survey. *JAMA, 289*(18), 2400-2406.

Evans K., Labbok M., & Abrahams S. (2011). WIC and breastfeeding support services: Does the mix of services offered vary with race and ethnicity? *Breastfeeding Medicine, 6*(6), 401-406.

Fox, S., & Duggan, M. (2012). Mobile health 2012. *Pew Research Center's Internet x0026 American Life Project.* Retrieved from http://www.pewinternet.org/2012/11/08/mobile-health-2012/

Gazmararian, J. A., Dalmida, S. G., Merino, Y., Blake, S., Thompson, W., & Gaydos, L. (2014). What new mothers need to know: Perspectives from women and providers in georgia. *Maternal and Child Health Journal, 18*(4), 839-851.

McCann, M. F., Baydar, N., & Williams, R. L. (2007). Breastfeeding attitudes and reported problems in a national sample of WIC participants. *Journal of Human Lactation, 23*(4), 314-324.

Mwamba, M. (2015, March). *What's dads got to do with it?* 10th Breastfeeding and Feminism International Conference at Chapel Hill, NC.

Ohlendorf, J. M., Weiss, M. E., & Ryan, P. (2012). Weight-management information needs of postpartum women. *MCN: The American Journal of Maternal/Child Nursing, 37*(1), 56-63.

Shieh, C., McDaniel, A., & Ke, I. (2009). Information–seeking and its predictors in low-income pregnant women. *Journal of Midwifery & Women's Health, 54*(5), 364-372.

Spencer, B. (2015, March). *A qualtitative description of african american men's experience as fathers of breastfed infants.* 10th Breastfeeding and Feminism International Conference at Chapel Hill, NC.

Tirado, M. (2011). Role of mobile health in the care of culturally and linguistically diverse U.S. populations. *Perspectives in Health Information Management/AHIMA, American Health Information Management Association, 8* (Winter).

U.S. Department of Health and Human Services, Centers for Disease Control and Prevention. (2011). *About Healthy People.* Retrieved from www.healthypeople.gov/2020/ about/default.aspx

CHAPTER 45

Engaging Youth in National Infant and Young Child-feeding Programs in a Resource-limited Setting Using Affordable Mobile Social Networks to Provide Breastfeeding Awareness

Dexter Chagwena, Bhekimpilo Sithole, Rutendo Masendu, Yemurai Mkondo, Anthony Chiromba, Monica Muti, Charity Zvandaziva, and Charles Maponga

P romotion of breastfeeding has been shown to be effective in improving child survival (Bhutta et al., 2008). Poor breastfeeding and child-feeding practices are prevalent in resource-limited countries (RLCs), yet implementation of infant and young child-feeding (IYCF) programs is centrally located in health centers targeting mothers as they attend antenatal clinics and community programs. This approach usually leaves out important groups, such as youth, men, and extended-family members involved in infant-feeding decision-making. Working women especially from urban areas are also usually left out, resulting in lack of IYCF knowledge, and poor child-feeding practices.

Poor breastfeeding practices are common in Zimbabwe, with prevalence of exclusive breastfeeding (EBF) continuing to be reported as very low, ranging from 6% to 41% per national health surveys conducted in the last five years (FNC & MoHCW 2010; ZIMSTAT & ICF International 2012; Zimbabwe National Statistics Agency [ZNSA], 2015). Poor child-feeding practices employed by caregivers of children are also common in the country (Ministry of Health and Child Welfare [MHCW], 2012; ZNSA, 2015), and this is mainly attributed to inadequate knowledge on optimal-breastfeeding practices, and lack of community support for women to confidently employ optimal child-feeding practices. Therefore, there is need to design nutrition interventions that reach all community members including youth, men, and working women who are usually left from child-feeding programs.

Mass media and social media have been shown to improve communication of health messages and support behavior change (Snyder, 2007; Wakefield, Loken, & Hornik, 2010). In Uganda, Lifecare initiative successfully utilized social media platforms to conduct nutrition programs that enhance healthy living in communities, and promote a family approach to nutrition and food security. There is sufficient evidence showing social media as an effective tool to promote good health behaviors. Social media makes information easily accessible, catchy, and provides a platform that enhance behavior change (Nomatotovu, 2014). Girerd-Barclay (2013) reported positive results in use of social media platforms that include use of the World Alliance for Breastfeeding Action (WABA) website used in improving awareness of breastfeeding among youth.

There seems to be a gap in breastfeeding promotion programs in Zimbabwe, as lack of breastfeeding and IYCF knowledge continue to be reported among women and communities. The aim of this paper is to evaluate the effectiveness of using an affordable mobile social communication platform in reaching young people to participate in national IYCF programs, and disseminate breastfeeding information.

Method

The Ministry of Health and Childcare in collaboration with Nutri@ ctive Zimbabwe, a youth organization designed a novel intervention aimed at mobilizing youth to participate in a breastfeeding awareness program utilizing an affordable mobile social communication platform, WhatsApp, and an edutainment street campaign during the 2014 World Breastfeeding Week (WBW) commemorations. Fifty youth volunteers (i.e., nutrition professionals and nutrition students), aged 19 to 25 years, were trained on IYCF prior the WBW to spearhead a breastfeeding campaign in Harare during the 2014 WBW, and the entire month of August.

An affordable mobile social communication platform, WhatsApp, was utilized to mobilize youth to participate in the program and disseminate breastfeeding-promoting messages. Following the training workshop, a WhatsApp group for youth volunteers was created to share short messages on breastfeeding during the WBW. Each member forwarded the messages to the public, targeting mainly youth, young men, and women. Messages highlighted the importance of breastfeeding, optimal-breastfeeding practices, feeding practices recommended for HIV-infected mothers, and mobilizing community individuals to attend the breastfeeding edutainment street campaign in Harare. Barriers and challenges to optimal-breastfeeding raised by the public through WhatsApp were discussed in the WhatsApp group and individuals provided follow-up support to these individuals. A breastfeeding Facebook page, and the Nutri@ctive website, were also utilized to provide more information on breastfeeding to the public, addressing barriers and challenges to optimal child-feeding (see Figure 1).

A breastfeeding street awareness campaign led by youth volunteers was held along Harare First Street from 21 to 23 August. A breastfeeding branded-van with youths providing edutainment traveled around Harare central business markets and streets encouraging young people to attend the street awareness campaign. Data were collected on number of young people reached and mobilized to actively participate in the national breastfeeding campaign program. Information on knowledge gaps and concerns regarding breastfeeding by the public was also recorded.

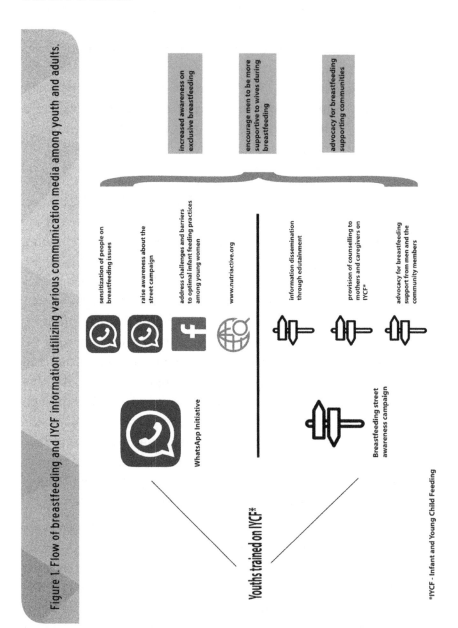

Figure 1. Flow of breastfeeding and IYCF information utilizing various communication media among youth and adults.

*IYCF - Infant and Young Child Feeding

Findings

The intervention was successful in mobilizing over 85 youth volunteers to spearhead a national breastfeeding campaign and WBW commemorations in Harare during the entire month of August 2014. More than 9,000 people were reached through WhatsApp and the street awareness campaign.

Approximately 2,000 youths were reached through this program actively participating on WhatsApp, where information on importance of breastfeeding and optimal breastfeeding practices was disseminated. Concerns were raised on EBF for 6 months, with participants reporting that it was not feasible, especially for working mothers. Other concerns raised include contradicting messages from health workers on recommended infant-feeding methods for HIV-infected mothers, lack of support, and male involvement in infant feeding. There was a misconception among the public that breastfeeding whilst pregnant was dangerous for the baby, it was reported to be culturally forbidden, as the breastfeeding child would get sick. This belief was common among young and older women.

Discussion

In the African culture, child-feeding decisions are not solely made by mothers, but the extended family play a significant role in this process (MHCW, 2012). In spite of this fact, most of our breastfeeding promotion interventions are centered at health centers targeting mainly pregnant and lactating women. This reduces chances of optimal infant-feeding practices being employed by mothers as they go back in the community and face pressure to adopt to cultural practices that hinder recommended feeding practices. Young women are mostly affected as they rely on advice they get from older women in the society, or what they are told by their husbands. The idea of targeting both men and women in promoting optimal breastfeeding and child-feeding practices is one way to ensure caregivers adhere to recommended child-feeding practices.

Implementation of this breastfeeding awareness program was successful in reaching young people, showing social media can be an effective tool to reach young people in IYCF and nutrition communication programs. Such platforms have not been explored in nutrition programming in Zimbabwe, but shows to be very promising in improving nutrition communication for behavior change among population groups. Our findings concur with other authors in that existing popular social platforms, such as Facebook, Twitter, Skype, email, and SMS have been shown to be useful, and can address issues of reach, engagement, and retention in health programs (Maher et al., 2014). Contribution of age has been reported to have an effect on adopting positive nutrition practices, as older people tend to think that messages from social media cannot be taken seriously (Girerd-Barclay, 2013). In our intervention, utilizing social media platforms in providing breastfeeding information targeting young people was effective in reaching a wider audience. The amount of time spent on social networks by youth makes social media a useful and effective tool in disseminating information. Thus, youths can be targeted to adopt and improve nutrition practices, such as promoting breastfeeding, healthy eating, and weight management. The methods used, however, have to be attractive and stimulate interest among individuals.

Through use of WhatsApp, we eliminated huge costs associated with breastfeeding promotion interventions. The application is very affordable, resulting in most individuals in resource-limited settings with mobile phones and electronic gadgets, such as tablets, using it. In Zimbabwe, approximately 60% of the population have access to mobile phones (POTRAZ, 2013). As most young people use social communication platforms, such as WhatsApp and Facebook, social media becomes an effective tool that can be used to reach many people at limited costs, as resources to implement nutrition communication programs are scarce.

In this intervention, impact of the awareness program on breastfeeding practices or knowledge on breastfeeding was not evaluated. However, previous studies have shown positive impact of social media on behavior change in health attitudes and stimulating self-efficacy (Flora, Maibach, & Maccoby, 1989; Girerd-Barclay, 2013). Cole-Lewis and Kershaw (2010) highlighted existence of evidence, suggesting mobile phones are a useful tool for interventions seeking improvement in health outcomes. The evidence supports text messaging being a useful tool for behavior change interventions, and they also show that the way a message is framed can affect whether a person is receptive to making a behavior change.

A study in Bangladesh reported limited knowledge among adolescent girls and young women's knowledge on IYCF recommendations, particularly those concerning early and exclusive breastfeeding, and feeding of appropriate nutrient-rich complementary foods (Hackett et al., 2012). This is one of the very few studies on assessment of IYCF knowledge among adolescents, highlighting the challenge that RLCs face in having future parents with limited knowledge on IYCF. This has a direct bearing on health among future generations.

On the other hand, Girerd-Barclay (2013) conducted an evaluation study of a WBW campaign in Penang, Malaysia among students. The author reported a successful program in increasing awareness, promotion, and discussions on breastfeeding among young people. Similar findings to our observations that young people were mostly interested in the edutainment activities and this drew their attention and interest in the breastfeeding awareness project. This study also showed that utilizing mass media together with other communication channels, such as social media, can have greater impact and stimulate interest in young people, ensuring their participation (Flora et al., 1989; Girerd-Barclay, 2013).

A study in rural Zimbabwe also reported the positive impact of road shows in improving knowledge of participants on EBF. The authors reported that individuals directly exposed to road shows were more informed compared to individuals indirectly exposed, as they were only likely to recall the entertainment aspects rather than key messages. Jenkins and colleagues also highlighted that such activities can be used to close the gap of EBF knowledge between men and women as road show exposure were more associated with EBF knowledge among men (Jenkins et al., 2012). In our intervention, men showed interest although only a few (7%) visited the breastfeeding tent to inquire more information about breastfeeding. Targeting young men will ensure adequate support to breastfeeding mothers and this helps to ensure appropriate decisions on IYCF are made.

Conclusion

Use of affordable social platforms and mass media strategies are effective in mobilizing and reaching young people to promote breastfeeding in a resource-limited setting. There is potential to improve breastfeeding knowledge and IYCF practices among difficult to reach population groups, such as young women, working women, and men.

References

Bhutta, Z. A., Ahmed, T., Black, R. E., Cousens, S., Dewey, K., Giugliani, E., Haider, B.A., Kirkwood, B., Morris, S.S., Sachdev, H.P.S., Shekar, M., & Maternal and Child Undernutrition Study Group. (2008). What works? Interventions for maternal and child undernutrition and survival. *The Lancet, 371*(9610), 417-440.

Cole-Lewis, H., & Kershaw, T. (2010). Text messaging as a tool for behavior change in disease prevention and management. *Epidemiologic Reviews, 32*(1), 56-69.

FNC & MoHCW (2010). *Zimbabwe National Nutrition Survey. Harare, Zimbabwe, Ministry of Health and Child Welfare; Food and Nutrition Council.* https://www.humanitarianresponse.info/sites/www. humanitarianresponse.info/files/assessments/Zimbabwe%20 Nutrition%20Survey%202010.pdf.

Girerd-Barclay, L. C. (2013). *The promotion of breastfeeding in malaysia. What works, what doesn't, and why?* (Doctoral dissertation, Colorado State University).https://dspace.library.colostate.edu/bitstream/ handle/10217/79052/GirerdBarclay_colostate_0053N_11569. pdf?sequence=1&isAllowed=y.

Hackett, K. M., Mukta, U. S., Jalal, C. S., & Sellen, D. W. (2015). Knowledge, attitudes and perceptions on infant and young child nutrition and feeding among adolescent girls and young mothers in rural Bangladesh. *Maternal & Child Nutrition, 11*(2), 173-189.

Jenkins, A. L., Tavengwa, N. V., Chasekwa, B., Chatora, K., Taruberekera, N., Mushayi, W., Madzima, R.C., & Mbuya, M. N. (2012). Addressing social barriers and closing the gender knowledge gap: Exposure to road shows is associated with more knowledge and more positive beliefs, attitudes, and social norms regarding exclusive breastfeeding in rural Zimbabwe. *Maternal & Child Nutrition, 8*(4), 459-470.

Flora, J. A., Maibach, E. W., & Maccoby, N. (1989). The role of media across four levels of health promotion intervention. *Annual Review of Public Health, 10*(1), 181-201.

Maher, C. A., Lewis, L. K., Ferrar, K., Marshall, S., De Bourdeaudhuij, I., & Vandelanotte, C. (2014). Are health behavior change interventions that use online social networks effective? A systematic review. *Journal of Medical Internet Research, 16*(2).

Ministry of Health and Child Welfare (2012). *Barriers and facilitators of optimal infant and young child feeding in Zimbabwe: Beliefs, influences and practices.* IYCF Formative Research Report prepared by Maguranyanga & Chigumira. Harare, Zimbabwe, MoHCW, UNICEF, CCORE & USAID/MCHIP Zimbabwe.

Nomatotovu, C. (2014). *Utilizing ICTs in breastfeeding and nutrition promotion.* Breastfeeding ICTs and Food Security. Retreived from http:// www.cto.int/media/events/pst-ev/2013/e-Gove/Christine%20 Namatovu.pdf.

POTRAZ (2013*). Postal and telecommunications regulatory authority of Zimbabwe December 2013 Report*, POTRAZ. Retreived from http://www.techzim.co.zw/2014/11/60-zimbabwean-population-connected-mobile-potraz/ www.potraz.gov.zw/index.php/ categorylinks/120-quarterly-reports.

Snyder, L. B. (2007). Health communication campaigns and their impact on behavior. Journal of *Nutrition Education and Behavior, 39*(2), S32-S40.

Wakefield, M. A., Loken, B., & Hornik, R. C. (2010). Use of mass media campaigns to change health behaviour. *The Lancet, 376*(9748), 1261-1271.

Zimbabwe National Statistics Agency. (2015). *Zimabbwe Multiple Indicator Cluster Survey 2014, Final Report.* Harare, Zimbabwe, ZIMSTAT.

Retreived from http://www.childinfo.org/files/Zimbabwe_2014_
KFR.pdf.

ZIMSTAT and ICF International. (2012). *Zimbabwe Demographic and
Health Survey, 2010-11.* Calverton, Maryland, Zimbabwe National
Statistics Agency (ZIMSTAT) and ICF International Inc.
Retrieved from http://www.zimstat.co.zw/dmdocuments/Census/
ZDHS2011/ZDHS2011.pdf

Improving Male Support
for Breastfeeding

CHAPTER 46

What do Men Believe About Breastfeeding? Results of a Formative Research Study from Northern Nigeria

Azeez Oseni

O f infant and young child feeding have great implications for progress in reducing malnutrition and improving child mortality statistics, especially in developing countries. As part of planning to develop a SBCC package for nutrition and hygiene on the USAID-funded "Support to Vulnerable Households for Accelerated Revenue Earnings (SHARE) project," a formative research was conducted in northern Nigeria's Sokoto State and the Federal Capital Territory to understand the determinants of nutrition and hygiene behavior. SHARE (now called Feed the Future Nigeria Livelihoods Project) is a 5-year, $20 million USD project aiming to help 42,000 vulnerable households improve their agricultural production, incomes, and nutrition through a multi-sector approach.

The study used a barrier analysis approach, and divided respondents into doers and non-doers of the specifically studied behaviors

(Kittle, 2013). Focus Group Discussions (FGDs) and Key Informant Interviews (KIIs) were conducted for non-doer fathers, and husbands of caregivers in order to determine the motivations for their current lack of practice of (or support for) appropriate nutritional behaviors. While the study was broad-based in its demographic reach, this summary focuses on the husband/father subgroup of respondents, and on the infant and young child feeding components.

Study Objectives

1. To describe current practices, and identify household and caregiver characteristics that influence negative and positive nutrition and hygiene behaviors.

2. To conduct barrier analysis for key high-impact Infant and Young Child Feeding (IYCF) and hygiene behaviors, where current adoption is low, including timely initiation of breast-feeding, exclusive breastfeeding, introduction of semisolid foods at 6 months, dietary diversification using at least four food types from 6 to 24 months, continued breastfeeding to 24 months, proper hand washing, and sanitary disposal of feces.

3. To identify primary and auxiliary child caregivers and key decision makers related to household nutrition, and key factors that influence their decision making around both adult and child feeding.

4. To determine the most appropriate modes of communication, and the best avenues to achieve behavior change.

5. To determine the most appropriate messages to be communicated to facilitate positive changes in nutrition and hygiene behaviors in the specific context.

Method

Study Area

Federal Capital Territory (FCT) and Sokoto State, Nigeria.

Study Design

The study was a cross-sectional descriptive study consisting of:

- **Barrier Analysis** of five nutrition-related and two hygiene-related behaviors. The nutrition behaviors assessed included child feeding parameters, such as timely initiation of lactation, exclusive breastfeeding, introduction of complementary feeding at 6 months, dietary diversification at 6 to 24 months, and continued breastfeeding up to 24 months. The hygiene-related indicators included proper hand washing and proper fecal disposal.

- **Qualitative Exploration** using FGDs, KIIs and Observation. Separate FGDs were organized for fathers and husbands, while the KIIs focused on traditional and religious leaders, and health workers. Other nutrition-related behaviors, such as nutritional value of foods currently consumed in the households, women's diet during pregnancy, decision making on adult and child feeding, spacing of pregnancy, as well as proper food handling by mothers/caregivers, including use of feeding bottles, boiling water before use, and use clean utensils were included in the thematic areas explored in the FGDs and KIIs.

Sampling

Purposive and multi-stage cluster sampling methods were used to determine the Local Government Area (LGA), clusters, households, and caregivers to be studied. In line with standard guidance for the barrier analysis methodology, a sample size (of 45 "doers" and 45 "non-doers" of each behavior) was determined for each LGA: one in FCT, and four in Sokoto.

Barrier Analysis

Each selected behavior or practice was explored using behavior questions to identify doers and non-doers. A questionnaire was developed for each behavior to explore eight core determinants: (1) Perceived susceptibility; (2) Perceived severity; (3) Perceived benefits (which includes perceived action efficacy); (4) Perceived barriers (which we will discuss as negative attributes of the action); (5) Cues for action; (6) Perceived self-efficacy; (7) Perceived social acceptability; and (8) Perception of divine will (Brieger, 2006).

Data Analysis

Data was analyzed after coding and entry into a Barrier Analysis Excel template, which was used to determine the relative significance of the determinants of studied behaviors in doers and non-doers.

Results

Exclusive Breastfeeding

Husbands/fathers reported the belief that Exclusive Breastfeeding (EBF) could result in malnutrition, starvation, and ill-health in the child. They also reported that EBF was difficult, tasking, and cruel to the child and nature itself.

Timely Initiation of Breastfeeding

Studied men reported that colostrum is harmful or poisonous, causes diarrhea, and should always be discarded. They also stressed that giving colostrum to a newborn was culturally unacceptable. Breast-feeding immediately after birth was also not encouraged for religious reasons, as certain "prayer mixtures" had to be given to the baby first.

Continued Breastfeeding to 24 Months

Men do not support this practice and believe that continued breast-feeding for too long makes children dull and unintelligent. While aware of the Islamic injunction to breastfeed up to 2 years, they felt it was diffi-cult, frustrating, and not agreeable to their culture. They recommended immediate stoppage of breastfeeding (at any age) if the woman becomes pregnant, again citing poisoned breastmilk as a reason.

Introduction of Semisolid Foods at 6 Months

Most respondents recognize that complementary foods can prevent malnutrition and promote growth, but do not agree on a specific time for introduction (this is related to their lack of belief in EBF). Bottle-feeding was acceptable to respondents for a good and convenient practice.

Dietary Diversification

Regarding dietary diversification using at least four food types from 6 to 24 months, most respondents agreed that this is ideal practice to prevent malnutrition and improve productivity in adult life. However, they identified certain barriers preventing implementation of the prac-tice: high cost of food, lack of knowledge of nutritious locally available food options, poverty, and the risk of spoiling the child.

Conclusions/Recommendations

- Men were overwhelmingly recognized as influencers of child-feeding behavior in studied northern Nigerian communities. Interventions should recognize and utilize this fact.

- In contexts where decision-making is heavily skewed in favor of men, gender programs and agenda should have a reverse focus: recognize men as the main agents of change, and leverage on their influence to achieve behavior change.

- Men's social networks are a viable platform for promoting optimal nutrition practices as the level of peer influence on expressed opinions seen during the FGDs was significant.

- Religious and traditional leaders play a key role in shaping beliefs, since they are the custodians of culture. Convincing them about optimal breastfeeding practices, like timely initiation of breastfeeding (within 30 minutes to 1 hour of birth), will go a long way towards shaping community opinion, and consequently, their child-feeding behavior.

- The findings of this study suggest that weak household economy can negatively influence the adoption of optimal child-feeding practices. Interventions designed to reduce poverty (particularly those focusing on empowering women) are well-positioned to improve nutrition behavior positively

- The specific findings will guide the creation of targeted and context-appropriate key messages for dissemination through men's social networks and community platforms

- Overall, involving and engaging men in child feeding will have a significant impact on improving positive behaviors, and empowering women to make more healthy choices for their children

References

Brieger, W.R. (2006). *Health belief model, social learning theory*. Baltimore, MD: Johns Hopkins University. Available at http://ocw.jhsph.edu/courses/SocialBehavioralFoundations/PDFs/Lecture5.pdf.

Kittle, B. (2013). *A practical guide to conducting a barrier analysis*. New York: Helen Keller International. Available at http://www.coregroup.org/storage/barrier/Practical_Guide_to_Conducting_a_Barrier_Analysis_Oct_2013.pdf.

What Men Got to Do with Breastfeeding Intervention?

Muswamba Mwamba

B reastfeeding is a global concern and a public health priority (U.S. Department of Health and Human Services, 2011). The Healthy People 2020 objectives call for an increase in the proportion of women who exclusively breastfeed in the Unites States (Avery & Magnus, 2011). Studies that include fathers show that they have a great deal of influence on women's early infant-feeding decisions. Fathers can provide emotional and practical support to new mothers (Freed, Fraley, & Schanler, 1992). As such, they are logical target for interventions that seek to increase breastfeeding duration.

WIC Program Culture

WIC, the Special Supplemental Nutrition Program for Women, Infants and Children, was established in 1972 as a 2-year pilot program with the goal of helping low-income mothers and young children receive proper nutritional care. The program was permanently authorized in 1974, and it has grown from serving 88,000 women and children, to currently aiding more than 9 million participants (Walker, 2002).

When WIC was established in 1972, it was designed to be run and staffed by women to primarily serve women and their children. Therefore, WIC processes were ill equipped to involve fathers. Today, WIC operations are still not inclusive of fathers, even though there have been changes in the American family social structure. The traditional family consisted of two parents in a heterosexual relationship with several children. The father worked, brought home the paycheck, and thereby provided economic security. The wife raised and nurtured the children, and provided social and psychological security. A social and cultural shift has occurred in which there are now diverse family structures, including single parents, divorced individuals raising children alone, divorced couples with joint custody of the children, blended families, and gay and lesbian couples with children. From a mostly female operation, there is a need to alter the WIC image to make it a more friendly to men.

Men Role in Breastfeeding Support

It is now well-established that the baby's father plays the largest role in providing all types of support for breastfeeding women (Arora, McJunkin, Wehrer, & Kuhn, 2000; Bar-Yam & Darby, 1997; Cohen, Lange, & Slusser, 2002). Understanding men's knowledge and attitudes about breastfeeding reveal reasons why men might support or discourage breastfeeding practices. Early studies involving fathers in breastfeeding decision dated back to 1992. Until 2005, the majority of studies were survey questionnaires that were handed or mailed to identify participants. Studies published after 2005 were cross-sectional designs and focus groups. From those studies, one of the most consistent findings is that sources of influence vary as a function of ethnicity. For White women, the most influential member of the social network appears to be the husband or partner. For Hispanic women, their mothers tend to exert the most influence, and for Black women, close friends are most important (Freed et al., 1992).

Many factors affecting breastfeeding initiation and duration, such as maternal education, mode of delivery, birthweight, socioeconomic status (SES), and support of the infant's father have studied. An important modifiable factor in initiation is the "support of the infant's father for breastfeeding." There is a general consensus that in many cultures, the father of the baby is one of the most influential persons to the mother concerning breastfeeding (Maycock et al., 2013). In a survey of 2,145 men from Texas, support by the fathers for breastfeeding was found to be related to ethnicity, country of origin, education level, and SES (Vaaler et al., 2011). This study found that men's attitudes to 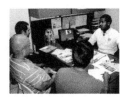 breastfeeding were formed early in life, and were related to ethnicity and SES. Although the evidence from observational epidemiological studies for the importance of fathers in breastfeeding is strong, the number of intervention studies is limited.

In 2002, an innovative pilot study in a Texas WIC program used a father-to-father peer counseling approach to improve breastfeeding rates among participants' wives and partners (Stremler & Lovera, 2004). The pilot not only demonstrated improved breastfeeding rates, but also showed improvements in fathers' knowledge about breastfeeding, and their beliefs that they could provide support to their breastfeeding partners. The City of Dallas Peer Dad program was modeled from the pilot study with the difference that the intervention was carried out by men only (see picture of male-to-male interaction below).

City of Dallas WIC Peer Dad Program

The WIC Peer Dad Program is a promotional and educational breastfeeding intervention program targeting men. Initially, the Peer Dad Program implementation was challenged on all fronts. By tradition, WIC program is predominantly run and accessed by females; it is a women's business, from participants to staff. Considering any contribution of male support in the decision to breastfeed was completely unheard of. Yet, the potential role of men for breastfeeding success in the WIC setting was already tested in Texas. Encouraging testimonies from early participating fathers, coupled with the framework distilled form the PEN-3 theoretical model, helped develop positive approaches

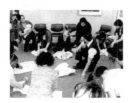

to involve men from the Dallas WIC community. In the 7 years the program has been in effect, it engaged well over 50,000 families in the Dallas WIC community, local high schools, hospitals and, everywhere fathers and future fathers would be found (see picture of Peer Dad (sitting on the floor) teaching a class to families).

Peer Dad Conceptual Model

The PEN-3 cultural model (Iwelunmor, Newsome, & Airhihenbuwa, 2014) consists of three primary domains: (1) Cultural Identity, (2) Relationships and Expectations, and (3) Cultural Empowerment. Each domain includes three factors that form the acronym PEN; Person, Extended Family, Neighborhood (Cultural Identity Domain); Perceptions, Enablers, and Nurturers (relationship and expectation domain); Positive, Existential, and Negative (Cultural Empowerment Domain).

The Cultural Identity Domain highlights the intervention points of entry. These may occur at the level of persons (e.g., expecting fathers), extended family members (grandfathers), or neighborhoods (communities). **With the Relationships and Expectations Domain**, perceptions or attitudes about the men breastfeeding concerns, the societal or structural resources, such as breastfeeding myths that promote or discourage effective lactation practices, as well as the influence of family and kin in nurturing decisions surrounding effective breastfeeding management are examined.

With the Cultural Empowerment Domain, health problems are explored first by identifying beliefs and practices that are positive, exploring and highlighting values and beliefs that are existential and have no harmful health consequences, before identifying negative health practices that serve as barriers. In this way, cultural beliefs and practices that influence health are examined, whereby solutions to health problems that are beneficial are encouraged, those that are harmless are acknowledged, before finally tackling practices that are harmful and have negative health consequences.

The PEN-3 cultural model offers an opportunity to promote the notion of multiple truths by examining cultures and behavior, and by beginning with and identifying the positives—fathers' breastfeeding support—before identifying the negative. In this way, the peer dad program intervention promotes more positive values as it is changing negative ones (see Figure 1).

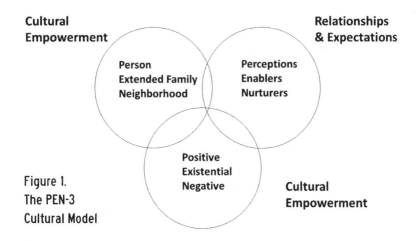

Cultural
Empowerment

Relationships
& Expectations

Person
Extended Family
Neighborhood

Perceptions
Enablers
Nurturers

Positive
Existential
Negative

Cultural
Empowerment

Figure 1.
The PEN-3
Cultural Model

Peer Dad Program Challenge

Breastfeeding initiation rates in Texas are high. A great deal of work needs to be done to increase breastfeeding duration and exclusivity to reap the maximal medical benefits of breastfeeding, and lower the cost of medical intervention. Changes need to occur in a variety of settings, including the family, community, health care sector, workplace, and society. Accessing men remains the challenge of the peer dad program. Partnerships with other male focused programs and groups have been established to provide fathers with more resources and platforms where they can interact. The idea is to address the entire community connected to WIC, not only to women. As the community is educated, it would be empowered to make healthy choices.

References

Arora, S., McJunkin, C., Wehrer, J., & Kuhn, P. (2000). Major factors influencing breastfeeding rates: Mother's perception of father's attitude and milk supply. *Pediatrics, 106*(5), e67-e67.

Avery, A., B., & Magnus, J., H. (2011). Expectant fathers' and mothers' perceptions of breastfeeding and formula feeding: A focus group study in three US cities. *Journal of Human Lactation, 27*(2), 147-154. doi:10.1177/0890334410395753.

Bar-Yam, N. B., & Darby, L. (1997). Fathers and breastfeeding: A review of the literature. *Journal of Human Lactation, 13*(1), 45-50.

Cohen, R., Lange, L., & Slusser, W. (2002). A description of a male-focused breastfeeding promotion corporate lactation program. *Journal of Human Lactation, 18*(1), 61-65.

Freed, G. L., Fraley, J. K., & Schanler, R. J. (1992). Attitudes of expectant fathers regarding breast-feeding. *Pediatrics, 90*(2 Pt 1), 224-227.

Iwelunmor, J., Newsome, V., & Airhihenbuwa, C. O. (2014). Framing the impact of culture on health: A systematic review of the PEN-3 cultural model and its application in public health research and interventions. *Ethnicity & Health, 19*(1), 20-46.

Maycock, B., Binns, C. W., Dhaliwal, S., Tohotoa, J., Hauck, Y., Burns, S., & Howat, P. (2013). Education and support for fathers improves breastfeeding rates: A randomized controlled trial. *Journal of Human Lactation, 29*(4), 484-490. doi:10.1177/0890334413484387 [doi].

Stremler, J., & Lovera, D. (2004). Insight from a breastfeeding peer support pilot program for husbands and fathers of texas WIC participants. *Journal of Human Lactation, 20*(4), 417-422. doi:20/4/417 [pii].

U.S. Department of Health and Human Services. (2011). *The Surgeon General's Call to Action to Support Breastfeeding.* Retrieved from http://www.surgeongeneral.gov/library/calls/breastfeeding/calltoactiontosupportbreastfeeding.pdf.

Vaaler, M. L., Castrucci, B. C., Parks, S. E., Clark, J., Stagg, J., & Erickson, T. (2011). Men's attitudes toward breastfeeding: Findings from the 2007 texas behavioral risk factor surveillance system. *Maternal and Child Health Journal, 15*(2), 148-157.

Walker, M. (2002). Expanding breastfeeding promotion and support in the special supplemental nutrition program for women, infants and children (WIC). *Journal of Human Lactation, 18*(2), 115-124.

CHAPTER 48

A Qualitative Description of African American Men's Experiences as Fathers of Breastfed Infants

Becky Spencer

Where do fathers fit in with breastfeeding and feminism? Lactivists use the term "dyad" to refer to the symbiotic relationship between a breastfeeding mother and her infant. Social, emotional, and physical support are important factors in the success of the breastfeeding dyad. Common categories of support include family, health care provider, workplace, peer, and government or policy support. The father of the baby tends to get grouped with family or general breastfeeding support. I would argue that the father of the breastfed infant is not an external support person separate from the dyad. A father is central to the breastfeeding relationship when he is actively engaged and feels included and important.

Research regarding the role of fathers in breastfeeding is relatively robust. Exploration of the impact of fathers on breastfeeding began to appear in the literature in the late 1970s to the early 1980s. What do we know from this body of literature that spans over 40 years and multiple disciplines, including medicine, nursing, nutrition, public health, and social science? Four main themes can be deduced: (a) fathers are one of the most influential voices in mothers' decision to breastfeed (Arora et al., 2000; Baronowski et al., 1983; Bentley et al. 1999; Beske & Garvis, 1982; Biscane, Continisio, Aldinucci, D'Amora, & Continisio, 2005), (b) mothers have higher initiation rates and longer duration of breastfeeding when fathers are included in breastfeeding education (Mitchell-Box & Braun, 2013; Özlüses & Çelebioglu, 2014; Redshaw & Henderson, 2013), (c) fathers of breastfed infants have reported feeling excluded, not important, and disconnected from the breastfeeding dyad (Brown & Davies, 2014; Gamble & Morse, 1992; Jordan & Wall, 1990), and (d) fathers of breastfed infants have expressed a strong desire to learn about breastfeeding, effectively provide breastfeeding support, and physically bond with their infants (Anderson, 1996; Barclay & Lupton, 1999; Schmidt & Sigman-Grant, 2000; Sherriff, Hall, & Pickin, 2009). The message from fathers is clear and consistent: they yearn to be a central influence and part of the mother-infant breastfeeding dyad, but they need education and preparation for their new role.

African American men are of particular interest in the examination of breastfeeding support by fathers. African American infants are less likely to have been breastfed than infants of any other racial minority in the United States (Table 1). Initiation rates and duration of breastfeeding in the African American community are improving, but a significant disparity remains when comparing breastfeeding rates to White, Asian, Hispanic/Latino, and Native American communities (Centers for Disease Control and Prevention, 2015). African American fathers' voices regarding breastfeeding are underreported in the published literature regarding fathers' experiences and roles in supporting the breastfeeding dyad. African American women have also reported that father support for breastfeeding was instrumental to their success in meeting breastfeeding goals (Spencer, Wambach, & Domian, 2015). A need exists to learn about African American men's thoughts and opinions regarding breastfeeding, and how they perceive father involvement and support of the breastfeeding dyad. This summary reports key findings from a qualitative descriptive study that explored African American men's experiences of fathering a breastfed infant.

Table 1. Comparison of Healthy People 2020 Breastfeeding Goals and Breastfeeding Rates in the African American (AA) Population from the National Immunization Survey (NIS) for 2000 and 2011

Initiation and Duration of Breastfeeding	Healthy People 2020 Targets	AA Rates 2000	Non-Hispanic Black or AA Rates 2011	White Rates 2011	Hispanic or Latino Rates 2011
Early Postpartum	89.1%	51%	61.6%	81.1%	83.8%
6 Months	60.6%	19%	35%	52.3%	48.4%
12 Months	34.1%	8%	16.4%	28.4%	24.8%
Exclusive at 3 Months	46.2%	*	26.9%	44.8%	38.3%
Exclusive at 6 Months	25.5%	*	13.7%	20.3%	17.1%

* Exclusive breastfeeding rates at 3 and 6 months were initially collected in the 2004 NIS

** The Non-Hispanic Black or African American demographic category was added to the NIS in 2003 (U.S. DHHS, 2011; U.S. DHHS, 2012)

Study Objectives

The specific aims for the study included to: (1) describe African American men's experiences as fathers of breastfed infants; (2) examine African American fathers' roles in the decision-making process to breastfeed; (3) examine African American fathers' roles in supporting and maintaining breastfeeding initiation and duration.

Method

A total of eight focus group interviews were conducted with 28 African American fathers. Ages of the fathers ranged from 18 to 56. All men had fathered at least one breastfed child. The educational preparation of the men ranged from high school to graduate degrees, and the annual income of the men ranged from less than $25,000 to $150,000 per year. Each participant received a $50 gift card for participation. Institutional review board committee approval from Baylor University was obtained prior to the initiation of the study.

Focus group interview questions began with asking the men to describe their experiences as fathers of breastfed infants. Probing questions addressed the decision-making process to breastfeed, challenges and benefits of breastfeeding, and what advice would they give to expectant fathers about breastfeeding.

Results

Four themes emerged from the data (a) lifting mom up, (b) being the shield, (c) bonding our family, and (d) sharing the goodness.

Lifting Mom Up

The men described a newfound respect and admiration for the mothers of their children through breastfeeding. They described amazement at women's ability to sustain and grow their children. The men also described extreme frustration and helplessness when mothers had difficulty with breastfeeding, especially within the first few weeks after birth.

Being a Shield

Many participants described protection as their most important role in breastfeeding support. Men described being a mediator between the mother and external stressors. Breastfeeding in public was described as a time when mothers needed their protection. Some men supported mothers' breastfeeding in public, while other men were concerned about mothers being scorned by others for breastfeeding in public.

Bonding the Family

Sharing their wife or partner's body with the infant was one of the most common challenges described by men in the focus groups. One father commented, "Another challenge was, uh, having to share the breasts with the baby. 'Cause that's – those are my toys, you know." Breastfeeding seemed to be symbolic of the transition from couple to family. While most men seemed to struggle with this transition, the struggle was temporary as they began to see the benefits of breastfeeding, including healthy growing children, and financial savings from not buying formula. Many men came to see breastfeeding as a source of bonding for their family. Another father commented, "We didn't have to worry about food because the baby could nurse from my wife. So it just felt natural. It was beautiful. This is what God intended."

Sharing the Goodness

All the fathers who participated in the focus groups considered themselves advocates for breastfeeding. They all agreed that breastfeeding should be promoted more in the African American community, and that fathers of breastfed infants should share their experiences. They also acknowledged that sharing about breastfeeding can be difficult because breastfeeding is not widely accepted in the African American community. One father shared an experience where he felt like his experience could have been valuable to a family.

> I know one of my good friends at – at church, uh, he
> and his wife, they spent a lot of money buying the extra
> special formula . . . and I kind of felt like it wasn't my

place to, you know, say, "You know what? You guys should really be breastfeeding." But I think it may have had an impact if I would have spoken up.

Men described African American churches and church groups as ideal places for men to share their support and experiences as fathers of breastfed infants. One father eloquently shared his advice for expectant African American fathers, "Just embrace it . . . Really put your wife and the baby before yourself."

Conclusions

The collaborative sharing of African American men's experiences of fathering a breastfed infant in the context of their day-to-day lives provides the basis for development of culturally relevant strategies that engage fathers in learning about and supporting breastfeeding. African American fathers desire more education on breastfeeding, and the support that mother's need to reach their breastfeeding goals. African American churches may be ideal places for fathers of breastfed children to connect and support one another. African American fathers clearly value the benefits of breastfeeding, and expressed a desire to support breastfeeding for their families. As health care providers, we need to provide specific education and guidance about the unique roles that fathers play in the success of breastfeeding. We need to actively engage fathers as early during pregnancy as possible, and continue to engage and support fathers in their support roles for breastfeeding after birth. We need to acknowledge mother-infant-father as a *triad*, rather than father as separate from the mother-infant dyad. This change in perspective will help support fathers as they transition from embracing the mother to embracing their family (Figure 1).

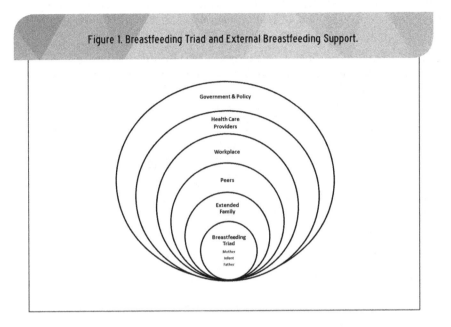

Figure 1. Breastfeeding Triad and External Breastfeeding Support.

References

Anderson, A. M. (1996). Factors influencing the father-infant relationship. *Journal of Family Nursing, 2*, 306-324. doi:10.1177/107484079600200306.

Arora, S., McJunkin, C., Wehrer, J., & Kuhn, P. (2000). Major factors influencing breastfeeding rates: Mother's perception of father's attitude and milk supply. *Pediatrics, 106(5)*, e67-e67. http://dx.doi.org/10.1542/peds.106.5.e67.

Abbass-Dick, J., Stern, S.B., Nelson, L.E., Watson W., & Dennis, C. (2015). Co-parenting breastfeeding support and exclusive breastfeeding: a randomized controlled trial. *Pediatrics, 135(1)*.

Baronowski, T., Bee, D. E., Rassin, D. K., Richardson, C. J., Brown, J. P., Guenther, N., & Nader, P. R. (1983). Social support, social influence, ethnicity and the breastfeeding decision. *Social Science & Medicine, 17(21)*, 1599-1611. doi:10.1016/0277-9536(83)90306-4.

Barclay, L., & Lupton, D. (1999). The experiences of new fatherhood: A socio-cultural analysis. *Journal of Advanced Nursing, 29(4)*, 1013-1020. doi:10.1046/j.1365-2648.1999.00978.x.

Beske, E. J., & Garvis, M. S. (1982). Important factors in breast-feeding success. *MCN: The American Journal of Maternal/Child Nursing, 7*(3), 174-179. doi:10.1097/00005721-198205000-00017.

Bentley, M. E., Caulfield, L. E., Gross, S. M., Bronner, Y., Jensen, J., Kessler, L. A., & Paige, D.M. (1999). Sources of influence on intention to breastfeed among African American women at entry to WIC. *Journal of Human Lactation, 15,* 27-34. http://dx.doi.org/10.1177/089033449901500109.

Brown, A., & Davies, R. (2014). Fathers' experiences of supporting breastfeeding: Challenges for breastfeeding promotion and education. *Maternal & Child Nutrition, 10*(4), 510-526. doi:10.1111/mcn.12129.

Centers for Disease Control (2015). *Breastfeeding.* Retrieved from http://www.cdc.gov/breastfeeding/data/NIS_data/index.htm.

Gamble, D., & Morse, J. M. (1992). Fathers of breastfed infants: Postponing and types of involvement. *Journal of Obstetric, Gynecologic, and Neonatal Nursing, 22*(4), 358-365. doi:10.1111/j.1552-6909.1993.tb01816.x.

Jordan, P. L., & Wall, V. R. (1990). Breastfeeding and fathers: Illuminating the darker side. *Birth, 17*(4), 210-213. doi:10.1111/j.1523-536x.1990.tb00024.x.

Mitchell-Box, K.M., & Braun, K.L. (2013). Impact of male-partner-focused interventions on breastfeeding initiation, exclusivity, and continuation. *Journal of Human Lactation, 29*(4), 473-479. doi:10.1177/0890334413491833.

Özlüses, E., & Çelebioglu, A. (2014). Educating fathers to improve breastfeeding rates and paternal-infant attachment. *Indian Pediatrics, 51*(8), 654-657. doi:10.1007/s13312-014-0471-3.

Pisacane, A., Continisio, G. I., Aldinucci, M., D'Amora, S., & Continisio, P. (2005). A controlled trial of the father's role in breastfeeding promotion. *Pediatrics, 116*(4), e494-e498. http://dx.doi.org/10.1542/peds.2005-0479.

Redshaw, M., & Henderson, J. (2013). Fathers' engagement in pregnancy and childbirth: Evidence from a national survey. *BMC Pregnancy and Childbirth, 13*(1), 70. doi:10.1186/1471-2393-13-70.

Schmidt, M. M., & Sigman-Grant, M. (2000). Perspectives of low-income fathers' support of breastfeeding: An exploratory study. *Journal of Nutrition Education, 32*(1), 31-37. doi:10.1016/s0022-3182(00)70507-3.

Sherriff, N., Hall, V., & Pickin, M. (2009). Fathers' perspectives on breastfeeding: Ideas for intervention. *British Journal of Midwifery, 17*(4), 223. http://dx.doi.org/10.12968/bjom.2009.17.4.41670.

Spencer, B., Wambach, K., & Domain, E. W. (2014). African American women's breastfeeding experiences cultural, personal, and political voices. *Qualitative Health Research, 25*(7), 974-987. doi:1049732314554097.

Engaging Men to Promote and Support Exclusive Breastfeeding: A Review of Results and Strategies in USAID's Child Survival and Health Grants Program 2003-2013

Jennifer Yourkavitch, Jeniece Alvey, Debra Prosnitz,
Miriam Labbok, and Jim Thomas

Mothers need support to optimally breastfeed, but the most effective delivery methods and frequency of support in different contexts remains largely unknown. Exclusive breastfeeding (EBF) rates either gain slowly or continue to lag in most developing countries (Cai, Wardlaw, & Brown, 2012). Since 1985, the United States Agency for International Development's Child Survival and Health Grant Program (CSHGP) has provided funding and technical assistance to more than 400 programs implemented by nearly 60 different non-governmental organizations (NGOs) in more than 60 countries to improve maternal, newborn, and child health outcomes (USAID, 2015). Various community-based strategies, including peer support and promotion, have been developed for increasing EBF in CSHGP and other project areas. The role of men in promoting and supporting EBF at the community level has not been systematically evaluated across different countries.

Only a few studies have evaluated interventions involving men in EBF promotion or support. A study by Brown and Davies (2014) found that new fathers in the United Kingdom (UK) encouraged breast-feeding, and wanted to be supportive, but often felt left out of the relationship and helpless. An intervention, including educational mate-rials, along with individual, couple, and group counseling, addressing breastfeeding among other health issues was tested in South Africa and India. It had no effect on breastfeeding (Kraft, Wilkinds, Morales, Widyono, & Middlestadt, 2014). A test of a hospital-based co-parenting class in Canada found an increase in breastfeeding duration, fathers' breastfeeding efficacy, and maternal report of paternal support, but did not show a significant difference for EBF (Abbass-Dick et al., 2015). An intervention study conducted in Vietnam provided fathers with educational materials and counseling during household visits to pro-mote EBF at the 4th and 6th month postpartum, and found higher EBF prevalence among mothers whose partners received the intervention (Bich, Hoa, & Malgvist, 2014).

Given the mixed evidence, we sought to examine the relationship of male engagement and EBF practice in several countries, comparing changes in EBF prevalence in CSHGP project areas, where men were engaged in EBF promotion and support, to changes in areas where men were not engaged, and to describe strategies that were used to promote and support EBF.

Data

NGOs that implement CSHGP projects conduct standardized, popula-tion-based Knowledge, Practice and Coverage surveys, which capture key maternal, newborn, and child health indicators at the beginning and end of each project. EBF was measured as the percentage of infants 0 to 5 months, who were exclusively breastfed in the 24 hours prior to the survey.[1] For this study, data from the CSHGP database, and final evaluation reports were used to determine EBF prevalence and strategies used to engage men in EBF promotion or support.[2] All CSHGP projects beginning and ending between 2003 and 2013 were selected (*N*=78). Those that promoted or supported EBF in low- and middle-income countries, as specified in the their final evaluation report (*N*=57), and had complete data (i.e., prevalence estimates, and 95% confidence intervals), with no indication of data collection problems were included in the final study sample (*N*=51).

Method

This study compared the EBF prevalence change in project areas where men were engaged in EBF promotion or support *(n=28)* to the EBF prevalence change in project areas where men were not engaged *(n=23)*. We also examined regional differences and compared EBF prevalence changes in project areas to national EBF prevalence trends. We further categorized male engagement strategies by level of intensity based on information we extracted from each final evaluation report. **High Intensity:** Projects that engaged men in a small group or one-on-one setting; **Low Intensity:** Projects that engaged men in large group settings; or **None**.

We calculated EBF prevalence differences with confidence intervals, overall and by region. We also compared EBF prevalence differences in project areas to national estimates from the Demographic and Health Surveys (DHS), where available within two years of project estimates *(n=21)*. We used logistic regression to model the relationship between EBF final prevalence greater than the median value and male engagement, adjusting for funding, region, and population size.

---

1 These standard questionnaires and indicators can be found at www.mchipngo.net
2 Project data are available at www.mchipngo.net

We also modeled the association for the sub-Saharan Africa, and South and Central Asia regions. We qualitatively examined and described different strategies that were used to promote and support EBF in the project countries that engaged men, and in those that did not. Keyword searches were conducted in each final evaluation report using primary search terms: men, husband(s), father(s), exclusive, breastfeeding, LAM; and secondary search terms: family, partner, male, decision maker, or other synonymous project-specific terms. We created a matrix, and thematically analyzed these according to intensity of male engagement.

Results

Overall, the mean EBF prevalence difference in areas where men were engaged was 0.26 (95% CI: 0.16 – 0.36), and where men were not engaged was 0.20 (95% CI: 0.11 – 0.29). In sub-Saharan Africa, the prevalence difference was 0.36 (95% CI 0.22 – 0.40) where men were engaged versus 0.28 (95% CI 0.12 – 0.44) where they were not. Project areas in the South and Central Asia region, where men were engaged had an average prevalence difference of 0.14 (95% CI 0.05 – 0.23); where men were not engaged had an average prevalence difference of 0.06 (95% CI 0.03 – 0.09). The Latin America and Southeast Asia regions had too few projects to analyze separately.

Figure 1 shows prevalence differences in project areas that engaged men, and Figure 2 shows prevalence differences in project areas that did not engage men in EBF promotion and support. Figures 3 and 4 show prevalence estimates for CSHGP projects, alongside national estimates, indicating that most project areas had a greater prevalence difference than what was observed nationally, regardless of male engagement. A multivariable model of the association between intensity of male engagement and odds of EBF prevalence greater than or equal to the final prevalence median value (74%), adjusted for funding, population size and region, yielded OR 0.98 (95% CI 0.25, 3.78) for high-intensity compared to no male engagement, and OR 0.10 (95% CI 0.01, 0.98) for low-intensity compared to no male engagement. A logistic regression model for sub-Saharan Africa (median final prevalence 73%) yielded odds of final prevalence greater than or equal to the median where there were high-intensity activities at 2.46 (95% CI: 0.40 – 15.27) times the odds of final prevalence greater than or equal to the median where men were not engaged, adjusted for population size and funding. The odds for low-intensity activities was 0.34 (95% CI: 0.03 – 4.40) times the odds where men were not engaged, adjusted for population size and funding. The model for South and Central Asia did not converge.

Strategies to engage men in EBF promotion and support varied by region and intensity. Three illustrative strategies are described here for each level of male engagement. As a high-intensity male engagement approach, Project Hope in Uzbekistan established a New Parents School in health centers, which educated expectant parents about health issues, including EBF, and gave them take-home materials, a doll for practicing breastfeeding positioning, and educational posters. EBF prevalence increased by 27 percentage points (95% CI 0.17, 0.37), to reach 90 percent when the project ended.

A low-intensity strategy used by CARE in Sierra Leone included the creation of Community Health Clubs to mobilize communities with behavior change communication messages given during 2-hour interactive health lessons, which included EBF. Participants who attended 20 meetings received a certificate. This project area had a 60-point (95% CI 0.51, 0.69) prevalence increase in EBF, ending at 68 percent. Lastly, with no male engagement, Salvation Army World Services in Zambia used the Care Group strategy to engage women in small group meetings or home visits in discussion on various health topics, including EBF. This project area had a 38-percentage point increase (95% CI 0.26, 0.50) in EBF prevalence, ending at 85 percent.

Discussion

The CSHGP projects employed various context-specific approaches to EBF promotion and support. While inconclusive, our analyses suggest there may be greater prevalence increases where men were engaged than where they were not, and that engaging men in EBF promotion and support through high-intensity activities, may, on average, be associated with a higher EBF prevalence than not engaging men at all in sub-Saharan Africa. There may be residual confounding in our estimates due to factors related to male dominance in communities; therefore, it may be important for programs that seek to increase EBF practice to assess whether male engagement is appropriate before including it as a project strategy. If women indicate that male (partner) support is important to their breastfeeding practice, as Brown and Davies (2014) found in the UK, then high-intensity activities that have some individual or small-group male engagement may have a greater impact than general activities that engage men nominally (e.g., through health fairs or non-specific health communication efforts or materials).

It is important to evaluate the cost and intensity of male engagement strategies, and conduct multiple tests in different areas to determine if they are scalable to a national level. More comparative studies are need within countries to determine which strategies are most effective with different populations. Contextual information about female autonomy should also be considered: where female autonomy is limited, can men be engaged in EBF promotion and support in a way that does not reinforce gender dynamics that are detrimental to women?

Limitations to this study include a small sample size, and unmeasured factors that may influence the relationship between male engagement and EBF prevalence in project areas. Prevalence difference, as an effect measure, may not tell the full story (e.g., a project area that moves from 60% to 80% EBF prevalence has still experienced an important success, even though its prevalence difference (20 points) is lower than a project area that moves from 20% to 50%). A higher final prevalence may, in fact, be more sustainable, since it indicates the normalization of EBF in an area. In addition, it may be ineffective, from a policy standpoint, to compare strategies employed among highly diverse populations. However, it is important to explore this relationship, and this study makes some suggestions regarding considerations for male engagement in EBF promotion and support.

Conclusion

While inconclusive, our analyses suggest greater change in EBF prevalence where men were engaged, and that engaging men in EBF promotion and support through high-intensity activities, may, on average, be associated with a higher EBF prevalence than not engaging men at all, in sub-Saharan Africa. We recommend that program implementers investigate the role of men as influencers of infant feeding practices, and engage men in EBF promotion and support where appropriate.

References

Abbass-Dick, J., Stern, S.B., Nelson, L.E., Watson W., & Dennis, C. (2015). Co-parenting breastfeeding support and exclusive breastfeeding: a randomized controlled trial. *Pediatrics*, 135(1).

Brown, A., & Davies, R. (2014). Fathers' experiences of supporting breastfeeding: Challenges for breastfeeding promotion and education. *Maternal Child Nutrition*, 10(4), 510-526.

Brown, A., & Lee, M. (2011). An exploration of the attitudes and experiences of mothers in the United Kingdom who chose to breastfeed exclusively for 6 months postpartum. *Breastfeeding Medicine*, 6(4), 197-204.

Bich, T., Hoa, D., & Malqvist, M. (2014). Fathers as supporters for improved exclusive breastfeeding in Vietnam. *Maternal Child Health Journal*, 18, 1444-1453.

Cai, X. Wardlaw T, & Brown D. (2012) Global trends in exclusive breastfeeding. *International Breastfeeding Journal*, 7, 12.

Kraft, J.M., Wilkinds, K.G., Morales, G.J., Widyono, M., & Middlestadt, S.E. (2014) An evidence review of gender-integrated interventions in reproductive and maternal-child health. *Journal of Health Communication*, 19(Suppl1), 122-141.

USAID. (2015). *Maternal and child health integrated program*. Available at www.mchipngo.net.

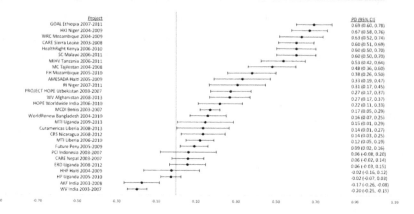

Figure 1: Prevalence Differences in Projects that Engaged Men in EBF Promotion.

Project	PD (95% CI)
GOAL Ethiopia 2007-2011	0.69 (0.60, 0.78)
HKI Niger 2004-2009	0.67 (0.58, 0.76)
WRC Mozambique 2004-2009	0.63 (0.52, 0.74)
CARE Sierra Leone 2003-2008	0.60 (0.51, 0.69)
HealthRight Kenya 2006-2010	0.60 (0.50, 0.70)
SC Malawi 2006-2011	0.60 (0.50, 0.70)
MIHV Tanzania 2006-2011	0.53 (0.42, 0.64)
MC Tajikistan 2004-2008	0.48 (0.36, 0.60)
FH Mozambique 2005-2010	0.38 (0.26, 0.50)
AMESADA Haiti 2005-2009	0.33 (0.19, 0.47)
RI Niger 2007-2011	0.31 (0.17, 0.45)
PROJECT HOPE Uzbekistan 2003-2007	0.27 (0.17, 0.37)
WV Afghanistan 2008-2013	0.27 (0.17, 0.37)
HOPE Worldwide India 2006-2010	0.22 (0.11, 0.33)
MCDI Benin 2003-2007	0.17 (0.05, 0.29)
WorldRenew Bangladesh 2004-2010	0.16 (0.07, 0.25)
MTI Uganda 2009-2013	0.15 (0.01, 0.29)
Curamericas Liberia 2008-2013	0.14 (0.01, 0.27)
CRS Nicaragua 2008-2012	0.14 (0.03, 0.25)
MTI Liberia 2006-2010	0.12 (0.05, 0.19)
Future Peru 2005-2009	0.09 (0.02, 0.16)
PCI Indonesia 2003-2007	0.06 (-0.08, 0.20)
CARE Nepal 2003-2007	0.06 (-0.02, 0.14)
ERD Uganda 2008-2012	0.06 (-0.03, 0.15)
HHF Haiti 2004-2009	-0.02 (-0.16, 0.12)
HP Uganda 2005-2010	-0.02 (-0.07, 0.03)
AKF India 2003-2008	-0.17 (-0.26, -0.08)
WV India 2003-2007	-0.20 (-0.25, -0.15)

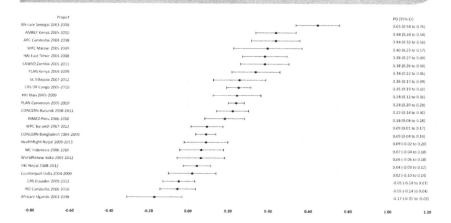

Figure 2: Prevalence Differences in Projects that Did Not Engage Men in EBF Promotion.

Project	PD (95% CI)
Africare Senegal 2003-2008	0.65 (0.54 to 0.76)
AMREF Kenya 2005-2010	0.44 (0.34 to 0.54)
ARC Cambodia 2004-2008	0.44 (0.32 to 0.56)
WRC Malawi 2005-2009	0.40 (0.23 to 0.57)
HAI East Timor 2004-2008	0.38 (0.27 to 0.49)
SAWSO Zambia 2005-2011	0.38 (0.26 to 0.50)
PLAN Kenya 2004-2009	0.34 (0.22 to 0.46)
SC Ethiopia 2007-2012	0.26 (0.13 to 0.39)
CRS DR Congo 2005-2010	0.25 (0.19 to 0.31)
HKI Mali 2005-2009	0.24 (0.12 to 0.36)
PLAN Cameroon 2005-2010	0.24 (0.20 to 0.28)
CONCERN Burundi 2008-2013	0.22 (0.14 to 0.30)
INMED Peru 2006-2010	0.18 (0.08 to 0.28)
WRC Burundi 2007-2012	0.09 (0.01 to 0.17)
CONCERN Bangladesh 2004-2009	0.09 (0.04 to 0.14)
HealthRight Nepal 2009-2013	0.09 (-0.02 to 0.20)
MC Indonesia 2006-2010	0.07 (-0.04 to 0.18)
WorldRenew India 2007-2012	0.06 (-0.06 to 0.18)
HKI Nepal 2008-2012	0.04 (-0.03 to 0.17)
Counterpart India 2004-2009	0.02 (-0.10 to 0.14)
CHS Ecuador 2009-2013	-0.05 (-0.14 to 0.03)
IRD Cambodia 2006-2010	-0.05 (-0.14 to 0.04)
Africare Uganda 2003-2008	-0.17 (-0.31 to -0.03)

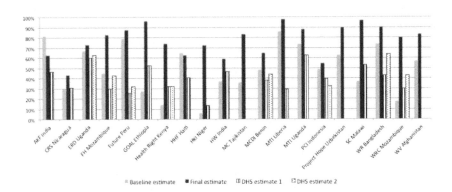

Figure 3: EBF prevalence by high intensity male engagement for CSHGP projects with corresponding DHS data, 2003-2013; n=20.

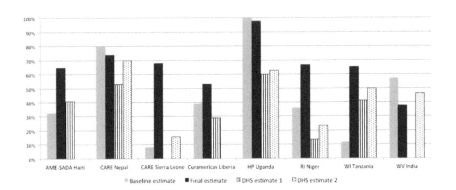

Figure 4: EBF prevalence by low intensity male engagement for CSHGP projects with corresponding DHS data, 2003-2013; n=5.

Concluding Comments

Paige Hall Smith and Miriam Labbok

We feel privileged and honored have been part of the Breastfeeding and Feminism International Conference for the past
decade. As the only breastfeeding conference that focuses on the
gendered, sociocultural, economic, health, and political impacts on,
and of, women's infant feeding decisions, BFIC attracts wide diversity
of participants from different academic disciplines, practice locals,
and cultural arenas. We hope the four books published from conference presentations have helped to broaden the dissemination of the
high-quality research, practice, and policy initiatives that are being
conducted by these participants. We are also pleased to have had the
opportunity collaborate with Praeclarus Press for this three-part series
from the 2013, 2014, and 2015 conferences.

The enthusiasm we experience from the eclectic body of participants leads us to us to conclude that the conference will be around
another 10 years. The theme for this year's conference, Social Justice
and Equity, is likely to remain a central part of the work presented
and discussed at BFIC going forward. The broad range of topics that
we hope to be covered in the forthcoming years include a continued
focus on how the complexities of women's experiences shape their
feeding decisions, how gender intersects with sexuality, ethnicity, race,
culture, and socioeconomic status to create new patterns and intricacies to breastfeeding decision-making and practice, how breastfeeding

may shape, or be shaped by, other important health-related facets of women's lives including contraception, medication, and mental and physical health. We are also interested in how feminism, and feminist perspectives, can embolden and/or interfere with breastfeeding. Finally, we want to know how we can improve the range of breastfeeding practice, promotion, and support strategies in ways that privilege women's experiences, and recognize the value of caregiving and parent-child relationships, advancing effective strategies across the social ecology.

We encourage you to submit and abstract and join us!

Contributing Authors

Miki Akiyama, PhD, is an Associate Professor of Environment and Information Studies at Keio University.

Jeniece Alvey, MPH, has over 5 years of experience in global maternal-child health and nutrition research, and program evaluation. She currently works as a Research Assistant for the Measurement, Learning, and Evaluation Project for the Urban Reproductive Health Initiative at the UNC Carolina Population Center, where she analyzes the use of LAM as a postpartum family planning method in Nigeria. Her research interests are in global maternal, newborn, and child health, infant and young child feeding, breastfeeding, family planning, and program evaluation. Jeniece completed her MPH at the Gillings School of Global Public Health at the University of North Carolina at Chapel Hill, where she also completed the CGBI Mary Rose Tully Training Initiative for her IBCLC certification.

Kathleen L. Anderson, MEd, CLC is director of Community Breastfeeding at The Carolina Global Breastfeeding Institute where she implements a statewide Breastfeeding-Friendly Child Care project and coordinates a project studying breastfeeding services from day 2 to week 12 postpartum. She also facilitates a national collaborative on advancing breastfeeding in child care. Kathleen has a Master's degree in Education with focus on Early Intervention and Family Support. She is a Certified Lactation Counselor and La Leche League Leader.

Erin Austen, PhD, is an Assistant Professor in the Department of Psychology at St. Francis Xavier University in Nova Scotia. One of her research interests is the perception of breastfeeding among young adults. She is interested in possible techniques to improve comfort levels with breastfeeding. Her research uses objective measures, such as eye movements, to assess reactions to breastfeeding. She is particularly interested in whether negative reactions to breastfeeding impact memory for print information that accompanies breastfeeding images. Erin is one of the founding members of a local community initiative called BaBE (Building a Breastfeeding Environment). She and her student researchers collaborate with individuals from Public Health and La Leche League; they recently created a breast-feeding support video targeted at young adults that has been widely accessed.

Erica Hesch Anstey, PhD, CLC works for McKing Consulting Corporation in the Nutrition Branch of the Centers for Disease Control and Prevention (CDC) where she works with the Infant Feeding Team on translating research into guidance. She received her PhD in public health from the University of South Florida in Tampa, where she worked on the study presented in these conference proceedings. She also has an MA in women's studies and is a certified lactation counselor (CLC). Erica has long been interested in becoming a leader in Maternal and Child Health (MCH), and is a member of the Editorial Review Board for the *Journal of Human Lactation*. Her research interests include breastfeeding management issues, tongue-tie, breast-feeding disparities, and family-centered care. She has worked on several studies related to breastfeeding including a community needs assessment for a university-led clinical lactation program, and her dissertation on International Board Certified Lactation Consultants' (IBCLCs') perceived professional barriers to managing early breastfeeding problems. Erica is particularly interested in bridging the disciplines of feminist studies and public health as a way to improve maternal and child health outcomes and delivery of care.

Helen Ball obtained her PhD in Biological Anthropology at the University of Massachusetts, Amherst in 1992. Her undergraduate degree was in Human Biology, and her interests span both biology and anthropology. She established the Parent-Infant Sleep Lab at Durham University in 2000, was promoted to Professor in 2007 and became Head of the Anthropology Department in 2013. Broadly defined, her research examines the sleep ecology of infants, young children, and their parents. This encompasses attitudes and practices regarding infant sleep, behavioral and physiological monitoring of infants and their parents during sleep, infant sleep development, and the discordance between cultural sleep preferences and biological sleep needs. She conducts research in hospitals and the community, and contributes to national and international policy and practice guidelines on infant care (see www.dur.ac.uk/sleep.lab/). She oversees the translation of academic research on infant sleep into evidence for use by parents and healthcare staff via ISIS -- the Infant Sleep Information Source website (www.isisonline.org.uk).

Cecilia E. Barbosa, PhD, MPH, MCP is principal, cBe consulting. She received a PhD in social and behavioral health from Virginia Commonwealth University in December 2014; her dissertation was on infant feeding barriers and facilitators among low-income African American women in Richmond. She has worked for over 20 years in public health in Virginia, as an independent consultant, as Director, Division of Child and Adolescent Health and as Director of Planning and Evaluation, Division of Maternal and Child Health, Virginia Department of Health. She received Master of Public Health and Master of City Planning degrees from the University of California at Berkeley. She serves on the Governor of Virginia's Latino Advisory Board, the Virginia Department of Health Institutional Review Board, the Mayor of Richmond's Breastfeeding Taskforce, and Virginia Public Health Association board. She is fluent in Portuguese, Spanish, and French.

Micheline Beaudry, PhD, MNS, PDt - Following a doctorate in international nutrition from Cornell University (1971), her career in Public nutrition—community, public health, international—unfolded with two universities (Moncton and Laval), and two international agencies (PAHO/WHO and UNICEF), until her retirement in 2006. Early on, her international experience led her to recognize the crucial role that breastfeeding plays—and the even greater role it could play—throughout the world. This has fuelled much of her work. She has published several scientific papers, given many conferences and scientific communications and supervised several graduate students, mainly on issues related to infant feeding, breastfeeding, and household food security. In 2006, she co-authored a book for health professionals *Biologie de l'allaitement – Le sein, le lait, le geste,* a first in French which rapidly required three reprints. In 2009, she was a founding member of the *Mouvement allaitement du Québec (MAQ),* where she is still very active. She also coordinated the work of the *Commission on health, living conditions and social services* of *Québec solidaire* (2008-2012), where she remains an active member.

Vivian Black is a medical doctor with a master's of Science in infectious Disease. Dr. Black works for the Wits Reproductive Health and HIV Institute, and ran the maternal health and HIV programs within the inner city of Johannesburg for over 10 years. Part of her role was developing, implementing and evaluating health systems strengthening initiatives in health districts (rural, semi-urban, and densely populated urban environments) in South Africa. She assists the South African National Department of Health on the antiretroviral treatment guidelines committee, PMTCT committee (which she chaired). She draft-wrote the 2008, 2010, and 2014 South African PMTCT guidelines. Together, with a Department of Health HIV Director, she co-chaired the South African National AIDS Council Treatment and Care Technical Task Team. She assists local government with programmatic advice and sits on their PMTCT and Training working groups.

Elizabeth Brooks JD, IBCLC, FILCA, is a lawyer (since 1983), and private practice lactation consultant (since 1997), who brings to life the connection between lactation consultation and the law. IBCLCs face a maze of ethical, moral and legal requirements in their day-to-day practice, no matter what their work setting. With plain language and humor, Liz explains the laws affecting IBCLCs, so the lactation consultant can work ethically and legally. She offers pragmatic tips that can immediately be used in daily practice. She recently served as the President of the International Lactation Consultant Association (ILCA) (2012-2014), and is a Board member for the United States Breastfeeding Committee (USBC) (2014-2016) and Human Milk Banking Association of North America (HMBANA)(2015-2018). She wrote the only textbook focusing on IBCLC ethics and law, and is a well-received writer and lecturer in her field.

Lorraine Burrage is the Coordinator of the Newfoundland and Labrador Provincial Perinatal Program, St. John's, Newfoundland and Labrador, Canada.

Katherine Carroll, PhD, is a medical sociologist and qualitative researcher in the Faculty of Health Sciences at Mayo Clinic, USA. She has researched human milk donation and the use of donated human milk for preterm infants hospitalized in NICU using ethnographic and interview methods in the USA and Australia. Her postdoctoral research has been funded by the Australian Research Council, Endeavour Fellowship, and University of Technology, Sydney Early Career Research Award. Katherine has recently collaborated with stakeholders from Australian milk banks and NICUs to produce Australia's first national statement on milk donation after neonatal death. Her research on breastmilk and human milk donation is published in various book chapters and journal articles across both the social and health science disciplines. She is continuing her work on human milk donation at Mayo Clinic.

Kellie E. Carlyle, PhD, MPH, is Associate Professor and Program Director in the Department of Social and Behavioral Health in the School of Medicine and affiliate faculty in the Center for Media and Health, and Institute for Women's Health, at Virginia Commonwealth University. She holds a PhD in Social and Behavioral Sciences, and MPH in Health Behavior and Health Promotion from The Ohio State University. Dr. Carlyle was named a Centennial Professor for excellence in teaching, mentoring, and community engagement in her previous position at Arizona State University, and has received multiple Community Engagement grants from VCU. She publishes and teaches in the areas of health behavior theory; campaign design, implementation and evaluation; women's health; violence prevention; and sexual health promotion.

Aynmarie Carter, MPH, is a Health Educator at the Virginia Department of Health where she provides lactation education and support to pregnant and breastfeeding women by facilitating monthly breastfeeding classes, support groups, and individual counseling sessions. She received her MPH in public health from the University of South Florida in Tampa in 2014.

Dianne Cassidy is a Lactation Consultant in Rochester, New York with Advanced Lactation Certification. Dianne works in Private Practice, and in a busy Pediatrician office supporting mothers and babies. She also teaches prenatal breastfeeding and childbirth in the hospital setting. In the fall of 2013, Dianne completed her MA in Health and Wellness/Lactation. She is dedicated to serving mothers and babies, and has the unique ability to identify with the needs and concerns of new mothers. Dianne has worked extensively with women who have survived trauma, babies struggling with tongue-tie, birth trauma, milk supply issues, attachment, identifying latch problems, returning to work, and breastfeeding multiples. Dianne has three biological children, including twins, three stepchildren, and a wonderful husband. Dianne is an author and public speaker, and enjoys teaching caregivers how to support new families through breastfeeding struggles.

Brittany D. Chambers, MPH, CHES, is currently a doctoral student in the public health education department at the University of North Carolina, Greensboro. Ms. Chambers works under the mentorship of Dr. Paige Hall Smith on various projects addressing reproductive health issues among women in Greensboro, NC, including breastfeeding support for adolescent mothers. Her career objectives are to decrease reproductive and sexual health disparities experienced by marginalized group of women through the development and implementation of structural interventions.

Dexter Chagwena is a Nutrition postgraduate candidate at the University of Zimbabwe and an Adjunct Faculty Instructor at the State University of New York at Buffalo, School of Pharmacy and Pharmaceutical Sciences. A pre-doctoral fellow in the National Institutes of Health Fogarty International Center (NIH FIC) UB-UZ AITRP program. Dexter is a goal-oriented nutrition scientist involved in spearheading nutrition implementation research at Nutri@ctive Zimbabwe, a group of young nutrition professionals with passion in driving the agenda of nutrition implementation science Zimbabwe. Dexter is also a member of the Majority World Global Implementation Network Group. He believes the solution to global nutrition-related concerns lies in a new breed of nutrition scientists with the ability of translating laboratory and population-based research findings into implementation programs that provide public health solutions to communities.

Jodine Chase is a public relations and communications consultant, specializing issues and crisis management news analysis. Jodine is a long-time breastfeeding advocate who, as a volunteer, has worked for many breastfeeding-related causes, including advocating for the re-establishment of donor human milk banks in Canada, and amending policies and legislation to protect breastfeeding rights. She has been involved with the Breastfeeding Action Committee of Edmonton (BACE), the Best for Babes Foundation, the Alberta Breastfeeding Committee, ILCA's Social Media Alert team, INFACT Canada, Protect Alberta Breastfeeding, Protect Breastfeeding in Canada, The Facebook vs. Breastfeeding Alliance, Friends of the WHO Code, World Milksharing Week, and the Best for Babes NIP Hotline's Canadian arm. Although, Jodine is more often found behind the scenes assisting others to reach their communication goals, her various involvements include mainstream and social media and public speaking outreach. She is actively live-tweeting and blogging about the breastfeeding events and conferences she attends, and she sometimes accepts honoraria for social media support and for public speaking engagements.

Ellen Chetwynd BSN, MPH, IBCLC is a PhD candidate at the University of North Carolina at Chapel Hill and a lactation consultant at an out of hospital birth center. She has been a lactation consultant for fifteen years, and worked extensively in maternal and child health as a clinician and in management. The education she is receiving in epidemiologic methods allows for direct translational research from the clinical setting to the academic and scientific spheres as well as the application of implementation science in the study of and advocacy for systems of breastfeeding support. Her publications cover topics in advocacy for the profession of lactation consulting, as well as explorations of breastfeeding difficulties, breastfeeding support systems, and the biological make up of human milk. She is an adamant supporter of diverse breastfeeding populations, and has published on the intricacies of two mother families, as well as working on several projects engaging minority populations. Her dissertation work will explore the association between breastfeeding and metabolic health in a large cohort of African American women.

Sylvie Chiasson, MA, BSc - A biologist with a Master's degree in Communication and mother of three breastfed children, she was a breastfeeding support mother for over 20 years before becoming a lactation consultant. Co-author of *Biologie de l'allaitement – Le sein, le lait, le geste,* a book in French for health professionals (PUQ, 2006 : 624 pp). She was also a founding member of the *Mouvement allaitement du Québec (MAQ),* where she has remained very active in its training committee.

Rajshree Das is a post graduate in Social Work from Raipur University, India. She is also trained on disaster management, international perspective on participatory monitoring and evaluation and participatory training methodology. She has been associated in the development sector for over 15 years in different parts of India. Rajshree has served in renowned development organizations like CARE, Catholic Relief Services, and Project Concern International in India. She has designed, led, and managed implementation of large portfolio projects in the sector of livelihoods, health, women and child protection and disaster management. She has worked in government supported women empowerment and community mobilization projects in India. In her current role as the deputy chief of party, she is leading the implementation of a community mobilization project amongst the most marginalized communities in Bihar, India. This project aims at empowering the most marginalized communities for changing behaviors linked with Maternal and Child health and improving access to health services and entitlements.

Susan DeYoung recently retired from the University of Exeter, UK, where she taught and researched in the fields of childhood studies, early childhood education and music education. She trained originally as a pianist and worked as a school teacher before gaining her first university position more than 20 years ago. She has a PhD from the University of Surrey, which focuses on spontaneous music play in early childhood. Determined to lead an active retirement, she enrolled on a further post-graduate research degree in anthropology at the University of Bristol. The focus of this degree on infant feeding among Somali women in the city brings together many long-standing interests; in infancy, in the refugee and recently arrived Muslim communities in the UK and in breastfeeding; all of which she has prior experience through research projects and teaching carried out in her university position.

Joan E. Dodgson, PhD, MPH, FAAN, is an Associate Professor at Arizona State University and the Executive Director of the Southwest Clinical Lactation Education Program. Her research interests include infant feeding, breastfeeding, effects of culture, perinatal nursing, community-based, qualitative methods, Asia, and nursing philosophy.

Aimee R. Eden, PhD, MPH is a medical anthropologist and qualitative researcher at the American Board of Family Medicine (ABFM). She earned her PhD in applied anthropology and MPH with a maternal and child health concentration, and holds a master's degree in International Development. She has conducted qualitative research domestically and internationally on reproductive and maternal-child health topics including breastfeeding and the maternal-child health care workforce. She has served on the International Board of Lactation Consultant Examiners (IBLCE) board of directors since 2010, and chairs the Care of Infants and Children Group of the Society of Teachers of Family Medicine (STFM).

Dr. Katherine Foss is an Associate Professor at Middle Tennessee State University. She has studied breastfeeding discourse across media—the research of her forthcoming book. Her work has also been published in *Health Communication, Women and Health, Critical Studies in Media Communication, Disability Studies Quarterly*, and other peer-reviewed journals. The first book of Dr. Foss (2014), *Television and Health Responsibility in an Age of Individualism*, connects discourse in fictional medical dramas to public perceptions of health care. Dr. Foss earned her PhD in Mass Communication from the University of Minnesota.

Hannah E. Fraley, PhD(c), RN, IBCLC is a PhD Candidate in Population Health Nursing at the University of Massachusetts Boston and an Instructor at Salem State University College of Health and Human Services. Hannah has an extensive background in Perinatal Nursing, is an International Board Certified Lactation Consultant, and is an advocate for vulnerable populations of women and children.

Susan Gallagher has a Baccalaureate Degree in Nursing. Susan has been a nurse for 25 years, and employed with Toronto Public

Health (TPH) for over 16 years as a Public Health Nurse. At TPH she has worked with families in the prenatal, postnatal, and parenting programs. Recently she has been part of the team that help TPH achieve Baby-Friendly Initiative (BFI) designation in January 2013. She is currently working as a Public Health Nurse in a Breastfeeding Designated Assignment facilitating implementation of TPH's BFI sustainability plan.

Quinn Gentry is Founder and CEO of Messages of Empowerment Productions, LLC (TEAM-MOE) where she serves as the principal investigator for several social and health projects focusing primarily on women and girls. A behavioral, scientist by training, Dr. Gentry completed a post-doctoral fellowship at The Johns Hopkins University's Bloomberg School of Public Health in the Urban Health Institute. Dr. Gentry is the author of *Black Women's Risk for HIV: Rough Living* (Taylor & Francis), which is based upon her clinical HIV prevention research with high-risk African American women from 1999-2002. From 2005-2007, Dr. Gentry was a National Institute of Health-sponsored clinical researcher where she built evaluation capacity for AID Atlanta's HIV prevention services and programs. Dr. Gentry has over a decade of experience in programs, evaluation, and research on the social determinants of health with a primary emphasis on intervention development to address health inequities. From a substantive perspective, Dr. Gentry is a subject matter expert on women and girls in the following areas: teen reproductive health, HIV/AIDS, substance abuse risk and treatment, domestic violence, juvenile delinquency, child welfare, mental health, and urban family dynamics.

Sara Gill, RN, PhD, IBCLC, FAAN, is a Professor and the PhD Program Director at the University of Texas Health Science Center San Antonio School of Nursing. She is the Director of Research and Special Projects for the International Lactation

Consultant Association. Dr. Gill oversees the lactation program for University Health System, San Antonio. Practice has provided an opportunity to identify, design, and test strategies to support vulnerable breastfeeding families.

Janet Murphy Goodridge, RN, MN, IBCLC, is the Provincial Breastfeeding Consultant with the Newfoundland and Labrador Provincial Perinatal Program and Chair of the Baby-Friendly Council of Newfoundland and Labrador, St. John's, Newfoundland and Labrador, Canada.

Virginia Guidry, PhD, MPH, is a postdoctoral fellow in the Department of Epidemiology at the University of North Carolina at Chapel Hill. She studies the impact of air pollutants on communities with a focus on environmental justice and community-based research. Her current research is examining the respiratory health effects experienced by children who attend schools near industrial livestock operations.

Manami Hongo is in the MD program of the Faculty of Medicine at the University of Toyama in Japan. She has been a member of WABA YOUth since 2008, and attended the U.S. Commission on the Status of Women-55 as a youth representative from Japan through United Methodist Women. She also has a BA in Policy Management from Keio University.

Barbara Hormenoo is an alumna of the University of North Carolina at Greensboro, with a Bachelor of Science degree in Public Health, with a concentration in Community Health Education. She is the 2014-2015 recipient of the Loretta M. Williams Undergraduate Research Award in the Center for Women's Health and Wellness, UNC Greensboro.

Kathryn Houk/Wouk is a third-year doctoral student in the Maternal and Child Health Department of the Gillings School of Global

Public Health at the University of North Carolina at Chapel Hill. She is a Reproductive, Perinatal, and Pediatric Epidemiology Predoctoral Trainee, and has worked previously as a Research Assistant at the Carolina Global Breastfeeding Institute. She is Secretary Elect of the APHA Breastfeeding Forum, and is currently studying to become a lactation consultant student through the Mary Rose Tully Training Initiative at UNC.

Wafa Khasawneh is currently a PhD student at Arizona State University, School of Nursing and Health Innovation, Phoenix, USA. Her dissertation research focuses on breastfeeding experiences of immigrant Muslim mothers. She holds a Master of Science in Nursing degree from University of Windsor, Canada, and is a certified lactation consultant. Mrs. Khasawneh has over 10 years of experience in assisting mothers to maximize success in breastfeeding, and motivated nursing faculty with enthusiasm for teaching and learning. She has a wide range of experience in the areas of breastfeeding, nursing education, and health research.

Miriam Labbok, MD, MPH, IBCLC, is the Carolina Global Breastfeeding Institute Professor and Director in the Department of MCH at the University of North Carolina, Chapel Hill. Her previous work at Georgetown and Hopkins Universities, UNICEF and USAID on breastfeeding and family planning global issues and more recent work in North Carolina have been recognized with honors from her alma maters, and by LLLI, ILCA, and USAID, as well as with the 2012 Carl Taylor Lifetime Achievement Award from APHA, 2013 NC-GSKF Lifetime Achievement Award, and Award for Evidence-Based Leadership in Breastfeeding, ILCA/JHL 2014. She has published >100 peer-reviewed articles, > 40 chapters, co-edited three books, with two, in preparation, dozens of monographs, and 100s of scientific presentations. Dr. Labbok is pleased to serve as the co-director of the Breastfeeding and Feminism International Conference.

Julie Lauzière, Msc, PDt, is a doctoral student in Health Science Research (Community Health) at the Université de Sherbrooke, Quebec, Canada. She has been working primarily with public health organizations, universities, and research centers on projects related to breastfeeding promotion and support, and young child nutrition. She is a co-founder of the *Quebec Breastfeeding Movement,* and she is the co-responsible of its committee on training, which has the mandate to improve the health professionals' training on breastfeeding. Her research interests also include family support, healthy environments, and sociocultural factors influencing health.

Juliette LeRoy, MD, from Université Claude Bernard, Lyon, France, she has undertaken osteopathy in Quebec and is also a lactation consultant (IBCLC) since 2005. She is currently undertaking a master degree at the Université de Sherbrooke, Quebec, Canada, on the efficiency of osteopathy for babies with suckling dysfunctions. Juliette is part of the *Quebec Breastfeeding Movement* from 2010, member of its training committee for future health professionals. During her first life in France, she was involved in many projects such as: the creation of the first breastfeeding resource center; the French part of the European Blueprint for action a regional training for daycare to support mothers going back to work; and actions to support breastfeeding for low-income mothers. Now she lives in Canada, and continues to be involved in clinical practice, while she works in a mother-to-mother support group.

Isabelle Michaud-Létourneau, PhD, MPH, PDt, is a nutritionist from Quebec, Canada. She holds a Bachelor's degree in nutrition, a Masters in Public Health (in Maternal and Child Health) from the University of North Carolina at Chapel Hill, and a doctorate in international nutrition from Cornell University. She also pursued peace and conflict resolution studies, at UNC Chapel Hill, jointly with Duke University, as a Rotary World Peace fellow. Isabelle has undertaken international projects in Cuba, Bolivia, Senegal, Brazil, and Mozambique. She is now developing a large evaluation and research project in seven countries in Southeast Asia, and two African countries to strengthen the theory and practice of infant and young-child feeding advocacy and policy change. More locally, Isabelle is a member of the *Quebec Breastfeeding Movement,* where she is co-responsible for the committee on training whose mandate is to improve and harmonize the health professionals' training on breastfeeding.

Marie Dietrich Leurer, RN, PhD, Assistant Professor, College of Nursing, University of Saskatchewan. Marie is an Assistant Professor with the College of Nursing, University of Saskatchewan, Canada. She is an RN with a PhD in Community Health and Epidemiology. Prior to teaching, Marie worked as a public health nurse for over 25 years in rural Saskatchewan providing, among other services, breastfeeding support to new mothers. Her research interests include public-health nursing education and practice, early childhood nutrition and development, and knowledge translation to assist in the development of policies and programs that promote community health. Marie is currently serving on the Canadian Association of Schools of Nursing Public Health Task Force, and on the Community Health Nurses of Canada Standards and Competence Standing Committee.

Hannah Luedtke graduated from the University of North Carolina – Greensboro with a Master's degree in Women's and Gender Studies. Her recent research has included a project on Gender

Disappointment in mothers, as well as her thesis discussing books on breastfeeding. She is a mother to two wonderful little boys. Hannah hopes to pursue IBCLC training in the near future.

Professor CC Maponga, B. Pharm (Hons), Pharm D., MHPE, is a Professor and Director of the School of Pharmacy within the University of Zimbabwe's College of Health Sciences. He is also seconded as Technical Director for the National Nanotechnology Programme within the Ministry of Higher and Tertiary Education, Science and Technology Development. He provides an essential collaborative link between Health Sciences training and research programs in Zimbabwe. He also holds a visiting faculty position in the University at Buffalo, Buffalo, New York's School of Pharmacy. He holds several responsibilities including membership of the national medicines regulatory body, Medicines Control Authority Zimbabwe. He is the principal investigator for the recently approved AIDS Clinical Trials Group Harare Site's International Pharmacology Specialty Laboratory (UZ-IPSL) in the University of Zimbabwe, College of Health Sciences. His major goal is to build human capacity particularly within the pharmaceutical sector, and promote public sector to private sector partnerships in the adoption of emerging technologies including, biotechnology, information communication technology, and nanotechnology for socioeconomic development.

Saba Masho, MD, MPH, DrPH, is Associate Professor of Family Medicine and Population Health and Obstetrics and Gynecology at Virginia Commonwealth University (VCU) with expertise in Maternal and Child Health Epidemiology. She is the director of Community Based Participatory Research at the VCU Institute of Women's Health, a Federally designated Center of Excellence in Women's Health. Dr. Masho is a principal investigator and co-investigator of multiple federally funded research projects in the area of perinatal health, provision of comprehensive care to underserved pregnant women, and youth violence. She has authored numerous peer-reviewed manuscripts, and given several national scientific presentations. Her recent article examining the association between BMI and breastfeeding was featured in the *Breastfeeding Medicine.*

Alysha McFadden is a certified public health nurse in British Columbia, Canada who has studied and worked in the United States, Northern Canada, and Haiti. She recently completed a Master of Science degree at Simon Fraser University in the Faculty of Health Sciences, specializing in medical anthropology, breastfeeding, and nursing practices. Due to her diverse education, work, and volunteer experiences, Alysha has developed unique perspectives on global, and local, health disparities and inequities, which continue to inform her clinical practice and research interests. Her goal is to improve public and population health programs and services, specifically by completing a PhD in Nursing, and becoming an expert in the area of infant, child, and maternal health, with a specialization in breastfeeding and health equity. She aims to translate nursing research into practice by making it accessible to policy makers, health care providers, as well as the general public. Currently, Alysha is a Clinical Associate at UBC School of Nursing providing clinical instruction for students in their population health rotation.

Kelly McGlothen graduated with a BSN from the University of Texas Health Science Center at San Antonio, School of Nursing in 2012, and is currently a PhD student at UTHSCSA. Her research interests include the influence of contextual and cultural experiences of mothers on the transition to motherhood, mother-infant attachment, and the social-emotional development of the child. Her research and clinical practice aims are to work with vulnerable families to increase parenting efficacy, encourage the development of positive mother-infant relationships, and encourage optimal child development. She hopes to utilize this research to create culturally and developmentally appropriate maternal-child behavior promotion programs. Ms. McGlothen became an International Board Certified Lactation Consultant and Certified Infant Massage Instructor in 2013, and currently works in this capacity at University Hospital in San Antonio, Texas.

Eunice Misskey is a Freelance Public Health Nutritionist. She is an RD with a Masters in Continuing Education. Eunice most recently worked with the Saskatchewan Ministry of Health as the Provincial Public Health Nutrition Consultant, and for many years in a number of capacities at the regional level in Southeast Saskatchewan, including A/Manager of Health Promotion. Her interests have focused on the development of provincial nutrition and growth standards for the early childhood population, breastfeeding policy, food security, and related community research. Eunice has contributed to many provincial and national committees and boards serving in leadership positions including two three-year terms as the Dietitians of Canada Liaison on the Nutrition and Gastroenterology Committee of the Canadian Paediatric Society.

Muswamba Mwamba, IBCLC, MPH, is a Breastfeeding and Peer Dad Coordinator for the WIC program of the City of Dallas, Texas. As such, he prepares, equips, and empowers men through a peer perspective to be supportive of their partners' breastfeeding choice and practice. He is also currently working on his PhD in Leadership in Public Health at the University of Chapel Hill, and considers breastfeeding to be a public health priority as the foundation of good nutrition.

Julia Temple Newhook, PhD, conducted this research as a Canadian Institutes of Health Research Postdoctoral Fellow. She is presently a Pediatrics Research Associate in the Faculty of Medicine at Memorial University in St. John's, Newfoundland and Labrador, Canada.

Leigh Anne Newhook, MD, MSc, FRCPC, is a Pediatrician with Eastern Health and an Associate Professor of Pediatrics at Memorial University, in St. John's, Newfoundland and Labrador, Canada.

Rachel Newhouse MSN, CNM, is currently studying for a PhD at the University of Illinois at Chicago following a Master's in Nursing specializing in Nurse-Midwifery. Newhouse's clinical practice focuses on outpatient gynecology including birth control management, STD treatment, and routine well-woman care. Her research focuses on how to improve U.S. policies and practice norms that influence women's lives after they give birth. For her dissertation, she will be completing a comparative historical analysis about the development of postpartum policies and practices between New Zealand and the United States.

Deidre Orriola, MPH, CLC, graduated from the University of South Florida (USF) with her MPH 2006. Her position as faculty at the College of Public Health began in 2010. In 2015, she earned her CLC credentials, was promoted to Faculty Instructor II, and began teaching study abroad courses that focus on public health.

Dr. Azeez Oseni has over seven years of experience in the non-profit sector and earned a Master's degree in Public Health from the University of Liverpool in Liverpool, United Kingdom, and a Bachelor's degree in Medicine and Surgery from the

University of Ilorin in Nigeria. Working as Nutrition Team Lead, he leads the nutrition component of a large multi-sector USAID project aiming to improve the livelihoods of 42,000 vulnerable farming households in three states of Nigeria. Previously, he worked with Save the Children where he led an EU-funded project to reduce the burden of acute malnutrition in Northern Nigeria. He has also worked with APIN-Plus/ Harvard PEPFAR (AIDS Prevention Initiative in Nigeria) as a Treatment and Care Coordinator working to reduce the impact of HIV/AIDS in Benue State, Nigeria. Azeez has an interest in nutrition interventions, maternal and child health, and management of health systems.

Catherine Palmer graduated from Elon University in May of 2015 with a BA in Public Health. A semester of studying and interning at the Brooklyn Chest Tuberculosis Hospital in Cape Town, South Africa left Catherine with a passion for community health, and a desire to work with mothers facing barriers to health care. In addition to extensive community work in Alamance County, Catherine has also served as an intern for her university's Kernodle Center for Service-Learning and Community Engagement, promoting student service and leadership, and developing educational material on current social justice issues. An internship at Peacehaven Community Farm honed Catherine's horticultural skills and knowledge of intellectual disabilities, and provided valuable experience working in a non-profit. Catherine has spent the last four years learning how to work in communities, and is looking forward to starting a career in maternal health and gender-equity advocacy.

Aunchalee Palmquist, PhD, Assistant Professor of Sociology and Anthropology at Elon University, is a medical anthropologist and International Board Certified Lactation Consultant

(IBCLC). She received her PhD at the University of Hawaii at Manoa in 2006. Before arriving at Elon, she held a two-year appointment as Postdoctoral Associate and Lecturer at Yale University, Jackson Institute for Global Affairs, Global Health Initiative. She completed a postdoctoral fellowship at the National Institutes of Health-National Human Genome Research Institute, Social and Behavioral Research Branch from 2007-2009. Dr. Palmquist has conducted research on a wide range of topics, from healing systems in Palau, to family communication about genetic test results in the U.S. She has worked in clinical, community-based, and interdisciplinary settings. She has done ethnographic fieldwork in Hawaii, Palau, and Thailand. Her current research addresses social inequalities in health, infant and child health, women's and gender studies, and science and technology studies.

Laura Rosa Pascual, MD, PhD, IBCLC, is a physician and a lactation consultant. From 1990 to 2007, she was a professor and researcher at the Faculty of Medical Sciences, National University of Cordoba, Argentina, where, in 2003, she developed a 40-hour course on breastfeeding as a joint project between UNICEF-Argentina, and the Association of Faculties of Medicine of Argentina. The course is still offered in several Faculties of Medicine of the country. Since settling in Canada with her family in 2008, she remains involved with breastfeeding. In 2009-2010, she collaborated with the Office of International Relations and the WHO/PAHO Collaborating Centre of the Faculty of Medicine and Health Sciences of the University of Sherbrooke. Between 2009-2012, she was a lecturer for the Master of Clinical Sciences in the same faculty. From Oct 2010 to Jan 2014, and since May 2015, she has been responsible for the Baby-Friendly Initiative at the University Hospital of Sherbrooke. She is a member of the *Quebec Breastfeeding Movement,* and of its committee on training which she coordinated from

2010 to 2014, a committee whose mandate is to improve and harmonize health professionals' training on breastfeeding.

Melanie Pringle, BA, is finishing her MA in Women's and Gender Studies at the University of North Carolina at Greensboro in May 2016. She has been the Graduate Assistant for the Center for Women's Health and Wellness for three years, and helped to plan and facilitate the BFIC for each of those years, a formative experience. She is currently an intern with the Director of Philanthropy at Planned Parenthood, and is looking forward to a lifetime of work in reproductive justice and women's reproductive health.

Debra Prosnitz, MPH, is a global health professional with experience in maternal and child health, community health, malaria, integrated community case management (iCCM), and gender. Since 2013, she has served as the Project Manager for M&E Support to the WHO RAcE Program, and previously served as the Program Manager for the U.S. President's Malaria Initiative (PMI) Malaria Communities Program. Debra is skilled in providing technical assistance to NGOs and local partners to design, implement, monitor, and evaluate community-based programs. She has also written guidance and provided support for integrating gender into program design, monitoring, and evaluation.

Clare Relton, PhD, is a Senior Research Fellow in Public Health at ScHARR (Sheffield School of Health & Related Research), University of Sheffield, UK. After 10 years as a homeopath, Clare retrained, completing her MSc (Health Service Research) in 2004, and PhD (Practical randomized controlled trial (RCT) design) in 2009. Building on her innovative methodological thesis on trial design, she specializes in practical and rigorous comparative effectiveness trial design. Clare is an external expert on the UK's Cross Government Trials Advice Panel. Clare currently leads the team exploring the potential of offering financial incentives to breastfeed to women living in areas with low breastfeeding rates in the UK: https://www. sheffield.ac.uk/scharr/sections/ph/research/breastmilk. This study received national and international media coverage in November 2013 when the feasibility of offering women shopping vouchers to breastfeed began to be field tested. The intervention is now being tested in 88 clusters, with 12,000 women included in the randomized controlled trial.

Bhekimpilo G Sithole is a Zimbabwean based Nutritionist with Nutri@ctive Zimbabwe, and the Ministry of Health and Child Care. He has a keen interest in implementation research on diverse community nutrition intervention strategies. He has an inborn passion for nutrition work, especially maternal and young child nutrition in emergencies.

Hollie Sue Mann is a professor of Political Science at University of North Carolina at Chapel Hill. She specializes in ethics of care, feminist and queer theory, and politics and animal life. She has published on a range of subjects, including John Stuart Mill's feminism, the bodily work of caregiving, and Aristotelian virtue. Presently, she is teaching courses in advanced feminist theory and animal rights. Hollie Sue is also a mother of four, a yoga teacher, and an avid long-distance runner. When she is not working or playing with her kids, she can usually be found meditating or running in the woods with her best dog friend.

Paige Hall Smith, MSPH, PhD, is professor of Public Health Education and the Director of the Center for Women's Health and Wellness, at the University of North Carolina at Greensboro, where she also has a faculty appointment in the Women's and Gender Studies Program. In 2004, Dr. Smith was the recipient of the Linda Arnold Carlisle Professorship in Women's and Gender Studies at UNCG. She is founder, and now co-director, of the Breastfeeding and Feminism International Conference, and is also the co-coordinator of the Gender Working Group of the World Alliance for Breastfeeding Action. She is editor of three books that have emerged from presentations at the BFIC. She has received federal, state, and local funding for her research on breastfeeding, violence against women, and women's reproductive health.

Deborah McCarter-Spaulding, PhD, RN, is an Associate Professor of Nursing at Saint Anselm College, and International Board Certified Lactation Consultant (IBCLC). Her current research is addressing an educational intervention provided by postpartum nurses and its effect on postpartum depression symptoms. She is also looking at the relationship between postpartum depression and breastfeeding. Her previous research work has also been related to breastfeeding, particularly breastfeeding confidence (self-efficacy). She is also interested in women's health, gender issues, and global health, particularly in interdisciplinary context.

Becky Spencer, PhD, RN, IBCLC, is an Assistant Professor at Texas Woman's University in the College of Nursing. She received her PhD in nursing from the University of Kansas in 2012. Dr. Spencer has over 20 years of experience in nursing practice with pediatric, neonatal, and maternity populations. She currently teaches in the graduate nursing program at Texas Woman's University, and provides nursing research consultation services to Medical City Hospital in Dallas, Texas. Her research interests include health disparities affecting women and children and breastfeeding promotion and education in underserved populations. She is an active member of the International Lactation Consultant Association, Association of

Women's Health, Obstetric, and Neonatal Nurses, the Texas Nurses Association, and Sigma Theta Tau.

Courtenay Sprague (PhD, University of the Witwatersrand, South Africa; joint-MA, Boston University) is an Associate Professor of Global Health at the University of Massachusetts Boston. Her research engages health equity and social justice concerns affecting socially marginalized women, primarily HIV and intimate partner violence. For the last decade, she has focused on the provision of timely combination antiretroviral treatment (cART) for women's own health and programs to prevent mother to child HIV transmission (PMTCT)—in the high HIV prevalence setting of southern Africa, where women's health outcomes are some of the poorest globally. She was a faculty member at the University of the Witwatersrand in South Africa for seven years, and held research and program posts at Harvard University and Carnegie Corporation of New York. She has conducted health and HIV research, and work for UNAIDS, WHO, UNDP, and USAID, and is a research fellow with UNDP.

Alison Stuebe MD, MSc, FACOG, FABM, completed her Obstetrics and Gynecology residency at Brigham and Women's Hospital, and Massachusetts General Hospital in Boston. She completed fellowship training in Maternal Fetal Medicine at Brigham and Women's, and she earned a Masters in Epidemiology from the Harvard School of Public Health. She has published more than 80 peer-reviewed articles. She is currently an associate professor, and board-certified maternal-fetal medicine subspecialist at the University of North Carolina School of Medicine, and Distinguished Scholar of Infant and Young Child Feeding at the Gillings School of Global Public Health. She is a Fellow of the Academy of Breastfeeding Medicine. She serves on the board of directors for the Academy of Breastfeeding Medicine, and edits the Breastfeeding Medicine Blog. In the clinical arena, she is Medical Director of Lactation Services at UNC Health Care, and she works with an interdisciplinary team of faculty and staff to enable women to achieve their infant feeding goals. Her current research focuses on clinical management of breastfeeding complications, and the role of oxytocin in women's health.

Elizabeth Thomas worked with breastfeeding mothers for eight years as a La Leche League Leader and International Board Certified Lactation Consultant, and was a finalist for "Best Lactation Consultant" in the 2012 Austin Birth Awards. She has also advocated for childbearing women as a board member of Texans for Midwifery and birth doula. Elizabeth is currently a Master's student in the Department of Maternal and Child Health at the Gillings School of Public Health at UNC.

Dr. James Thomas, PhD, MPH, has over 30 years of experience working in the field of public health. He earned a Bachelor of Science in Nutrition from the University of California, Davis, and then masters and doctoral degrees in epidemiology from the University of California, Los Angeles (UCLA). Over the course of his career, Dr. Thomas has been a policy advisor, nutritionist, program implementer, professor, researcher, technical advisor, manager, and founder of two nonprofit organizations. He has lived in the Democratic Republic of the Congo and Kenya, and has worked in many countries of Africa and Asia. As a professor of epidemiology at the University of North Carolina, his principal interests are in the social epidemiology of HIV/AIDS, and public health ethics and human rights. In addition to his many scholarly articles, he was an editor and author of a textbook on epidemiologic methods in the study of infectious diseases, and principal author of the American Public Health Association's Code of

Ethics. As Director of MEASURE Evaluation, a $180 million five-year program funded by the United States Agency for International Development, Dr. Thomas is leading a global team that is advancing the capacity of countries and communities to strengthen capacity in developing countries to gather, interpret, and use data to improve health. Dr. Thomas brings to this effort a particular interest in complexity science and systems thinking. Two examples from his own work are organizational network analysis to improve coordination of disease control efforts, and the evaluation of structural interventions.

Dr. Cecilia Tomori is an anthropologist, trained at the University of Michigan, specializing in sociocultural and medical anthropology. Her book, *Nighttime Breastfeeding: An American Cultural Dilemma* (2014, New York, London: Berghahn Books), examines the cultural contradictions surrounding breastfeeding and infant sleep. She has presented her research at numerous conferences for anthropological, public health, medical, and lay audiences. Dr. Tomori is currently a Research Associate at the Johns Hopkins Bloomberg School of Public Health.

Laurie Twells, PhD, is an Associate Professor with the School of Pharmacy, and Faculty of Medicine, Memorial University, St. John's, Newfoundland and Labrador, Canada.

Kristin Tully is a Research Associate at the Center for Developmental Science, and Carolina Global Breastfeeding Institute at the University of North Carolina at Chapel Hill, United States. She obtained her PhD in Biological Anthropology from Durham University, United Kingdom, in 2010. Dr. Tully was a Postdoctoral Fellow in the Carolina Consortium on Human Development, supported by the Eunice Kennedy Shriver National Institute of Child Health and Human Development from 2010-2013. Her interest is in investigating provider care and parenting decisions in the domains of childbirth and infancy. She aims to contribute to nursing science, advance developmental theory, and improve family well-being. Dr. Tully's research disentangles factors underlying perinatal outcomes such as mode of childbirth, breastfeeding rates, and parent-infant sleep practices.

Sarah Verbiest, DrPH, MSW, MPH, is a Clinical Associate Professor at the School of Social Work and the Executive Director of the Center for Maternal and Infant Health at the University of North Carolina at Chapel Hill. She is the CDC Senior Consultant for the National Preconception Health and Health Care Initiative, and the cofounder of the Every Woman Southeast Coalition, a regional preconception health initiative. Dr. Verbiest coordinates the NC Recurring Preterm Birth Prevention Program, a statewide smoking cessation program for pregnant and new mothers, and several projects serving high-risk pregnant women, new mothers and their infants. She serves on the Governor's NC Child Fatality Task Force, chairs the NC Perinatal Health Committee, and serves on AMCHP's Best Practice Review Committee. She earned her graduate degrees at UNC-CH, including a Master's in Social Work, Master's in Public Health in Maternal and Child, and a Doctorate in Public Health Leadership from the Department of Health Policy and Management. She is the mom of two teenagers, and is active in her faith community.

Amanda Watkins, PhD, RD, LDN, IBCLC, is the Director for the Southwest Clinical Lactation Education Program at Arizona State University's College of Nursing and Health Innovation. She has a doctorate in Nursing and Health Innovation, a Master's degree in Nutrition, is a Registered Dietitian, and a practicing IBCLC. During her 20 years working in maternal and child health, she has provided consultations and taught college-level professional lactation courses. Dr. Watkins' research interests include breastfeeding educational interventions for health care providers and community-based breastfeeding decisions.

Anise Gold-Watts, Jennifer Lawall, Marielle Matthews, and **Jewels Rhode** graduated from the MPH program at the University of North Carolina's Gillings School of Global Public Health in May of 2015. In lieu of a Master's thesis, they were involved in a Capstone project with IntraHealth International guided by Girdhari Bora (ICT Advisor), Dr. David Potenziani (Senior Informatics Advisor), Dykki Settle (HRIS Leader), and Dr. Kathryn Muessig (Assistant Professor, UNC Gillings). Ms. Gold-Watts' research interests center on strategies that integrate traditional culture and evidence-based public health practices in developing countries. Ms. Lawall focuses on behavioral components of vaccine and infectious disease epidemiology. Ms. Matthews is passionate about rural health and equitable access to health services. Finally, Ms. Rhode is interested in chronic disease prevention and management and eliminating racial/ethnic health disparities. In this Capstone project, these students focused on mitigating barriers to breastfeeding among low-income African American women through mobile health.

Jacqueline H. Wolf is Professor of the History of Medicine in the Department of Social Medicine at Ohio University. She specializes in the history of women's and children's health and medicine and the history of public health. Her research focuses on the history of birth and breastfeeding practices in the United States. Her articles have appeared in many venues including the *American Journal of Public Health, Women and Health, Journal of Social History, Journal of Women's History, Signs, Journal of Human Lactation, Breastfeeding Medicine* and, most recently, *The Mil-*

bank Quarterly, which ran her article about her mother's death as a featured article in the December 2013 issue. She is the author of two books, *Don't Kill Your Baby: Public Health and the Decline of Breastfeeding in the 19th and 20th Centuries* (Ohio State University Press, 2001), and *Deliver Me from Pain: Anesthesia and Birth in America* (Johns Hopkins University Press, 2009). She is currently working on a book-length social history of cesarean section in the United States, to be published by Johns Hopkins University Press. Her current research is supported by a three-year National Institutes of Health Scholarly Works in Medicine and Health grant.

Jennifer Yourkavitch, MPH, CLC, is an epidemiologist with more than 15 years of experience with maternal and child health, malaria and HIV/AIDS projects, and is a seasoned manager, trainer, and facilitator. She has supervised or contributed to health projects funded by USAID, USDA, CDC, foreign governments and private donors, in partnership with local government, international and local NGOs, and communities. She is skilled in building the capacity of NGOs and local partners to design, implement, monitor and evaluate health projects. She has created various technical and management tools, and authored publications about breastfeeding, data quality, control of diarrheal disease and the sustainability of health outcomes. Her professional objective is to research maternal and child health issues, with a particular focus on lactation, maternal experience, gender, equity and sustainability, in order to ultimately translate research into policy and programmatic guidance for improved health outcomes.

Amanda Zabala obtained her Masters of Public Health degree in Maternal and Child Health at the University of North Carolina at Chapel Hill, where her research focused on preconception, pregnancy, postpartum, and women's health. She also received a

Certificate in Interdisciplinary Health Disparities, and provides consultative support to the North Carolina Office of Minority Health and Health Disparities, and the University of North Carolina's Center for Maternal and Infant Health on issues related to maternal, child, and minority health. She currently serves as a CDC/CSTE Applied Epidemiology Fellow at the Ohio Department of Health, where she promotes injury prevention strategies for recreational waters, and analyzes the impact of waterborne diseases on women and children's health.

Lauren Zalla, MSc-GH, is a mixed-methods researcher in the Department of Epidemiology at the University of North Carolina at Chapel Hill. Her research interests include the social determinants and cultural context of health, with a particular focus on nutrition and reproductive health. As a Foreign Language and Area Studies Fellow at Duke University, she studied the social context of exclusive breastfeeding and its association with infant nutritional status in Haiti.

Charity Zvandaziva is a Public Health Nutritionist with 18 years of experience in the field of Health and Nutrition. Currently working for United Nations for Children's Fund. She holds a Bachelor of Science degree in Nutrition, Masters in Public Health and Postgraduate diploma in Maternal and Child Health. Charity has hands on experience in spearheading innovative approaches for alleviating malnutrition.

We would also like to acknowledge the following contributing authors Anthony Chiromba, Patrice van Cleemput, Rutendo Masendu, Jill Mather, Yemurai Mkondo, Monica Muti, Mary Renfrew, Elaine Scott, Mark Strong, Catherine E. Taylor, Kate Thomas, Barbara Whelan, and Heather Whitford.